Advances in Neuroimaging of the Fetus and Newborn

Editors

SANGAM KANEKAR
SARAH SARVIS MILLA

CLINICS IN PERINATOLOGY

www.perinatology.theclinics.com

Consulting Editor
LUCKY JAIN

September 2022 • Volume 49 • Number 3

ELSEVIER

1600 John F. Kennedy Boulevard • Suite 1800 • Philadelphia, Pennsylvania, 19103-2899

http://www.theclinics.com

CLINICS IN PERINATOLOGY Volume 49, Number 3
September 2022 ISSN 0095-5108, ISBN-13: 978-0-323-84884-8

Editor: Kerry Holland
Developmental Editor: Karen Solomon

Clinics in Perinatology (ISSN 0095-5108) is published quarterly by Elsevier Inc., 360 Park Avenue South, New York, NY 10010-1710. Months of issue are March, June, September, and December. Business and Editorial Offices: 1600 John F. Kennedy Blvd., Ste. 1800, Philadelphia, PA 19103-2899. Customer Service Office: 3251 Riverport Lane, Maryland Heights, MO 63043. Periodicals postage paid at New York, NY and additional mailing offices. Subscription prices are $331.00 per year (US individuals), $823.00 per year (US institutions), $376.00 per year (Canadian individuals), $860.00 per year (Canadian institutions), $448.00 per year (international individuals), $860.00 per year (international institutions), $100.00 per year (US and Canadian students), and $195.00 per year (International students). International air speed delivery is included in all Clinics subscription prices. All prices are subject to change without notice. **POSTMASTER:** Send address changes to *Clinics in Perinatology*, Elsevier Health Sciences Division, Subscription Customer Service, 3251 Riverport Lane, Maryland Heights, MO 63043. **Customer Service: Telephone: 1-800-654-2452** (U.S. and Canada); **1-314-447-8871** (outside U.S. and Canada). **Fax: 1-314-447-8029. E-mail: journalscustomerservice-usa@elsevier.com** (for print support); **journalsonlinesupport-usa@elsevier.com** (for online support).

Reprints. For copies of 100 or more, of articles in this publication, please contact the Commercial Reprints Department, Elsevier Inc., 360 Park Avenue South, New York, NY 10010-1710. Tel. 212-633-3874; Fax: 212-633-3820; E-mail: reprints@elsevier.com.

Clinics in Perinatology is also published in Spanish by McGraw-Hill Interamericana Editores S.A., P.O. Box 5-237, 06500 Mexico D.F., Mexico.

Clinics in Perinatology is covered in *MEDLINE/PubMed (Index Medicus) Current Contents, Excepta Medica, BIOSIS and ISI/BIOMED.*

Contributors

CONSULTING EDITOR

LUCKY JAIN, MD, MBA
George W. Brumley Jr Professor and Chairman, Emory University School of Medicine, Department of Pediatrics, Chief Academic Officer, Children's Healthcare of Atlanta, Executive Director, Emory + Children's Pediatric Institute, Atlanta, Georgia

EDITORS

SANGAM KANEKAR, MD
Professor of Radiology and Neurology, Vice Chair, Radiology Research, Chief, Division of Neuroradiology, Penn State Health, Penn State College of Medicine, Hershey, Pennsylvania

SARAH SARVIS MILLA, MD, FAAP
Professor of Radiology and Pediatrics, University of Colorado School of Medicine, Vice Chair of Radiology, University of Colorado Anschutz Medical Campus, Department of Radiology, Pediatric Radiologist and Neuroradiologist, Chief of Radiology, Children's Hospital Colorado, Aurora, Colorado

AUTHORS

COREY S. BREGMAN, MD
Attending Pediatric Neuroradiologist, Ann & Robert H. Lurie Children's Hospital of Chicago, Chicago, Illinois; Assistant Professor of Radiology, Northwestern University Feinberg School of Medicine

JING CHEN, MD
Department of Radiology, Penn State Health, Penn State College of Medicine, Hershey, Pennsylvania

PATRICIA CORNEJO, MD
Department of Radiology, Phoenix Children's Hospital, Clinical Assistant Professor Radiology, University of Arizona College of Medicine, Clinical Assistant Professor Radiology, Creighton University School of Medicine, Barrows Neurological Institute, Phoenix, Arizona; Assistant Professor in Radiology, Mayo Clinic, Scottsdale, Arizona

LAURA Z. FENTON, MD
Department of Diagnostic Radiology, Professor of Radiology, University of Colorado School of Medicine, Children's Hospital Colorado, Aurora, Colorado

JUDITH A. GADDE, DO, MBA
Attending Pediatric Neuroradiologist, Ann & Robert H. Lurie Children's Hospital of Chicago, Chicago, Illinois; Director of Academic Innovation, Medical Imaging Department, Assistant Professor of Radiology, Northwestern University Feinberg School of Medicine

LUIS F. GONCALVES, MD
Department of Radiology, Phoenix Children's Hospital, Clinical Professor Radiology, University of Arizona College of Medicine, Clinical Assistant Professor Radiology, Creighton University School of Medicine, Phoenix, Arizona; Professor in Radiology, Mayo Clinic, Scottsdale, Arizona

SANGAM KANEKAR, MD
Professor of Radiology and Neurology, Vice Chair, Radiology Research, Chief, Division of Neuroradiology, Penn State Health, Penn State College of Medicine, Hershey, Pennsylvania

ABIGAIL LOCKE
Department of Radiology, Penn State Health, Penn State College of Medicine, Hershey, Pennsylvania

JOHN A. MALONEY, MD
Department of Radiology, Children's Hospital Colorado, University of Colorado Anschutz Medical Campus, Aurora, Colorado

ERIN MCNAMARA, MD, MPH
Instructor in Surgery, Harvard Medical School, Department of Urology, Boston Children's Hospital, Boston, Massachusetts

SARAH SARVIS MILLA, MD, FAAP
Professor of Radiology and Pediatrics, University of Colorado School of Medicine, Vice Chair of Radiology, University of Colorado Anschutz Medical Campus, Department of Radiology, Pediatric Radiologist and Neuroradiologist, Chief of Radiology, Children's Hospital Colorado, Aurora, Colorado

DAVID M. MIRSKY, MD
Associate Professor, Department of Radiology, Director of Fetal Neuroimaging and Pediatric Neuroradiology Fellowship, Children's Hospital Colorado, University of Colorado School of Medicine University of Colorado, Aurora, Colorado

ALI MOOSAVI
Division of Neuroradiology, Penn State Health, Penn State College of Medicine, Hershey, Pennsylvania

ILANA NEUBERGER, MD
Assistant Professor, Department of Radiology, Director of Radiology Informatics, Children's Hospital Colorado, University of Colorado School of Medicine, University of Colorado Anschutz Medical Campus, University of Colorado, Aurora, Colorado

CHUKWUDI OKAFOR, MD
Department of Radiology, Division of Neuroradiology, Penn State Health, Penn State College of Medicine, Hershey, Pennsylvania

ANDREA C. PARDO, MD, FAAP
Medical Director, Ruth D. and Ken M. Davee Pediatric Neurocritical Care Program, Attending Neurologist, Ann & Robert H. Lurie Children's Hospital of Chicago, Associate Professor of Pediatrics and Neurology, Northwestern University Feinberg School of Medicine, Chicago, Illinois

ANDRIA M. POWERS, MD
Associate Professor, Children's Hospital and Medical Center, University of Nebraska Medical Center, Omaha, Nebraska

KARTIK M. REDDY, MD
Assistant Professor of Radiology and Imaging Sciences, Children's Healthcare of Atlanta
and Emory University School of Medicine, Atlanta, Georgia

MAURA E. RYAN, MD
Attending Pediatric Neuroradiologist, Ann & Robert H. Lurie Children's Hospital of
Chicago, Chicago, Illinois; Associate Professor of Radiology, Northwestern University
Feinberg School of Medicine

DEBORAH STEIN, MD
Assistant Professor of Pediatrics, Harvard Medical School, Department of Pediatrics,
Boston Children's Hospital, Boston, Massachusetts

NICHOLAS V. STENCE, BS, MD
Associate Professor, Department of Radiology, Director of Pediatric Neuroradiology,
Children's Hospital Colorado, University of Colorado School of Medicine University of
Colorado, Aurora, Colorado

ANNA V. TROFIMOVA, MD, PhD
Assistant Professor of Radiology and Imaging Sciences, Children's Healthcare of Atlanta
and Emory University School of Medicine, Atlanta, Georgia

JENNIFER A. VAUGHN, MD
Department of Radiology, Phoenix Children's Hospital, Clinical Assistant Professor of
Radiology, University of Arizona College of Medicine, Clinical Assistant Professor of
Radiology, Creighton University School of Medicine, Barrows Neurological Institute,
Phoenix, Arizona

CHRISTINA WHITE, DO
Assistant Professor, Radiology, Children's Hospital Colorado, University of Colorado
Anschutz Medical Campus, University of Colorado, Aurora, Colorado

Contents

Fetal MRI is a safe, noninvasive examination of the fetus and placenta, a complement to ultrasonography. MRI provides detailed CNS evaluation, including depicting parenchymal architecture and posterior fossa morphology, and is key in prenatal assessment of spinal dysraphism, neck masses, and ventriculomegaly. Fetal MRI is typically performed after 22 weeks gestation, and ultrafast T1 and T2-weighted MRI sequences are the core of the exam, with advanced sequences such as diffusion weighted imaging used for specific questions. The fetal brain grows and develops rapidly, and familiarity with gestational age specific norms is essential to MRI interpretation.

Brain formation is a continuous and complicated process that is historically categorized by the timing of development. The earliest disorders of dorsal induction occur in the first month of gestation and include anencephaly and cephalocele. Disorders of ventral induction occur during the second month of gestation and include the holoprosencephaly and septo-optic dysplasia spectrums. The third and longest timeframe include the disorders of neuronal migration and proliferation (gestational weeks eight-25) and include malformations of cortical development: lissencephaly, polymicrogyria, schizencephaly, gray matter heterotopia, and corpus callosal dysgenesis. This review will highlight the neuroimaging of these malformations.

Advances in pre and postnatal neuroimaging techniques, and molecular genetics have increased our understanding of the congenital malformation of the brain. Correct diagnosis of these malformations in regards to embryology, and molecular neurogenetics is of paramount importance to understand the inheritance pattern and risk of recurrence. Lesions detected on prenatal imaging require confirmation either with postnatal ultrasound and/or with MR imaging. With the advent of the faster (rapid) MRI techniques, which can be conducted without sedation, MRI is commonly used in the evaluation of congenital malformation of the brain. Based on neuroimaging pattern, the congenital malformations of the posterior fossa are classified into 4 main categories: (a) predominantly cerebellar, (b) cerebellar and brainstem, (c) predominantly brainstem, and (d) predominantly midbrain malformations.

Imaging of Congenital Spine Malformations

Christina White, Sarah Sarvis Milla, John A. Maloney, and Ilana Neuberger

Congenital malformations of the spine and spinal cord reflect a diverse collection of clinical and phenotypic malformations resulting from aberrations in embryologic development. The term "spinal dysraphism" is often used broadly in the clinical setting but should be reserved for mishaps in primary neuralation. For the sake of completeness, this article will also discuss imaging features of other abnormalities demonstrating incomplete midline closure of mesenchymal, osseous, and nervous tissue, occurring at any point during embryologic development. In addition, this article will review normal spinal embryology, a clinical approach for classification of congenital spine malformations, and recommendations for appropriate imaging.

Imaging of Premature Infants

Abigail Locke and Sangam Kanekar

According to the World Health Organization (WHO), 15 million babies are born preterm each year. Preterm infants are those born at less than 37 weeks, while extremely and very preterm neonates include those born at 22 to less than 32 weeks gestational age. Infants that fail to make it to term are missing a key part in neurodevelopment, as weeks 24 to 40 are a critical period of brain development. Neonatal brain injury is a crucial predictor for mortality and morbidity in premature and low birth weight (<1500 g) infants. Although the complications associated with preterm birth continue to be the number one cause of death in children under 5, the survival rates are increasing (Volpe, 2019). Despite this, the incidence of comorbidities, such as learning disabilities and visual and hearing problems, is still high. The functional deficits seen in these infants can be contributed to the white matter abnormalities (WMA) that have been found in 50% to 80% of extremely and very preterm neonates. While numerous, the etiology of the neonatal brain injury is essential for determining the mortality and morbidities of the infant, as there is an increased risk for both intraventricular hemorrhage (IVH) and periventricular leukomalacia (PVL), which can be attributed to their lack of cerebrovascular autoregulation and hypoxic events. Neuroimaging plays a key role in detecting and assessing these neurologic injuries that preterm infants are at risk for. It is essential to diagnose these events early on to assess neurologic damage, minimize disease progression, and provide supportive care. Brain MRI and cranial ultrasound (CUS) are both extensively used neuroimaging techniques to assess WMA, and it has become ever more important to determine the best imaging techniques and modalities with the increasing survival rates and high incidence of comorbidities among these infants.

Inherited metabolic disorders represent a large group of disorders of which approximately 25% present in neonatal period with acute metabolic decompensation, rapid clinical deterioration, and often nonspecific imaging findings. Neonatal onset signifies the profound severity of the metabolic abnormality compared with cases with later presentation and necessitates rapid diagnosis and urgent therapeutic measures in an attempt to decrease the extent of brain injury and prevent grave neurologic sequela or death. Here, the authors discuss classification and clinical and imaging findings in a spectrum of metabolic and endocrine disorders with neonatal presentation.

Perinatal ischemic stroke is a common cause of lifelong disability.

One of the most common definitions of microcephaly cited is that of an occipitofrontal circumference (OFC) of the head that is less than two standard deviations below the average for age (or gestational age, if identified prenatally) and sex. Similarly, severe microcephaly is defined as an OFC that is less than three standard deviations below the average. Microcephaly is not a diagnosis, but rather, a finding that is secondary to a multitude of etiologies that can be categorized as prenatal versus postnatal, genetic versus environmental, and congenital versus acquired.

Macrocephaly is a common diagnosis in the pediatric population, particularly in the infantile time period. There is a wide range of causes of macrocephaly, from benign to malignant, for which imaging plays a key role in the diagnosis and clinical guidance. Our aim is to review the distinct and prevalent neuroimaging findings in the evaluation of the macrocephalic infant.

Hypoxic-ischemic injury (HII) is a major worldwide contributor of term neonatal mortality and long-term morbidity. At present, therapeutic hypothermia is the only therapy that has demonstrated efficacy in reducing severe disability or death in infants with moderate to severe encephalopathy. MRI and MRS performed during the first week of life are adequate to assess brain injury and offer prognosis. Patterns of injury will depend on the gestation age of the neonate, as well as the degree of hypotension.

> Imaging plays an important role in evaluating patients with suspected intrauterine and perinatal infections. Advances in fetal imaging including both ultrasound and MRI allow for increasingly more specific diagnosis if the radiologist is familiar with specific imaging features and patterns. Early imaging of neonates with suspected central nervous system infection is valuable to enable prompt treatment and differentiate infection from other conditions which can clinically present similarly. Ultrasound is a useful initial modality to screen for abnormalities however MRI with and without contrast remains the optimal examination to characterize infection, evaluate for potential surgical targets, and provide prognostic information.

> Craniofacial malformation is one of the most commonly encountered birth defects in the prenatal and postnatal periods. Higher-resolution and 3D antenatal ultrasonography and multidetector computed tomographic scan with 3D reformatted images have improved the definition of the soft tissue and bone structures of the craniofacial anatomy and its malformations. Early diagnosis of these conditions is important to make the clinical decisions and more so in understanding the possibility of malformation recurring in the next pregnancy, which is one of the major concerns for the parents and the treating physicians.

> Congenital anomalies of the kidneys and urinary tract (CAKUT) are some of the most common abnormalities detected on prenatal imaging assessment. It is estimated that CAKUT comprises 20% to 30% of all major birth defects. More than 200 clinical syndromes currently include CAKUT as a component of the phenotype. This chapter outlines the evaluation and management of the most common forms of CAKUT.

PROGRAM OBJECTIVE
The goal of *Clinics in Perinatology* is to keep practicing perinatologists, neonatologists, obstetricians, practicing physicians and residents up to date with current clinical practice in perinatology by providing timely articles reviewing the state of the art in patient care.

TARGET AUDIENCE
Perinatologists, neonatologists, obstetricians, practicing physicians, residents and healthcare professionals who provide patient care utilizing findings from *Clinics in Perinatology*.

LEARNING OBJECTIVES
Upon completion of this activity, participants will be able to:
1. Recognize imaging as an evidence-based practice and standard of care for characterizing, identifying, diagnosing, and planning treatment for fetuses with structural anomalies of the spine, cranium, and soft tissue, neurologic injury, or metabolic disorder.
2. Discuss the importance of a multidisciplinary team approach with the use of imaging techniques to identify, diagnose, determine a prognosis, plan treatment, and decrease the risk of recurrence of soft tissue, spine, and cranial anomalies, as well as neurologic injury, and metabolic disorders in the fetus in a timely manner.
3. Examine the indications for the use of imaging of anatomical structures such as soft tissue, spine, and cranial anomalies, as well as neurologic injury and metabolic and endocrine disorders in a fetus, both pre-and postnatally.

ACCREDITATION
The Elsevier Office of Continuing Medical Education (EOCME) is accredited by the Accreditation Council for Continuing Medical Education (ACCME) to provide continuing medical education for physicians.

The EOCME designates this journal-based CME activity for a maximum of 13 *AMA PRA Category 1 Credit*(s)™. Physicians should claim only the credit commensurate with the extent of their participation in the activity.

All other health care professionals requesting continuing education credit for this enduring material will be issued a certificate of participation.

DISCLOSURE OF CONFLICTS OF INTEREST
The EOCME assesses conflict of interest with its instructors, faculty, planners, and other individuals who are in a position to control the content of CME activities. All relevant conflicts of interest that are identified are thoroughly vetted by EOCME for fair balance, scientific objectivity, and patient care recommendations. EOCME is committed to providing its learners with CME activities that promote improvements or quality in healthcare and not a specific proprietary business or a commercial interest.

The planning committee, staff, authors, and editors listed below have identified no financial relationships or relationships to products or devices they or their spouse/life partner have with commercial interest related to the content of this CME activity:
Corey S. Bregman, MD; Jing Chen, PhD; Patricia Cornejo, MD; Laura Z. Fenton, MD; Judith A. Gadde, DO, MBA; Luis F. Goncalves, MD; Lucky Jain, MD, MBA; Erin McNamara, MD, MPH; Sangam Kanekar, MD; Abigail Locke; John A. Maloney, MD; Sarah Sarvis Milla, MD, FAAP; David M. Mirsky, MD; Ali Moosavi, DO; Ilana Neuberger, MD; Chukwudi Okafor, MD; Andrea C. Pardo, MD, FAAP; Andria Powers, MD; Kartik M. Reddy, MD; Maura E. Ryan, MD; Deborah Stein, MD; Nicholas V. Stence, MD; Jeyanthi Surendrakumar, BE; Doreen Thomas-Payne, MSN, BSN, RN, PMHNP-BC; Anna V. Trofimova, MD, PhD; Jennifer A. Vaughn, MD; Christina White, DO

UNAPPROVED/OFF-LABEL USE DISCLOSURE
The EOCME requires CME faculty to disclose to the participants:
1. When products or procedures being discussed are off-label, unlabelled, experimental, and/or investigational (not US Food and Drug Administration [FDA] approved); and
2. Any limitations on the information presented, such as data that are preliminary or that represent ongoing research, interim analyses, and/or unsupported opinions. Faculty may discuss information about pharmaceutical agents that is outside of FDA-approved labelling. This information is intended solely for CME and is not intended to promote off-label use of these medications. If you have any questions, contact the medical affairs department of the manufacturer for the most recent prescribing information.

TO ENROLL

To enroll in the *Clinics in Perinatology* Continuing Medical Education program, call customer service at 1-800-654-2452 or sign up online at http://www.theclinics.com/home/cme. The CME program is available to subscribers for an additional annual fee of USD 265.00.

METHOD OF PARTICIPATION

In order to claim credit, participants must complete the following:
1. Complete enrolment as indicated above.
2. Read the activity.
3. Complete the CME Test and Evaluation. Participants must achieve a score of 70% on the test. All CME Tests and Evaluations must be completed online.

CME INQUIRIES/SPECIAL NEEDS

For all CME inquiries or special needs, please contact elsevierCME@elsevier.com.

CLINICS IN PERINATOLOGY

SERIES OF RELATED INTEREST

Obstetrics and Gynecology Clinics of North America
https://www.obgyn.theclinics.com

THE CLINICS ARE AVAILABLE ONLINE!
Access your subscription at:
www.theclinics.com

CLINICS IN PERINATOLOGY

FORTHCOMING ISSUES

December 2022
Advances and Updates in Fetal and Neonatal Surgery
KuoJen Tsao and Hanmin Lee, Editors

March 2023
Neurological and Developmental Outcome of High-Risk Infants
Nathalie Maitre and Andrea F. Duncan, Editors

June 2023
Quality Improvement
Heather C. Kaplan and Munish Gupta, Editors

RECENT ISSUES

June 2022
Neonatal and Perinatal Nutrition
Akhil Maheshwari and Jonathan R. Swanson, Editors

March 2022
Current Controversies in Neonatology
Susan S. Cohen and Robert M. Kliegman, Editors

December 2021
Advances in Respiratory Management
Manuel Sanchez Luna, Editor

SERIES OF RELATED INTEREST

Obstetrics and Gynecology Clinics of North America
https://www.obgyn.theclinics.com/

THE CLINICS ARE AVAILABLE ONLINE
Access your subscription at:
www.theclinics.com

Foreword

Improving the Precision of Neonatal Neuroimaging

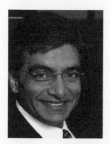

Lucky Jain, MD, MBA
Consulting Editor

Like in many other areas of medicine, much has changed in the field of neonatal neuro-imaging. In caring for a neurologically impaired newborn, the clinician relies heavily on imaging techniques to guide clinical care and prediction of long-term outcomes. Diagnostic modalities include ultrasound, magnetic resonance imaging (MRI), electroencephalogram (EEG), near-infrared spectroscopy, and more. Each is useful in specific circumstances; however, the future lies in combining these techniques into clinical algorithms derived from large databases and artificial intelligence (AI) to refine the diagnostic and predictive value.[1] Such approaches form the basis of precision medicine and can go a long way in helping families make key decisions when confronted with challenging diagnoses, such as hypoxic ischemic encephalopathy, neonatal stroke, and intracranial hemorrhage. After the critical initial period is over, questions invariably shift from survival to anxiety about longer-term sequelae, such as cerebral palsy and cognitive impairment. Our greatest hope lies in using machine learning and AI to improve the ability of these tests to more accurately predict longer-term outcomes by harnessing the extensive data on all available diagnostic approaches (**Fig. 1**).[1]

Indeed, many neonatal intensive care units assign multidisciplinary teams that are dedicated to brain-oriented care for neonates admitted to their specialized neuro-intensive care units. In addition to their focus on brain protection, neonates cared for in these dedicated areas have easier access to on-site and advanced neurologic assessments, such as MRIs, EEGs, general movement assessments, and diagnostic scales, such as the Hammersmith Infant Neurological Examination. These techniques can predict long-term sequelae, such as cerebral palsy, with remarkable accuracy even in very young infants.[2]

MRI has also become an indispensable tool for imaging fetal congenital malformations. Advanced MRI techniques and data can provide images with stunning clarity in disorders like spina bifida (**Fig. 2**).[3] These approaches can better predict severity

Clin Perinatol 49 (2022) xv–xvii
https://doi.org/10.1016/j.clp.2022.07.007
0095-5108/22/© 2022 Published by Elsevier Inc.

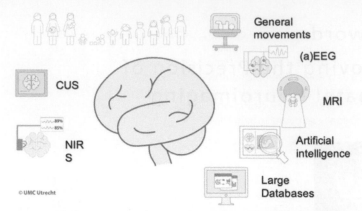

Fig. 1. Precision medicine for brain-oriented care. CUS, cranial ultrasound; MRS, magnetic resonance spectroscopy. (*From* Tataranno ML, Vijlbrief DC, Dudink J, Benders MJNL. Precision Medicine in Neonates: A Tailored Approach to Neonatal Brain Injury. Front Pediatr. 2021 May 19;9:634092.)

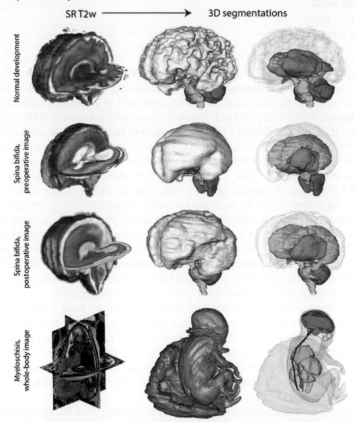

Fig. 2. Superresolution (SR) reconstruction of fetal MRI. For each case (normal development, preoperative, and postoperative images of spina bifida fetus undergoing fetal surgery and myeloschisis), the SR T2-weighted MRI (*left images*) and 2 surface reconstructions that were based on the segmentation of the reconstructed image (*right images*) are demonstrated. 3D, 3-dimensional; T2w, T2-weighted. (From Jakab A, Payette K, Mazzone L, Schauer S, Muller CO, Kottke R, Ochsenbein-Kölble N, Tuura R, Moehrlen U, Meuli M. Emerging magnetic resonance imaging techniques in open spina bifida in utero. Eur Radiol Exp. 2021 Jun 17;5(1):23.)

of the lesion and known complications, such as hydrocephalus; they are also better at predicting motor function later in life.

In this issue of the *Clinics in Perinatology*, Drs Kanekar and Milla have brought together an impressive lineup of authors and topics that address critical issues in neuroimaging. As always, I am grateful to the publishing staff at Elsevier, including Kerry Holland and Karen Justine Solomon, for their support in allowing us to bring a broad range of clinically relevant topics to you.

Lucky Jain, MD, MBA
Emory University School of Medicine, and
Children's Healthcare of Atlanta
1760 Haygood Drive, W409
Atlanta, GA 30322, USA

E-mail address:
ljain@emory.edu

REFERENCES

1. Tataranno ML, Vijlbrief DC, Dudink J, et al. Precision medicine in neonates: a tailored approach to neonatal brain injury. Front Pediatr 2021;9:634092. https://doi.org/10.3389/fped.2021.634092.
2. Bosanquet M, Copeland L, Ware R, et al. A systematic review of tests to predict cerebral palsy in young children. Dev Med Child Neurol 2013;55:418–26.
3. Jakab A, Payette K, Mazzone L, et al. Emerging magnetic resonance imaging techniques in open spina bifida in utero. Eur Radiol Exp 2021;23:1–10.

Preface

Advances in Neuroimaging of the Fetus and Newborn

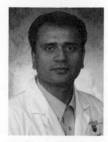 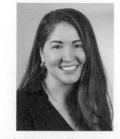

Sangam Kanekar, MD   Sarah Sarvis Milla, MD, FAAP
Editors

The prenatal and infancy periods are critical to the development of the child. Any insult during these stages of life may lead to a host of congenital malformations. Congenital brain malformations may result from inherited genetic defects, spontaneous mutations within the embryo's genes, or damage to the fetus caused by the mother's exposure to toxins, infection, trauma, or drug use. It is challenging for clinicians to suspect or diagnose these malformations or abnormalities clinically. Non–radiation imaging techniques, such as ultrasound and MRI, play a vital role in diagnosing and characterizing the severity of these conditions.

This *Clinics in Perinatology* issue focuses on advances in neuroimaging of the fetus and newborn. It is curated to expose the neonatology community to clinically relevant updates in diagnostic imaging. This issue has a total of 12 articles and is balanced with conventional and high-end modalities in diagnosis and characterization of these congenital anomalies and abnormalities encountered during the prenatal and infancy stages. The first article introduces the fetal MRI by focusing on techniques and neuroanatomy. The next three articles provide a practical approach to congenital malformation imaging of the brain and spine. The rest of the issue spans perinatal conditions, such as hypoxic ischemic injury and infections to postnatally recognized malformations and metabolic disorders. In addition, we present a microcephalic and macrocephalic imaging approach, a clinically relevant topic. The last article describes genetic and imaging approaches to congenital craniofacial anomalies and syndromes.

We thank all the authors for their excellent contributions that make this issue an outstanding and comprehensive review on neuroimaging of the fetus and newborn. We would like to thank the Consulting Editor, Dr Lucky Jain, and the Elsevier staff

Clin Perinatol 49 (2022) xix–xx
https://doi.org/10.1016/j.clp.2022.06.007
0095-5108/22/© 2022 Published by Elsevier Inc.

for giving us an opportunity to guest edit this issue and present this topic to a wider audience. Finally, we thank our families for their love and support. Happy reading!

Sangam Kanekar, MD
Penn State Health
Penn State College of Medicine
Mail Code H066
500 University Drive
Hershey, PA 17033, USA

Sarah Sarvis Milla, MD, FAAP
University of Colorado School of Medicine
Children's Hospital Colorado
7108 East Lowry Boulevard, #4100
Denver, CO 80230, USA

E-mail addresses:
skanekar@pennstatehealth.psu.edu (S. Kanekar)
sarah.milla@childrenscolorado.org (S.S. Milla)

Fetal MRI Neuroradiology
Indications

Andria M. Powers, MD[a],[*], Christina White, DO[b],
Ilana Neuberger, MD[b], John A. Maloney, MD[b],
Nicholas V. Stence, MD[b], David Mirsky, MD[b]

KEYWORDS

- Fetal • MRI • Neuroimaging fetal development • MRI safety

KEY POINTS

- Fetal MRI is a safe, noninvasive exam used together with obstetrical ultrasound to add diagnostic confidence to the evaluation of the fetus.
- Fetal MRI is especially helpful in CNS abnormalities, offering detailed depiction of brain parenchyma, posterior fossa structures, and often providing etiologic insight to fetuses with ventriculomegaly.
- Fetal MRI is typically performed after 22 weeks gestation, and can be performed through third gestation.
- The fetal brain grows and develops rapidly, and interpretation of fetal neuroimaging requires familiarity with the expected gestation related changes.

PURPOSE/VALUE ADDED BY MRI

Fetal MRI is a noninvasive imaging examination that provides useful information in the evaluation of the fetus and placenta and is complementary to obstetric ultrasonography. As such, fetal MRI is considered a second-line imaging study that is performed after the routinely obtained anatomic ultrasonography. Fetal MRI is used in select pregnancies for fetal and/or uterine evaluation when ultrasonography is inadequate, or the abnormality is incompletely visualized according to practice parameters described jointly by the American College of Radiology and Society of Pediatric Radiology.[1] MRI becomes a particularly powerful tool when ultrasonography is limited by poor acoustic windows and suboptimal sound penetration of fetus.[2] Factors that can impede ultrasound evaluation of the uterus include:

The authors have nothing to disclose.
[a] Children's Hospital and Medical Center, University of Nebraska Medical Center, 8200 Dodge Street, Omaha, NE 68114, USA; [b] Department of Radiology, Children's Hospital Colorado, University of Colorado, 13123 E. 16th Avenue, Box 125, Aurora, CO, 80045, USA
* Corresponding author.
E-mail address: anpowers@childrensomaha.org

Clin Perinatol 49 (2022) 573–586
https://doi.org/10.1016/j.clp.2022.05.001
0095-5108/22/© 2022 Elsevier Inc. All rights reserved.

- Large maternal body habitus
- Anterior placenta
- Oligohydramnios
- Difficult fetal lie or descent of fetal head into pelvis
- Intervening bowel gas/other artifact-producing anatomy

Myriad indications for fetal MRI exist, with the most common central nervous system (CNS) indications being ventriculomegaly, absent cavum septum pellucidum, posterior fossa malformation or cyst, supratentorial parenchymal lesion or destruction, skull deformity, suspected craniosynostosis, face/neck mass, neural tube defects, sacrococcygeal teratoma, and cleft lip/palate.

Fetal MRI adds value by increasing diagnostic certainty, allowing for detailed care and delivery planning, and providing details necessary for possible antenatal therapy.[1] Fluid and soft tissue are well defined on MRI, and the abundance of fluid surrounding the fetus allows for direct visualization of many fetal structures that can be difficult to evaluate with ultrasonography. With ultrasonography, the viewing window is focused on an individual anatomic structure. With MRI, the entire fetus can be visualized in a single image and relationships between structures and abnormalities better depicted. The differences in signal intensity between amniotic fluid and fetal tissue can allow surface rendering.[3]

Inherent contrast resolution between various soft tissues by MRI improves the ability to distinguish fetal organs from each other.[4,5] Many studies have shown that this increased contrast resolution of MRI is particularly useful in evaluating CNS abnormalities due to the better delineation and depiction of brain parenchyma and subplate morphology; this adds diagnostic accuracy in the evaluation of structural abnormalities, including posterior fossa deformities, corpus callosum morphology, and identification of findings such as heterotopia, manifestations of tuberous sclerosis, and congenital cytomegalovirus infection.[6–27] Specialized sequences, such as echoplanar imaging (EPI) and diffusion-weighted imaging (DWI), aid in the identification and confirmation of brain hemorrhage and ischemia, respectively. These findings can be particularly prognostically relevant in many conditions, including vein of Galen malformation.[20,21,24,28] Another common reason for MRI referral is in the setting of ventriculomegaly, where it often identifies additional brain abnormalities and provides etiologic insight.[29] The added detail of fetal MRI increases diagnostic confidence with improved prognostic accuracy and better-informed patient counseling, which then impacts care decisions.[11–13]

Fetal MRI is key in the evaluation of spinal dysraphism, and all candidates for prenatal surgery are required to obtain a preoperative fetal MRI, in conjunction with an ultrasonography.[30] Fetal MRI provides accurate assessment of the size and location of the spinal defect, as well as complete brain evaluation, including degree of hindbrain herniation, presence of hemorrhage, and severity of ventriculomegaly.[31] This information aids presurgical assessment and guides intrauterine surgical treatment.[18,31,32] In the head and neck region, MRI adds detail in the evaluation of craniofacial anomalies, improving the accuracy of assessment for degree of posterior palate involvement and lateral extent of the cleft lip and palate.[26,33] In fetuses with neck masses, such as cervical teratoma, MRI provides important information for delivery and presurgical planning due to the improved soft tissue contrast resolution, clear visualization of fluid within the airway, and ability to predict pulmonary hypoplasia.[25] Validated prenatal MRI predictors for neonatal morbidity and the need for an Ex Utero Intrapartum Treatment (EXIT) procedure include mass effect on the trachea and largest vertical pocket of amniotic fluid.[34,35]

LIMITATIONS

For all the benefits that fetal MRI can provide in prenatal assessment, there are limitations. Some implanted medical devices are contraindicated in the MRI environment, which prohibits some patients from undergoing MRI. All patients are screened before every MRI encounter, in line with current safety recommendations.

Access to MRI technologists who are experienced with fetal imaging and its unique challenges, such as fetal movement and nonstandard imaging planes, is required for high-quality imaging. Interpretation of fetal MRI should be performed by radiologists with experience and/or dedicated training in fetal MRI.

Large maternal size can present a challenge with regard to table weight limits, which vary by MRI machine, and/or if maternal abdominal diameter is too great for the MRI bore size. Standard MRI bore diameter is 60 cm, whereas a wide-bore MRI diameter is 70 cm. A gap between the patient and MRI walls must be left for padding and safety requirements.

The bore of the MRI machine is a confined space, and some patients experience claustrophobia in this environment. Useful techniques to mitigate feelings of claustrophobia and increase examination success include wearing video goggles, headphones with music, supplemental oxygen, and fans for continuous airflow. Placing the mother in decubitus position or having a guest present can also aid in combating feelings of claustrophobia. Patient positioning and padding for comfort is paramount in the ability to tolerate the examination and minimize contributions of maternal motion.

Excessive fetal motion results in poor image quality, because structures cannot be well illustrated, decreasing sensitivity of the test and impeding completeness, in some cases. Polyhydramnios or young gestational age are settings in which fetal motion may be particularly problematic.

Cardiac evaluation by fetal MRI, although subject of much promising research, is not currently standard clinical practice, and fetal echocardiography remains the mainstay for evaluation of cardiac anatomy and congenital heart disease.

Timing of Fetal MRI

Fetal MRI is performed after the obstetric morphology ultrasonography, which typically occurs between 18 and 20 weeks' gestation, so most fetal MRI occurs around 22 weeks' gestation. MRI can be performed before 22 weeks' gestation; however, before 18 weeks it does not typically provide additional information compared with detailed ultrasonography.[36] In some instances, urgency of the MRI depends on the findings on the ultrasonography that may impact the course of pregnancy, if termination of pregnancy is something the family and providers wish to discuss.

With increasing gestational age comes increased utility of MRI, because fetal tissues become better developed and therefore better seen and evaluated.[37] The fetal brain grows and matures rapidly, and the MRI appearance changes dramatically over the prenatal period. Gestational age-related parenchymal and sulcation changes can be evaluated and compared with normative data to identify normal development or pathology.[38,39] Early third-trimester MRI is useful to evaluate malformations of cortical development, heterotopia, and evolution of previous ischemia or hemorrhage. Later gestation follow-up MRI is often performed of fetuses with myelomeningocele after repair to reevaluate ventricle size, the posterior fossa, and hindbrain herniation.[30] Fetuses with fetal neck masses or severe micrognathia may benefit from later gestation MRI to evaluate the fetal airway before delivery.

In some conditions, third-trimester MRI can provide unique prognostic data that add value to the usual second-trimester MRI. Third-trimester second-look MRI in fetuses with congenital diaphragmatic hernia provides reassessment of lung volumetric data to provide prognostic information for delivery planning and need for extracorporeal membrane oxygenation at birth.[40]

Basics of Fetal Examination Experience

No unique patient preparation is necessary before fetal MRI, but all patients need to undergo the standard MRI screening for ferromagnetic implants and devices before entry into the MRI room. There are no accepted guidelines for maternal instructions regarding preexamination meal or medication; there is no evidence that maternal meal (including caffeine intake) significantly impacts fetal motion and related image quality.[41] Studies have also shown that maternal pretreatment with valium does not affect degree of fetal motion.[41,42] No intravenous contrast is needed for the examination, because gadolinium contrast agents cross the placenta, are not recommended by the US Food and Drug Administration for use in pregnancy, and are not used in pregnant patients.[5] Examination length varies depending on factors that can impact image quality and the need to repeat sequences, such as fetal motion or artifact, and by the complexity of the fetal abnormality requiring additional and/or specialized sequences. In general, a time slot of 40 to 60 minutes is sufficient.

The mother is placed on the MRI table within the center of the MRI bore in a comfortable position, usually feet first and on her back. The position may need to be modified to side (decubitus), and pillows are used for support and pressure relief.[43]

Basic MRI Examination Technique

Initially, magnetic resonance images are obtained along 3 planes oriented to the mother (**Fig. 1**), which provide assessment of the maternal uterus, placenta, cervix, and ovaries. Other maternal structures in the field of view, such as the spine or bony pelvis, are also reviewed for incidental findings. Dedicated triplanar images of the fetal brain and body are then obtained.

Ultrafast T2-weighted (fluid-sensitive) sequences are the workhorse of fetal MRI, providing evaluation of fetal anatomy and pathology. Fluid and fluid-containing structures appear hyperintense (bright), soft tissue structures demonstrate intermediate intensity, and bony structures are hypointense (dark). Fast sequence T1-weighted images (**Fig. 2**) are important for evaluation of intrinsic hyperintense T1 signal in meconium, liver, and thyroid and are useful when evaluating potential hemorrhage or fat.[44]

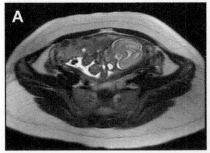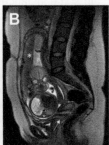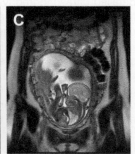

Fig. 1. Axial (*A*), sagittal (*B*), and coronal (*C*) magnetic resonance images oriented along the plane of the mother. This placenta (*asterisk*) is located anteriorly and the fetus is breech. Cervix (*arrow*) is assessed in sagittal view, where it can be seen in long axis and measured.

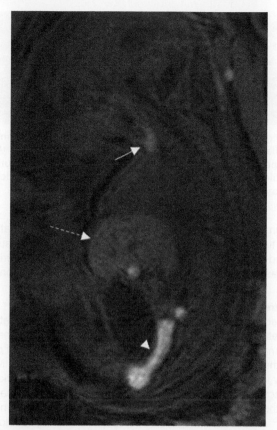

Fig. 2. Sagittal T1-weighted MR image of a 34-week fetus showing intermediate-signal-intensity liver (*dashed arrow*) and thyroid (*solid arrow*) and hyperintense meconium in the tubular rectum (*arrowhead*).

Steady-state free precession (SSFP) sequence, another fluid-sensitive sequence, provides a complementary look at fetal anatomy, with added benefit in evaluation of vasculature; SSFP renders vascular structures hyperintense, compared with their normal hypointense appearance on T2-weighted single shot ultrafast MRI technique (T2SS) (**Fig. 3**). T2-weighted cine sequences result in movielike clips, which provide dynamic assessment of moving structures. Cine sequence MRI can be helpful in some fetal conditions to assess fetal swallowing, bowel motion, or in face/neck where they assist in semiphysiologic assessment of upper airway obstructions or neck masses.[44] Advanced MRI sequences such as DWI and EPI can be useful in certain clinical settings, because they, respectively, evaluate for ischemic changes and blood products.[5,21]

FETAL MRI NEURORADIOLOGY: SAFETY
Safety Considerations in MRI Environment

Gestational age
No deleterious effects have been documented to fetuses exposed to MRI at any gestational age.[1] In general, fetal MRI is performed after 18 weeks due to the small

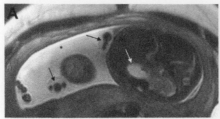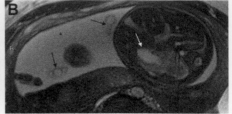

Fig. 3. Axial T2 single-shot turbo spin echo (TSE) (*A*) and SSFP (*B*) MR images through the fetal body at similar level in the same patient. Vascular structures of the umbilical cord (*black arrows*) appear hypointense on T2 single-shot TSE sequence but hyperintense on SSFP sequence. Fluid-containing fetal stomach (*white arrows*) and amniotic fluid (*asterisk*) are hyperintense on both sequences.

size of the fetus, immature development, and lower diagnostic yield at an earlier gestational age[43]; this timeframe also avoids theoretic risks of fetal exposure during organogenesis. Second-trimester MRI helps confirm or further characterize findings from the obstetric ultrasonography, and potentially identify additional abnormalities.

Magnetic field strength
MRI uses radiofrequency (RF) energy produced by an electromagnet. The strength of the electromagnet is measured in Tesla, which represents the magnetic field strength produced by the main component of the machine; in current clinical practice, the MRI machines are either 1.5 or 3 T. Electromagnetic radiation from the MRI machine deposits RF energy into the tissues, which is measured as the specific absorption rate (SAR). For all practical purposes, this increase in SAR reflects increased temperature of the tissues in the magnetic field environment. SAR is monitored and measured during MRI scans.[45] American College of Obstetricians and Gynecologists committee opinion on MRI during pregnancy reported negligible tissue heating near the uterus.[46] SAR values and local temperature increases have been shown to be within safety limits for imaging performed at 1.5 and 3.0 T.[47–50] Regulations in MRI machines for SAR monitoring and limits are in place during use in normal mode, and either 1.5 or 3 T can be used without patient concern.[51] Large studies of MRI outcomes during pregnancy (including 3T exposure) showed no increased risk of congenital anomalies, neoplasm, neonatal death, still birth, or low birth weight.[52,53]

Performing a fetal MRI at 3 T results in increased signal-to-noise ratio, which improves image clarity; tissue contrast and anatomic delineation are equal to improved.[19,45,47,49,51,54] On the other hand, the magnetic field is more heterogeneous with 3-T imaging, which can increase multiple artifacts that can decrease image quality. Artifacts seen at 3 T more than 1.5 T include the standing wave, shading, and susceptibility artifacts, especially in the setting of large maternal body habitus, polyhydramnios, or multiple gestations.[48]

Acoustic noise
Gradients are components of the MRI machine that shift and vary during scanning, and as a result produce loud sounds that can reach high decibel levels. To mitigate this, hearing protection is used by the patient during the scan. Maternal body and amniotic fluid surround the fetus, and fluid fills the external and inner ear structures, dampening sound to the fetal cochlea.[49,55] Both 1.5- and 3-T MRI during pregnancy have been studied and show no increased risk of postnatal hearing loss.[52,53,56]

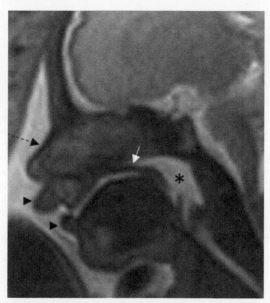

Fig. 4. Sagittal T2 single-shot TSE MR image of fetal face. Posterior palate appears as a hypointense curvilinear structure (*arrow*) above the tongue. T2-hyperintense fluid fills the fetal pharyngeal pouch (*asterisk*). Fetal nose (*dashed arrow*) and lips (*arrowheads*) seen in profile.

FETAL MRI NEURORADIOLOGY: BASIC ANATOMY

Growth of the fetal brain and spine has been well documented, with marked changes from early second trimester to the end of the third.

Skull ossification progresses throughout pregnancy, beginning at the basiocciput and orbital roofs. On fetal MRI, skull shape, size, and localized defects can be

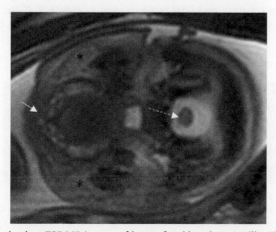

Fig. 5. Axial T2 single-shot TSE MR image of lower fetal head at maxilla. The typical curve of the alveolar ridge (*arrow*) contains multiple centrally T2-hyperintense tooth buds outlined in low signal. Buccal fat is symmetric (*asterisk*) and T2 hyperintense. Posteriorly, the lower brainstem (*dashed arrow*) is outlined by T2-hyperintense cerebrospinal fluid (CSF).

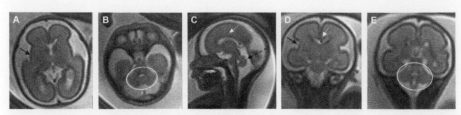

Fig. 6. Axial (*A, B*), sagittal (*C*), and coronal (*D, E*) T2-weighted single-shot TSE MR images of normal fetal brain anatomy at 25 weeks gestational age. The interhemispheric and sylvian fissures (*arrow*) are conspicuous at this stage, with relatively smooth appearance of brain surface otherwise. Bilobed cerebellum (*circled*) is well assessed in axial or coronal planes. The cerebellar vermis (*dashed arrow*) is best evaluated in sagittal plane, with typical reverse C morphology and fluid-containing triangular fourth ventricle apposed to the dorsal brainstem. Midline tissue of the corpus callosum (*white arrow*) is thin at this age, but typically visible on a midline sagittal image (*C*), and crossing midline in the coronal plane (*D*). T2-hyperintense fluid signal of the cavum septum pellucidum (*asterisk*) is also visible at the midline. Typical mild prominence of extra-axial fluid to brain parenchyma seen at this gestational age.

ascertained, aiding in evaluation of craniosynostosis syndromes, microcephaly, macrocephaly, and encephalocele anatomy/extent.[3] The orbits, facial bones, tongue base, lips and palate can be evaluated for abnormal development, with accurate depiction of the posterior palate (**Fig. 4**), an area that is difficult to visualize with ultrasonography due to acoustic shadowing.[3] The maxillary alveolar ridge is delineated in the axial plane, with identification of tooth buds (**Fig. 5**).

Fetal Brain

By late second to third trimesters, when most fetal MRI is performed, rapid growth of the brain occurs, with increasing gyral complexity/sulcation maturity, and myelination.[57] The structural organization of the brain is evaluated in the context of the gestational age and expected normal appearance at that stage (**Figs. 6** and **7**), with established normative data and fetal brain atlases available.[38,39] Parenchymal signal intensity changes with maturation and myelination of the fetal brain. Corpus callosum

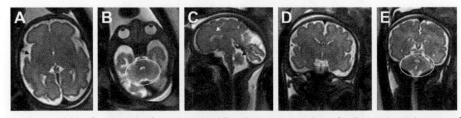

Fig. 7. Axial (*A, B*), sagittal (*C*), and coronal (*D, E*) T2-weighted single-shot TSE MR images of normal fetal brain anatomy at 32 weeks gestational age. There has been significant interval development of the fetal brain compared with **Fig. 6**A, with increased sulcation and relatively decreased extra-axial fluid to brain parenchyma. Ventricle morphology has not significantly changed. There is increased opercular coverage at the sylvian fissure (*black arrow*). Corpus callosum (*white arrow*), cavum septum pellucidum (*asterisk*), cerebellum (*circled*), and vermis (*dashed arrow*) for reference.

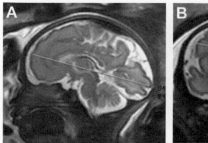
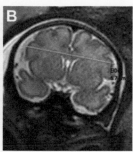
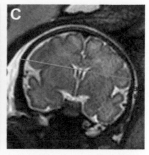

Fig. 8. Representative measurements of fronto-occipital diameter (FOD, *A*), cerebral biparietal diameter (c-BPD, *B*), and bone biparietal diameter (b-BPD, *C*) in the same fetus.

and the fluid-filled cavum septum pellucidum are typically identified on late second-trimester MRI at the midline (see **Figs. 6** and **7**).

Standard brain measurements

Normative data on fetal brain exist for each gestational age,[43] and the frontal-occipital diameter, cerebral biparietal diameter, and bone biparietal diameter are routinely measured (**Fig. 8**). Posterior fossa measurements include transverse cerebellar diameter, vermian height, and anteroposterior cerebellar length at the fastigium.

MRI and ultrasonography both define ventriculomegaly as greater than 10 mm in lateral ventricular atrial diameter. This definition is constant throughout gestation. This diameter can be measured in the coronal or axial planes. Axial measurements of the atria are obtained at the level of the thalami, noting that this may differ from ultrasonography by 1 to 2 mm. Lateral ventricle measurement in the coronal plane on MRI (**Fig. 9**) is obtained at the level of the choroid plexus and has a high concordance with ultrasonographic measurements.[58]

Fetal Spine

Vertebral bodies become visible on MRI by 11 to 12 weeks in the lower spine and at 19 weeks in the cervical spine[3] (**Fig. 10**). SSFP images are of great utility to visualize the fetal skeleton, due to the well-defined bone detail.[3] Typical timing of fetal MRI in

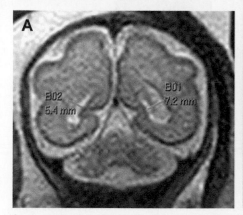
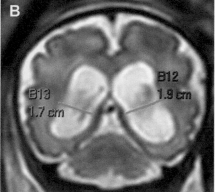

Fig. 9. Coronal T2 single-shot TSE MR images show typical lateral ventricle measurements at the level of choroid plexus in 2 patients; lateral ventricle measurements in a normal 28-week fetus (*A*) versus in a 35-week fetus with severe ventriculomegaly (*B*).

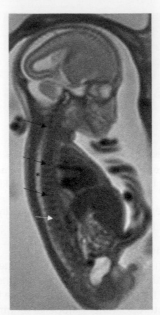

Fig. 10. Sagittal T2 single-shot TSE MR image of a 24.5-week fetus depicts the fetal spine. Hypointense vertebral bodies with typical rectangular morphology (*arrows*). The intervertebral disks (*white arrow*) are mildly T2 hyperintense, and the CSF in the spinal column is very T2 hyperintense (*asterisk*).

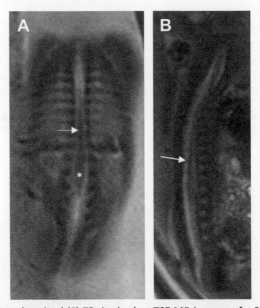

Fig. 11. Coronal (*A*) and sagittal (*B*) T2 single-shot TSE MR images of a 26-week fetus depict normal spinal canal containing T2-hyperintense CSF and homogeneous intermediate-signal-intensity spinal cord (*arrows*) with typical bulbous enlargement of distal cord and conus medullaris (*asterisk*), which ends at the level of lower kidneys (not included).

the second trimester is sufficient to evaluate for maldevelopment, most commonly a posterior dysraphism, such as a myelomeningocele, with the added benefit of MRI to evaluate the brain for expected associated findings. The spinal cord can be assessed for the presence of a syrinx and location of the conus medullaris **(Fig. 11)**.

REFERENCES

1. Halabi S, Epelman M, Pruthi S et al. ACR-SPR Practice Parameter for the safe and optimal performance of fetal magnetic resonance imaging (MRI). Revised 2020. Available at https://www.acr.org/-/media/ACR/Files/Practice-Parameters/MR-Fetal.pdf.
2. Manganaro L, Bernardo S, Antonelli A, et al. Fetal MRI of the central nervous system: state-of-the-art. Eur J Radiol 2017;93:273–83.
3. Chauvin NA, Victoria T, Khwaja A, et al. Magnetic resonance imaging of the fetal musculoskeletal system. Pediatr Radiol 2020;50(13):2009–27.
4. Frates MC, Kumar AJ, Benson CB, et al. Fetal anomalies: comparison of MR imaging and US for diagnosis. Radiology 2004;232(2):398–404.
5. Saleem SN. Fetal MRI: an approach to practice: a review. J Adv Res 2014;5(5): 507–23.
6. Birnbaum R, Ben-Sira L, Lerman-Sagie T, et al. The use of fetal neurosonography and brain MRI in cases of cytomegalovirus infection during pregnancy: a retrospective analysis with outcome correlation. Prenat Diagn 2017;37(13):1335–42.
7. Blondiaux E, Garel C. Fetal cerebral imaging - ultrasound vs. MRI: an update. Acta Radiol 2013;54(9):1046–54.
8. Frick N, Fazelnia C, Kanzian K, et al. The reliability of fetal MRI in the assessment of brain malformations. Fetal Diagn Ther 2015;37(2):93–101.
9. Girardi G. MRI-based methods to detect placental and fetal brain abnormalities in utero. J Reprod Immunol 2016;114:86–91.
10. Goel R, Aggarwal N, Lemmon ME, et al. Fetal and maternal manifestations of tuberous sclerosis complex: value of fetal MRI. Neuroradiol J 2016;29(1):57–60.
11. Griffiths PD, Bradburn M, Campbell MJ, et al. MRI in the diagnosis of fetal developmental brain abnormalities: the MERIDIAN diagnostic accuracy study. Health Technol Assess 2019;23(49):1–144.
12. Griffiths PD, Bradburn M, Campbell MJ, et al. Use of MRI in the diagnosis of fetal brain abnormalities in utero (MERIDIAN): a multicentre, prospective cohort study. Lancet 2017;389(10068):538–46.
13. Hart AR, Embleton ND, Bradburn M, et al. Accuracy of in-utero MRI to detect fetal brain abnormalities and prognosticate developmental outcome: postnatal follow-up of the MERIDIAN cohort. Lancet Child Adolesc Health 2020;4(2):131–40.
14. Irwin K, Henry A, Gopikrishna S, et al. Utility of fetal MRI for workup of fetal central nervous system anomalies in an Australian maternal-fetal medicine cohort. Aust N Z J Obstet Gynaecol 2016;56(3):267–73.
15. Kolbe AB, Merrow AC, Eckel LJ, et al. Congenital hemangioma of the face-Value of fetal MRI with prenatal ultrasound. Radiol Case Rep 2019;14(11):1443–6.
16. Manevich-Mazor M, Weissmann-Brenner A, Bar Yosef O, et al. Added value of fetal MRI in the evaluation of fetal anomalies of the corpus callosum: a retrospective analysis of 78 cases. Ultraschall Med 2018;39(5):513–25. https://doi.org/10.1055/s-0043-113820. Mehrwert der fetalen MRT bei der Beurteilung von Corpus-callosum-Anomalien beim Feten: Eine retrospektive Analyse von 78 Fallen.

17. Masselli G, Vaccaro Notte MR, Zacharzewska-Gondek A, et al. Fetal MRI of CNS abnormalities. Clin Radiol 2020;75(8):640 e1–640 e11.

18. Mirsky DM, Schwartz ES, Zarnow DM. Diagnostic features of myelomeningocele: the role of ultrafast fetal MRI. Fetal Diagn Ther 2015;37(3):219–25.

19. Priego G, Barrowman NJ, Hurteau-Miller J, et al. Does 3T fetal mri improve image resolution of normal brain structures between 20 and 24 weeks' gestational age? AJNR Am J Neuroradiol 2017;38(8):1636–42.

20. Putbrese B, Kennedy A. Findings and differential diagnosis of fetal intracranial haemorrhage and fetal ischaemic brain injury: what is the role of fetal MRI? Br J Radiol 2017;90(1070):20160253.

21. Sanapo L, Whitehead MT, Bulas DI, et al. Fetal intracranial hemorrhage: role of fetal MRI. Prenat Diagn 2017;37(8):827–36.

22. Schlatterer SD, Sanapo L, du Plessis AJ, et al. The role of fetal mri for suspected anomalies of the posterior fossa. Pediatr Neurol 2021;117:10–8.

23. van der Hoek-Snieders HEM, van den Heuvel A, van Os-Medendorp H, et al. Diagnostic accuracy of fetal MRI to detect cleft palate: a meta-analysis. Eur J Pediatr 2020;179(1):29–38.

24. Wagner MW, Vaught AJ, Poretti A, et al. Vein of galen aneurysmal malformation: prognostic markers depicted on fetal MRI. Neuroradiol J 2015;28(1):72–5.

25. Wolfe K, Lewis D, Witte D, et al. Fetal cervical teratoma: what is the role of fetal MRI in predicting pulmonary hypoplasia? Fetal Diagn Ther 2013;33(4):252–6.

26. Zemet R, Amdur-Zilberfarb I, Shapira M, et al. Prenatal diagnosis of congenital head, face, and neck malformations-Is complementary fetal MRI of value? Prenat Diagn 2020;40(1):142–50.

27. Diogo MC, Glatter S, Binder J, et al. The MRI spectrum of congenital cytomegalovirus infection. Prenat Diagn 2020;40(1):110–24.

28. Dai Y, Dong S, Zhu M, et al. Visualizing cerebral veins in fetal brain using susceptibility-weighted MRI. Clin Radiol 2014;69(10):e392–7.

29. Heaphy-Henault KJ, Guimaraes CV, Mehollin-Ray AR, et al. Congenital aqueductal stenosis: findings at fetal MRI that accurately predict a postnatal diagnosis. AJNR Am J Neuroradiol 2018;39(5):942–8.

30. Nagaraj UD, Kline-Fath BM. Imaging of open spinal dysraphisms in the era of prenatal surgery. Pediatr Radiol 2020;50(13):1988–98.

31. Nagaraj UD, Bierbrauer KS, Zhang B, et al. Hindbrain herniation in chiari II malformation on fetal and postnatal MRI. AJNR Am J Neuroradiol 2017;38(5):1031–6. https://doi.org/10.3174/ajnr.A5116.

32. Sherrod BA, Ho WS, Hedlund A, et al. A comparison of the accuracy of fetal MRI and prenatal ultrasonography at predicting lesion level and perinatal motor outcome in patients with myelomeningocele. Neurosurg Focus 2019;47(4):E4.

33. Manganaro L, Tomei A, Fierro F, et al. Fetal MRI as a complement to US in the evaluation of cleft lip and palate. Radiol Med 2011;116(7):1134–48.

34. Ng TW, Xi Y, Schindel D, et al. Fetal head and neck masses: mri prediction of significant morbidity. AJR Am J Roentgenol 2019;212(1):215–21.

35. Mirsky DM, Shekdar KV, Bilaniuk LT. Fetal MRI: head and neck. Magn Reson Imaging Clin N Am 2012;20(3):605–18.

36. Prayer D, Malinger G, Brugger PC, et al. ISUOG Practice Guidelines: performance of fetal magnetic resonance imaging. Ultrasound Obstet Gynecol 2017;49(5):671–80. https://doi.org/10.1002/uog.17412.

37. Haris K, Hedstrom E, Kording F, et al. Free-breathing fetal cardiac MRI with Doppler ultrasound gating, compressed sensing, and motion compensation. J Magn Reson Imaging 2020;51(1):260–72.
38. Gholipour A, Limperopoulos C, Clancy S, et al. Construction of a deformable spatio-temporal MRI atlas of the fetal brain: evaluation of similarity metrics and deformation models. Med Image Comput Comput Assist Interv 2014;17(Pt 2):292–9.
39. Gholipour A, Rollins CK, Velasco-Annis C, et al. A normative spatiotemporal MRI atlas of the fetal brain for automatic segmentation and analysis of early brain growth. Sci Rep 2017;7(1):476.
40. Style CC, Mehollin-Ray AR, Verla MA, et al. Timing of prenatal magnetic resonance imaging in the assessment of congenital diaphragmatic hernia. Fetal Diagn Ther 2020;47(3):205–13.
41. Yen CJ, Mehollin-Ray AR, Bernardo F, et al. Correlation between maternal meal and fetal motion during fetal MRI. Pediatr Radiol 2019;49(1):46–50.
42. Meyers ML, Mirsky DM, Dannull KA, et al. Effects of maternal valium administration on fetal MRI motion artifact: a comparison study at high altitude. Fetal Diagn Ther 2017;42(2):124–9.
43. Kline-Fath BM, Bulas DI, Bahado-Singh R. In: Beth M, Kline-Fath DI, Bulas RBS, editors. Fundamental and advanced fetal imaging : ultrasound and MRI. Philadelphia: Wolters Kluwer Health; 2015.
44. Coblentz AC, Teixeira SR, Mirsky DM, et al. How to read a fetal magnetic resonance image 101. Pediatr Radiol 2020;50(13):1810–29.
45. Welsh RC, Nemec U, Thomason ME. Fetal magnetic resonance imaging at 3.0 T. Top Magn Reson Imaging 2011;22(3):119–31.
46. Committee Opinion No. 723: guidelines for diagnostic imaging during pregnancy and lactation. Obstet Gynecol 2017;130(4):e210–6.
47. Krishnamurthy U, Neelavalli J, Mody S, et al. MR imaging of the fetal brain at 1.5T and 3.0T field strengths: comparing specific absorption rate (SAR) and image quality. J Perinat Med 2015;43(2):209–20.
48. Victoria T, Jaramillo D, Roberts TP, et al. Fetal magnetic resonance imaging: jumping from 1.5 to 3 tesla (preliminary experience). Pediatr Radiol 2014;44(4):376–86, quiz 373-5.
49. Victoria T, Johnson AM, Edgar JC, et al. Comparison between 1.5-T and 3-T MRI for Fetal imaging: is there an advantage to imaging with a higher field strength? Am J Roentgenol 2016;206(1):195–201.
50. Barrera CA, Francavilla ML, Serai SD, et al. Specific absorption rate and specific energy dose: comparison of 1.5-t versus 3.0-t fetal MRI. Radiology 2020;295(3):664–74.
51. Barth R, Victoria T, Kline-Fath B, et al. Society for pediatric radiology fetal imaging C. ISUOG guidelines for fetal MRI: a response to 3-T fetal imaging and limited fetal exams. Ultrasound Obstet Gynecol 2017;50(6):804–5.
52. Chartier AL, Bouvier MJ, McPherson DR, et al. The safety of maternal and fetal MRI at 3 T. AJR Am J Roentgenol 2019;213(5):1170–3.
53. Ray JG, Vermeulen MJ, Bharatha A, et al. Association between MRI exposure during pregnancy and fetal and childhood outcomes. JAMA 2016;316(9):952–61.
54. Weisstanner C, Gruber GM, Brugger PC, et al. Fetal MRI at 3T—ready for routine use? Br J Radiol 2017;90(1069). https://doi.org/10.1259/bjr.20160362.

55. Gowland, P. Safety of Fetal MRI Scanning. In: Prayer D, editor. Fetal MRI. Medical Radiology 2010; Springer: Berlin (Heidelberg). https://doi.org/10.1007/174_2010_122.

56. Jaimes C, Delgado J, Cunnane MB, et al. Does 3-T fetal MRI induce adverse acoustic effects in the neonate? A preliminary study comparing postnatal auditory test performance of fetuses scanned at 1.5 and 3 T. Pediatr Radiol 2019;49(1):37–45.

57. Choi JJ, Yang E, Soul JS, et al. Fetal magnetic resonance imaging: supratentorial brain malformations. Pediatr Radiol 2020;50(13):1934–47.

58. Garel C, Alberti C. Coronal measurement of the fetal lateral ventricles: comparison between ultrasonography and magnetic resonance imaging. Ultrasound Obstet Gynecol 2006;27(1):23–7.

Imaging of Congenital Malformations of the Brain

Laura Z. Fenton, MD

KEYWORDS

- Congenital • Brain • Cerebral • Malformation of cortical development

KEY POINTS

- Midline anomalies tend to occur together, thus when one midline brain anomaly is identified (ie, corpus callosum agenesis), investigate for others.
- Magnetic resonance imaging (MRI) is the most sensitive modality for the identification and characterization of congenital brain anomalies that may be first suspected on prenatal or postnatal ultrasound.
- MRI at 2 to 3 years of age may further elucidate often subtle malformations of cortical development that are occult earlier due to the degree of myelination in the neonatal and infant periods.

INTRODUCTION

Congenital brain malformations are anomalies of brain development caused by genetic and environmental influences. Advances in neuroimaging techniques and genetic research have led to a better understanding of the pathogenesis of many congenital brain malformations. This article highlights the neuroimaging appearance of common supratentorial congenital brain malformations.

BACKGROUND

Brain development involves a complex cascade of genetic signaling formation at critical time periods. The classification of congenital brain malformations is challenging because many brain structures develop simultaneously, and no 2 malformations are exactly alike. Thus, it is uncommon for one anomaly to occur in isolation and midline anomalies tend to occur together. Additionally, this process can be influenced and disrupted by genetic mutations as well as environmental factors. At times, certain patterns of multiple anomalies can suggest a genetic syndrome; other times the patterns are sporadic. The development of the nervous system involves the closure of the neuropore and eventually the neural tube. Cells in the neuroectoderm rely on signals to

Department of Diagnostic Radiology, University of Colorado School of Medicine, Children's Hospital Colorado, 13123 East 16th Avenue, Box 125, Aurora, CO 80045, USA
E-mail address: laura.fenton@childrenscolorado.org

Clin Perinatol 49 (2022) 587–601
https://doi.org/10.1016/j.clp.2022.05.002
0095-5108/22/© 2022 Elsevier Inc. All rights reserved.
perinatology.theclinics.com

initiate cell recognition and adhesion to proceed to the closure of the neural tube through the process of neurulation. Previous theories suggesting a stepwise cephalad to the caudal process have been refuted and replaced with the theory of simultaneous development with ultimate closure of the anterior neuropore at 25 days and posterior neuropore at 27 to 28 days gestational age. When the anterior neuropore closes, 3 subdivisions are formed: the prosencephalon (forebrain), mesencephalon (midbrain), and rhombencephalon (hindbrain).[1] Identifying intracranial congenital anomalies and understanding how the location and type of malformation affect brain, motor, or cognitive development can alter patient treatment, outcome and ultimately the quality of life.

DISORDERS OF DORSAL INDUCTION
Anencephaly

Anencephaly is the absence of the forebrain, midbrain, and hindbrain, as well as the skull and scalp. This malformation results when the cephalic end of the neural tube fails to close or reopens after closure and is not compatible with life.[2] Anencephaly affects females more often than males (3–4:1). Fetal ultrasound (US) is sufficient for diagnosis in most and shows the absence of the brain and skull above the orbits (**Fig. 1**) in combination with elevated maternal alpha-fetoprotein. Fetal magnetic resonance imaging (MRI) may play a role in assessing viability, for research purposes or to assess for the possibility of organ donation. There is infrequent postnatal imaging due to the high early mortality rate.

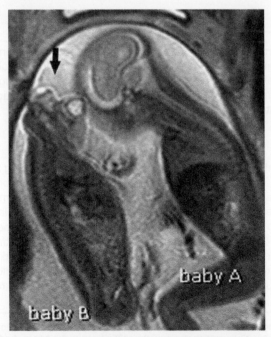

Fig. 1. Fetal anencephaly. Fetal MRI sagittal T2 weighted image performed on a twin gestation during the second trimester shows the absence of the fetal brain in baby B on the left side (*black arrow*). Note there is no brain present above the orbits. This examination was performed to evaluate baby A, who did not have any brain or body abnormality by fetal MRI.

Cephalocele

A cephalocele is a neural tube defect with focally deficient skull and dura through which there is an outward extension of intracranial structures. This term is synonymous with encephalocele when there is outward herniation of a portion of the brain through the defect. This is distinguished from meningocele which refers to the protrusion of meninges through an osseous defect (skull or posterior elements of the spine) that does not contain neural elements. Cephaloceles are named by the location of the bone defect with the most common location posterior in the occipital region (80%, **Fig. 2** A–D). Neuroimaging is performed to identify the skull and dural defect, the portion of brain herniated (which is often dysplastic), and additional brain anomalies. It is also important to assess for associated anomalous vasculature, especially dural venous sinus course, to assist in planning for neurosurgical resection.[3]

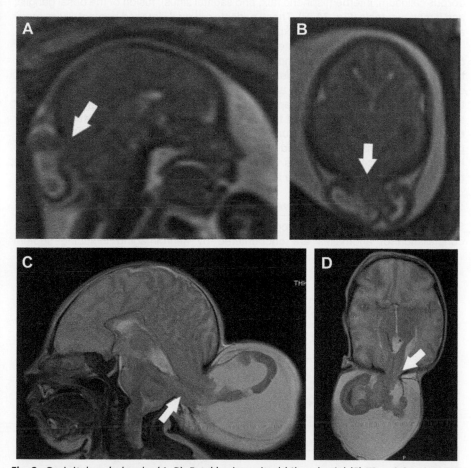

Fig. 2. Occipital cephalocele. (*A–D*). Fetal brain sagittal (*A*) and axial (*B*) T2 weighted MR images at 20 weeks gestation shows a midline occipital skull defect (*white arrow*) with outward herniation of brain. Postnatal sagittal (*C*) and axial (*D*) T2 weighted brain MR images show with better detail the herniated portions of the occipital lobes and cerebellum through the skull and dural defect (*white arrow*).

Disorders of Ventral Induction

Holoprosencephaly

Failure of midline cleavage of the prosencephalon (forebrain) results in the holoprosencephaly spectrum. *Holo*-means single and describes the failure of the division of the forebrain into 2 hemispheres. A genetic cause is confirmed in approximately 50% with mutations in the sonic hedgehog (*SHH*) gene the most prevalent.[4] Clinical presentation and prognosis vary depending on severity; therefore, subtypes are described on a continuum by the terms *alobar* (most severe), *semilobar* and *lobar* (least severe).

Alobar holoprosencephaly is the most common and most severe form with absent midline differentiation. Severe midline facial anomalies are often present including the presence of a midline proboscis instead of a nose, cyclopia (single fused globe), or hypotelorism-all reminiscent of the supporting statement "*the face predicts the brain.*" Fetal US is often sufficient for diagnosis with fetal MRI performed to confirm the diagnosis as indicated. Imaging shows the absence of midline structures (including the corpus callosum, interhemispheric falx, and sagittal sinus), fusion of the basal ganglia, and a monoventricle (**Fig. 3**A, B). These patients are rarely imaged postnatally as many are stillborn or have a short life expectancy.

In semilobar and lobar holoprosencephaly, the brain is more developed with milder or absent associated facial anomalies. In these milder forms of holoprosencephaly, there is partial midline differentiation and formation of the interhemispheric falx, corpus callosum, and ventricles, all to varying degrees from caudal to cranial (back to front). Semilobar holoprosencephaly has a posterior interhemispheric falx as well as temporal and occipital horns of the lateral ventricles and a characteristic dysplastic shortened posterior corpus callosum (splenium) only (**Fig. 4**A, B). Lobar holoprosencephaly (**Fig. 5**A–C) has a fully formed third ventricle and often dysplastic frontal horns. In lobar holoprosencephaly there is a fusion of the anterior frontal lobes across the midline due to the absence of the anterior portion of the interhemispheric falx.

Septo-Optic Dysplasia (Optic Nerve Hypoplasia Syndrome)

Septo-optic dysplasia is a heterogeneous disorder that is loosely defined when a constellation of anomalies are encountered by neuroimaging including septum

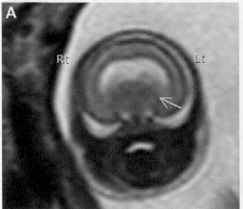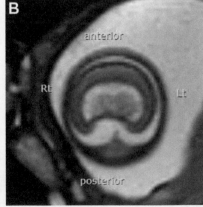

Fig. 3. Alobar holoprosencephaly. (*A, B*). Fetal brain coronal (*A*) and axial (*B*) T2 weighted MR images at 20 weeks gestation show absent division of the cerebral hemispheres with absent midline interhemispheric falx, fusion of the thalami (*green arrow* in *A*), and monoventricle.

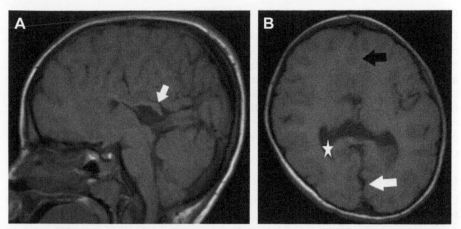

Fig. 4. Semilobar holoprosencephaly. (*A, B*). Postnatal brain MRI sagittal (*A*) T1 weighted image shows the incomplete formation of the corpus callosum with only the posterior splenium present (*white arrow*). Axial (*B*) T1 weighted image shows the presence of the posterior interhemispheric falx (*white arrow*), fusion of the frontal lobes across midline (*black arrow*), and separated occipital horns (*white star*) of the lateral ventricles. There is absence of the frontal horns.

pellucidum hypoplasia or absence, optic nerve hypoplasia, hypothalamic-pituitary abnormality, and/or cortical malformation.[1] If 2 of these 4 anomalies are encountered, it is worthwhile to suggest this diagnosis; however, the etiology is multifactorial and includes acquired and genetic causes. Children may present with nystagmus, decreased vision, seizures, and/or endocrinopathy. Neuroimaging shows a "boxcar" configuration of the frontal horns without midline separation due to the absence of the septum pellucidum, small optic nerve/s, an ectopic or absent posterior pituitary bright spot, and/or cortical malformation (**Fig. 6**A, B). Schizencephaly is the most frequent cortical malformation (**Fig. 7**A, B). Interestingly, a large review of reports on children with optic nerve hypoplasia noted a paucity of genetic findings and a striking preponderance of young mothers and primiparity suggesting a potential role for prenatal nutrition.[5]

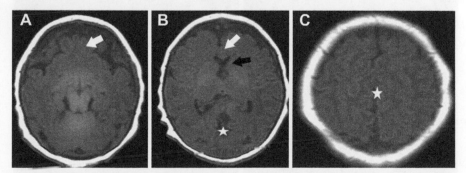

Fig. 5. Lobar holoprosencephaly. (*A–C*). Postnatal brain MRI axial images at the level of the lower frontal lobes (*A*), frontal horns of the lateral ventricles (*B*), and vertex (*C*). Note in A and B there is a fusion of the frontal lobes across the midline anteriorly (*white arrow*), dysplastic frontal horns in B (*black arrow*) and present of the superior portion of the interhemispheric falx in *B* and *C* (*white star*).

DISORDERS OF NEURONAL MIGRATION AND PROLIFERATION

Cerebral cortical development can be affected by diverse processes that inhibit neuronal or glial proliferation, migration, or cortical organization. This includes gene mutations, insults from infection or bleeding, exogenous toxins (alcohol or drug), and endogenous toxins (metabolic disorder).[6] More severe malformations may be identified via prenatal ultrasound at 18 to 20 weeks; however, less severe malformations may be subtle, even on postnatal MRI. Fetal and postnatal brain MRI are the most sensitive modalities to identify these malformations. Cortical malformations can be the cause of developmental delay, hypotonia, and seizures in infants and children.

Lissencephaly (Agyria-Pachygyria Spectrum)

Lissencephaly is a spectrum of neuronal migration disorders with a decrease in sulcal formation and diffusely thickened gyri. In the most severe type, agyria, there is a near complete absence of brain sulcal formation resulting in a smooth "figure of 8" brain, as in this extreme the sylvian fissure is the only well-formed sulcus (Fig. 8). A helpful clue to the presence of lissencephaly by MRI, to distinguish from other malformations of cortical development, is the presence of 4 alternating cortical zones (outer molecular layer, outer thin cortical layer, T2 hyperintense cell sparse zone, and an inner thick cortical layer) in the affected thickened cortex. Pathology shows a four-layer cortex instead of a normal six-layered cortex. Less severe in the lissencephaly spectrum is pachygyria, defined as thickened cortex with few broad flat gyri. Pachygyria is more likely to be localized and asymmetric and less commonly diffuse and bilateral (see Fig. 8, affecting the posterior brain). Band heterotopia, considered the mildest form of lissencephaly, is diagnosed by MRI by the identification of symmetric bands of gray matter located between the periventricular white matter and subcortical white matter (Fig. 9A, B). Band heterotopia may also occur to a lesser degree involving a single lobe of a cerebral hemisphere. The lissencephaly spectrum is associated with the

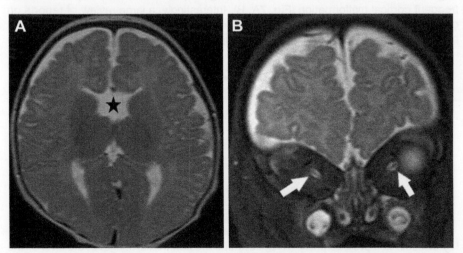

Fig. 6. Septo-optic dysplasia in a neonate. (A, B). Postnatal brain MRI axial (A) and coronal (B) T2 weighted images show "boxcar" configuration of the frontal horns due to the absence of the septum pellucidum in A (black star) and hypoplastic bilateral optic nerves in B (white arrows).

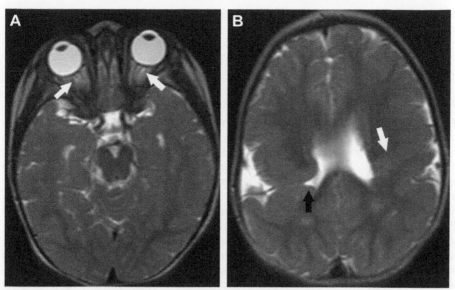

Fig. 7. Septo-optic dysplasia in a child with bilateral schizencephaly. (*A*, *B*). Postnatal brain MRI axial T2 weighted image at the level of the optic nerves (*A*) shows hypoplastic bilateral optic nerves (*white arrows*). At the level of bilateral frontal-parietal lobes (*B*) there is bilateral closed lip schizencephaly. Note the right lateral ventricular "dimple" at the level of the gray matter lined cleft (*black arrow*), and the abnormal gray matter extending through the left cerebral hemisphere (*white arrow*).

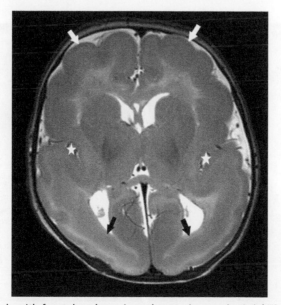

Fig. 8. Lissencephaly with frontal pachygyria and posterior agyria. Axial T2 weighted MR image in a 2-month-old boy shows a "figure 8" configuration of the brain with symmetric shallow sylvian fissures (*white stars*) and diffusely thickened cortex. Note anteriorly in bilateral frontal lobes, there are few, broad, flat gyri (pachygyria, *white arrows*) and posteriorly there are absent gyri with a smooth brain surface and zonal pattern (agyria, *black arrows*).

LIS1 or DCX gene mutations.[7] Patients typically have hypotonia, developmental delay, and seizures in the form of infantile spasms. Correlation of gestational age with the degree of gyral formation is imperative when evaluating for cortical malformations as premature newborns can appear to have a smooth brain and mimic the lissencephaly spectrum.

Polymicrogyria

Polymicrogyria is due to abnormal neuronal migration and distribution resulting in numerous small gyri with abnormal sulcation. This malformation can be focal, diffuse, unilateral, or bilateral but is most commonly located in and adjacent to the sylvian fissure (perisylvian). Polymicrogyria is distinguished from pachygyria in that the affected gyri do not follow typical anatomic naming, whereas pachygyria follows named gyri. Polymicrogyria is often the anatomic abnormality responsible for seizures. In the prenatal period, polymicrogyria is seen on MRI as focal irregular thickening of gyri (**Fig. 10**A, B). This is best appreciated when comparing the affected gyral thickness to the normal thin uniform gyri elsewhere in the brain. In the postnatal period, imaging of polymicrogyria on MRI varies from conspicuous to very subtle.[8] When conspicuous, polymicrogyria is visible as abnormally formed gyri with irregular thickened cortex and more numerous convolutions than are typically seen (**Fig. 11**A, B). As in the fetus, this is best appreciated when compared with the normal contralateral gyri or an age-matched normal control MRI. With age-appropriate myelination, polymicrogyria often becomes more conspicuous (**Fig. 12**A, B). However, polymicrogyria can also be difficult to visualize by MRI, visible only as subtle loss of gray-white matter differentiation. Hence, it is important to correlate the brain MRI abnormality with the site

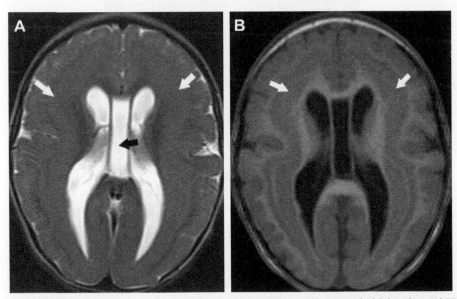

Fig. 9. Bilateral band gray matter heterotopia (mildest form of lissencephaly) (*A, B*). Axial T2 (*A*) and T1 (*B*) weighted Brain MR images show symmetric bands of gray matter between the periventricular white matter and subcortical white matter (*white arrows*). Incidentally noted is a patent cavum septum pellucidum et verge (cerebrospinal fluid space between the lateral ventricles), a normal variant (*black arrow* in A).

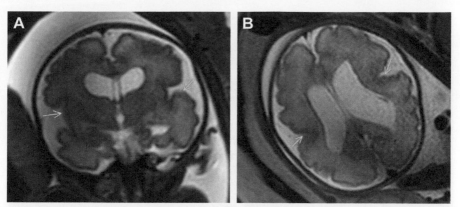

Fig. 10. Bilateral perisylvian polymicrogyria in a fetus (*A, B*). Fetal brain MRI coronal T2 (*A*) and axial T2 (*B*) weighted at 30 weeks gestation show irregular gyral thickening and nodularity in bilateral sylvian fissures (*thin green arrows*); this is best appreciated when compared to normal uniform thin gyral thickness in bilateral frontal lobes. Mild lateral ventriculomegaly is also present.

of known or suspected seizure focus by EEG and clinical semiology. An often-helpful clue to the presence of polymicrogyria is the prominence of the adjacent cortical veins, which have been implicated in pathogenesis.[9] In the setting of epilepsy, polymicrogyria may not be visible by imaging in infants and young children (less than 2 to 3 years of age) due to the degree of myelination. Thus, in the setting of a normal MRI in a young child with medically refractory epilepsy, repeat MRI at 2 to 3 years of age may reveal a previously occult cortical malformation.

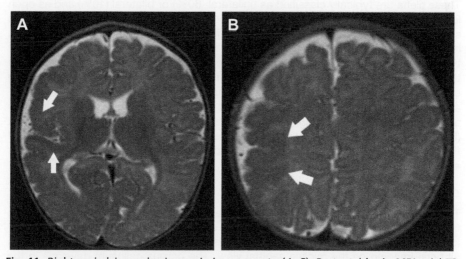

Fig. 11. Right perisylvian polymicrogyria in a neonate (*A, B*). Postnatal brain MRI axial T2 weighted images at the level of the third ventricle (*A*) and at the level of bilateral parietal lobes (*B*) performed at 2 weeks of age shows asymmetric nodular gyral thickening in the right perisylvian region (*white arrows*). Compare to normal thin, uniform gyral thickness in the left cerebral hemisphere.

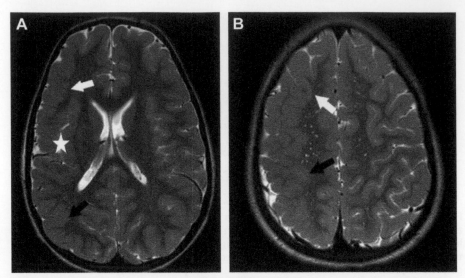

Fig. 12. Right perisylvian polymicrogyria in an older child (*A, B*). Brain MRI axial T2 weighted images at the level of the bodies of the lateral ventricles (*A*) and at the level of bilateral parietal lobes (*B*) show extensive asymmetric nodular thickening of gyri in the right perisylvian region (*white star*) extending to the right frontal lobe (*white arrow*) and right parietal lobe (*black arrow*).

Schizencephaly

Schizencephaly is a gray matter-lined cleft extending through the entire cerebral hemisphere from the ependymal surface of the lateral ventricle to the pial surface of the cortex. The lining gray matter is disorganized and dysplastic, most often polymicrogyria. These clefts are typically classified as unilateral (60%) or bilateral (40%) and as open lip (larger cerebrospinal fluid space) versus closed lip (barely visible). Most cases are sporadic with few familial cases described. Clinically, affected children have seizures, hemiparesis (related to the volume of brain missing, more extensive with open lip type), and variable developmental delay. Neuroimaging is often conspicuous with the open lip type as prominent cerebrospinal fluid fills the cleft (**Fig. 13**). In the setting of closed lip schizencephaly, the cerebrospinal fluid filled cleft may be indistinguishable, with outward "dimpling" of the lateral ventricle a helpful clue in addition to abnormal gray matter extending from the lateral ventricle edge to the peripheral cortex (**Fig. 14**A, B). MRI studies have reported evidence of prior hemorrhage in and around the cleft when schizencephaly are encountered in utero suggesting a prenatal vascular etiology.[10]

Corpus Callosal Dysgenesis

The cerebral white matter commissures connect the 2 cerebral hemispheres and form from the dorsal prosencephalon. The corpus callosum is the largest and most easily identified of the cerebral commissures and is a key imaging structure to identify in all brain imaging on the midline sagittal view. The corpus callosum develops in the fetus between 8 and 20 weeks and anomalies are common, occurring in 1.8 of 10,000 live births. The corpus callosum is divided into 5 sections from anterior to posterior: rostrum, genu, body, isthmus, and splenium. The incidence of corpus callosal dysgenesis is increased in newborns born prematurely, infants of diabetic mothers

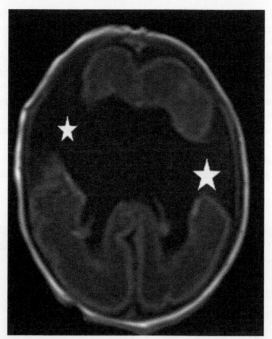

Fig. 13. Bilateral open lip schizencephaly in a premature neonate. Postnatal brain MRI axial T1 weighted image shows bilateral frontal cerebrospinal fluid-filled clefts (*white stars*). Note, the smooth appearance of the brain is due to prematurity, emphasizing the importance of correlating the degree of brain development with gestational age so as not to overcall a cortical malformation.

as well as in infants with genetic or other neurologic disorders.[11] Anomalies in the development of the corpus callosum range from partial to complete absence. Fetal US is used to screen for corpus callosal anomalies, however, has a reported false-positive rate of up to 20%.[12] Fetal MRI, therefore, adds value and sensitivity in this

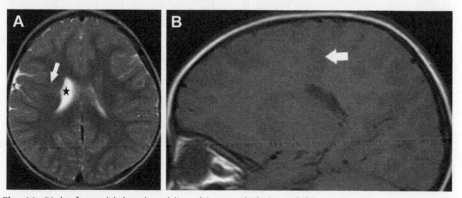

Fig. 14. Right frontal lobe closed lip schizencephaly in a child. Brain MRI axial T2 (*A*) and sagittal T1 (*B*) weighted images show a subtle gray matter lined cleft in the right frontal lobe (*white arrows*). Notice the presence of a ventricular dimple (*black star*) in the right lateral ventricle, a helpful clue to the presence of this malformation.

setting as well as screening for additional anomalies. With complete corpus callosal agenesis, neuroimaging shows parallel configuration of the lateral ventricles, "steer horn" shape of the frontal horns, a high riding third ventricle, and disproportionate enlargement of the occipital horns (known as colpocephaly) (**Fig. 15**A–D). Importantly, the presence of colpocephaly is rarely associated with increased intracranial pressure and is attributed to part of the callosal malformation. Intracranial anomalies associated with corpus callosal agenesis include interhemispheric cyst and lipoma as well as Chiari I malformation. Commonly associated syndromes with corpus callosal dysgenesis include Aicardi syndrome, cerebellar vermis hypoplasia-aplasia spectrum (also known as Dandy–Walker malformation), Chiari type II malformation, and fetal alcohol syndrome. Interestingly, a relatively thickened normally formed corpus callosum can be present in the setting of multiple malformations of cortical development.

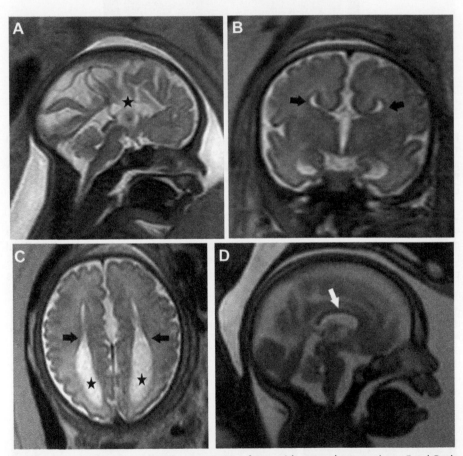

Fig. 15. Complete corpus callosal agenesis in a fetus with normal comparison. Fetal Brain MRI sagittal (*A*), coronal (*B*), and axial (*C*) T2 weighted images performed at 33 weeks gestational age show complete absence of the corpus callosum (*black star* in *A*) with steer horn configuration of the frontal horns on the coronal view (*black arrows* in *B*), parallel lateral ventricles (*black arrows* in *C*) and disproportionate dilation of the occipital horns (colpocephaly) on the axial view (*black stars* in *C*). Sagittal T2 (*D*) weighted MRI image in a different 29-week gestation fetus for comparison shows a normal corpus callosum (*white arrow*).

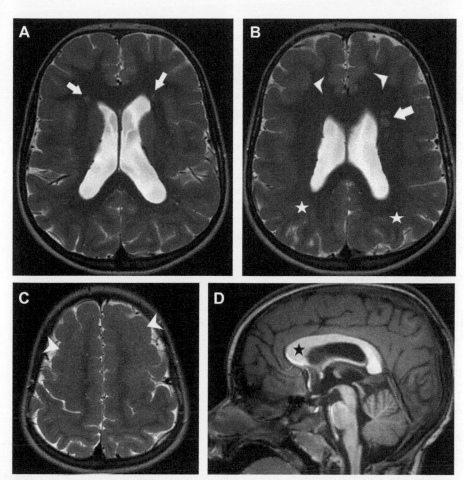

Fig. 16. Nodular periventricular gray matter heterotopia with bifrontal pachygyria and posterior band heterotopia. Brain MRI was performed on a 6-year-old boy with seizures and developmental delay. Axial T2 weighted images at the level of the lateral ventricular trigones (*A*), posterior frontal and parietal lobes (*B*) and near the vertex (*C*) show bifrontal nodules of gray matter signal intensity in the periventricular white matter (*white arrows*). Additionally, there is bifrontal-parietal smooth, broad, flat gyri (pachygyria, best seen in *B* and *C*, white *arrowheads*) and bilateral posterior bands of gray matter signal deep to the subcortical white matter (band heterotopia, *white stars*). Sagittal T1 weighted midline image (*D*) shows relative thickening of the corpus callosum (*black star*), which can coexist with extensive cortical malformations.

Gray matter heterotopia

Gray matter heterotopia is the collections of nerve cells in abnormal locations secondary to arrest in radial migration. There are two broad categories: nodular and band types. Note that the term heterotopia is pleural, referring to more than one abnormal focus, whereas heterotopia refers to a single focus (in the setting of nodular type). Patients may come to medical attention due to cognitive deficit, developmental delay, or seizures. Brain MRI shows nodular or band-shaped foci that follow gray matter signal on all pulse sequences, most often located in the periventricular or subcortical locations. Most patients have heterotopia that is asymmetric and single or few in number, most often located adjacent to the posterior lateral ventricular trigone. These heterotopia can be isolated or associated with other structural anomalies (**Fig. 16**A–D) such as Chiari II, cerebellar hypoplasia, cephaloceles, and other cortical malformations.[13] The band-type of heterotopia is better classified as a mild form of lissencephaly and is discussed previously in the lissencephaly section above.

SUMMARY

Congenital brain malformations are anomalies of brain development caused by genetic and environmental influences. Prenatal and postnatal brain MRI remain the gold standard for optimal identification and characterization of these malformations. When one malformation is identified, search for an additional malformation should be undertaken as these frequently coexist. It is essential for pediatric subspecialists to work together with neuroimagers to provide appropriate diagnostic and prognostic information to ultimately improve the quality of care for affected children and their families.

CLINICS CARE POINTS

- Brain MRI is the most sensitive imaging modality to identify congenital brain malformations.

DISCLOSURE

The author has no relevant financial or commercial conflict of interest, funding source, or other disclosure.

REFERENCES

1. Barkovich JA, Raybaud C. Congenital malformations of the brain and skull. In: Lippincott Williams & Wilkins, editor. Pediatric neuroimaging. 6th edition. Philadelphia: Wolters Kluwer; 2019. p. 405–632.
2. Calzolari F, Gambi B, Garani G, Tamisari L. Anencephaly: MRI findings and pathogenetic theories. Pediatr Radiol 2004;34(12):1012–6.
3. Kasprian GJ, Paldino MJ, Mehollin-Ray AR, et al. Prenatal imaging of occipital encephaloceles. Fetal Diagn Ther 2015;37:241–8.
4. Koussa YA, du Plessis AJ, Vezina G. Prenatal diagnosis of holoprosencephaly. Am J Med Genet C Semin Med Genet 2018;178(2):206–13.
5. Garcia-Filion P, Borchert M. Prenatal determination of optic nerve hypoplasia: review of suggested correlates and future focus. Surv Ophthalmol 2013;58:610–9.
6. Abdel Razek AA, Kandell AY, Elsorogy LG, et al. Disorders of cortical formation: MR imaging features. Am J Neuroradiol 2009;30(1):4–11.
7. Ghai S, Fong KW, Toi A, et al. Prenatal US and MR imaging findings of lissencephaly: review of fetal cerebral sulcal development. Radiographics 2006;26(2):389–405.
8. Stutterd CA, Leventer RJ. Polymicrogyria: a common and heterogeneous malformation of cortical development. Am J Med Genet C Semin Med Genet 2014;166C(2):227–39.
9. De Ciantis A, Barkovich AJ, Cosottini M, et al. Ultra-high-field MR imaging in polymicrogyria and epilepsy. Am J Neuroradiol 2015;36(2):309–16.

10. Nabavizadeh SA, Zarnow D, Bilaniuk LT, et al. Correlation of prenatal and post-natal MRI findings in schizencephaly. Am J Neuroradiol 2014;35:1418–24.
11. Tang PH, Bartha AI, Norton ME, et al. Agenesis of the corpus callosum: an MR imaging analysis of associated abnormalities in the fetus. Am J Neuroradiol 2009;30(2):257–63.
12. Santo S, D'Antonio F, Homfray T, et al. Counseling in fetal medicine: agenesis of the corpus callosum. Ultrasound Obstet Gynecol 2012;40(5):513–21.
13. Srour M, Rioux MF, Varga C, et al. The clinical spectrum of nodular heterotopias in children: report of 31 patients. Epilepsia 2011;52:728–37.

Congenital Malformations of Cerebellum

Ali Moosavi, Sangam Kanekar, MD*

KEYWORDS

- Cerebellum • Macrocerebellum • Rhombencephalosynapsis • Cerebral dysplasia
- Joubert Syndrome

KEY POINTS

- Malformations of the posterior cranial fossa may result from inherited (genetic) or acquired (disruptive) causes.
- The cerebellum is particularly vulnerable to metabolic and toxic insults as well as prenatal infections and hemorrhages, whereas it is less vulnerable to prenatal, perinatal, and postnatal hypoxic-ischemic events.
- Pontocerebellar hypoplasia is a group of autosomal recessive neurodegenerative disorders with prenatal onset, and are characterized by hypoplasia and variable atrophy of the cerebellum and pons.
- Unilateral cerebellar cleft is defined as a disruptive lesion affecting principally the cortical gray matter of one cerebellar hemisphere, extending from the hemisphere's surface into the parenchyma.

INTRODUCTION

Advances in pre and postnatal neuroimaging techniques, and molecular genetics have increased our understanding of the congenital malformations of the brain and have provided a better understanding of their pathogenesis. Correct diagnosis of these malformations in regards to morphology, embryology, and molecular neurogenetics is of paramount importance to inform the parents or the caregiver of the prognosis, inheritance pattern and risk of recurrence, as well as genetic counseling.

Malformations of the posterior cranial fossa may occur from any number of insults along the pathway from early embryogenesis to neural maturation. They may result from inherited (genetic) or acquired (disruptive) causes. Gene mutations causing malformations may be de novo or inherited (autosomal recessive, X linked) from the parents. Common disruptive causes include prenatal infection, hemorrhage, and ischemia. As compared with inherited causes, disruptive causes are without risk of

Radiology Research, Division of Neuroradiology, Penn State Health, Penn State College of Medicine, Mail Code H066 500 University Drive, Hershey, PA 17033, USA
* Corresponding author.
E-mail address: skanekar@pennstatehealth.psu.edu

Clin Perinatol 49 (2022) 603–621
https://doi.org/10.1016/j.clp.2022.04.003
0095-5108/22/© 2022 Elsevier Inc. All rights reserved.

recurrence. Clinically, posterior fossa malformations have heterogeneous presentation: ocular-motor apraxia, mental retardation, nystagmus, strabismus, abnormal speech and language development, and walking disabilities. Antenatal and postnatal imaging plays an important role in the diagnosis and classification of these malformations.

ANATOMY AND DEVELOPMENT

Development of the embryonic central nervous system begins in the fifth week of gestation with the formation of the primary neural tube, which is then divided to form 3 primary vesicles that will become the forebrain, midbrain, and hindbrain.[1] Cell-signaling interactions are responsible for maintaining these divisions during development. In particular, OTX2 expressed from the midbrain and GBX2 expressed from the hindbrain work to maintain this midbrain-hindbrain boundary.[2] The hindbrain is then further divided by the pontine flexure into secondary vesicles that develop into the metencephalon (which develops into the cerebellar hemispheres and pons) and the myelencephalon (which develops into the medulla).[3] HOX and KROX-20 transcription factors are responsible for dividing the embryonic hindbrain further into these differentiated segments, which are then maintained as separate elements through interactions between Eph ligands and their intrinsic Eph receptors.[2]

Once the neural tube is closed, the remaining neural canal posterior to the hindbrain becomes the fourth ventricle.[3] At approximately 6 weeks of gestation, there is bilateral thickening of the roof of the fourth ventricle to form the rhombic lips, which enlarge to form the cerebellar hemispheres.[4]

As the brainstem and cerebellum develop, the neuroectodermal roof plate secretes BMP and WNT signaling proteins which trigger the developing *posterior* brainstem and cerebellum to undergo *dorsal*-type differentiation. Conversely, prechordal plate secretes SHH, which triggers the *anterior* brainstem and cerebellum to undergo *ventral*-type differentiation.[2] By 9 weeks the cerebellar hemispheres growing from the rhomboid lips finally meet in the midline. It is the fusion of these hemispheres, as well as a contribution from the dorsal alar plate of the mesencephalon, that forms the cerebellar vermis.[4]

By 10 weeks, pontine flexure grows transversely to form the plica choroidalis to divide the fourth ventricle into the Anterior and Posterior Membranous areas.[5] The superior *Anterior* Membranous Area (AMA) forms the choroid plexus, while the inferior *Posterior* Membranous Area (PMA) fills with cerebrospinal fluid to form "Blake's pouch." Blakes pouch grows to communicate with the fourth ventricle and spinal subarachnoid space, then eventually regresses by 14 to 17 weeks to function as the foramen of Magendie.[3]

IMAGING MODALITIES

Ultrasound evaluation of the posterior cranial fossa is performed in the late first/early second trimester via the *transcerebellar* axial plane and uses the cisterna magna as a quantitative representation of its size. More qualitative evaluation of anatomy can be performed with *mid-sagittal* plane.[6] The advantage of ultrasound is in the visualization of fluid in the posterior cranial fossa, as increased or decreased fluid volume can prompt further evaluation/genetic screening. Typically starting at 11 weeks gestation, the hypoechoic brainstem and cerebellar hemispheres, anechoic fourth ventricle and cisterna magna, and the echogenic choroid plexus can be identified and differentiated sonographically.[3]

Detailed anatomic evaluation and more definitive radiological characterization of a posterior cranial fossa abnormality should be performed with MRI, Examination with MRI should be used for suspected posterior cranial fossa malformations only after 18 weeks, following the expected maturation of the cerebellum to avoid false-positive diagnosis.[7] The midline sagittal T1 or T2 weighted MRI sequences are best for the evaluation of the posterior cranial fossa structures, particularly of the cerebellar vermis, brainstem, and fourth ventricle.[8]

Lesions detected on prenatal imaging require confirmation either with postnatal ultrasound and/or with MR imaging. The anterior fontanelle provides a good acoustic window for the assessment of the anterior fontanelle and is able to detect most of the supratentorial anomalies such as lateral and third ventricular dilatation, cyst formation, parenchymal calcifications, abnormal cortical sulcation patterns, and midline extra-axial fluid collections. Visualization of the posterior fossa structures is limited due to the increased distance between the transducer and the area of interest and due to the high echogenicity of the tentorium and the vermis. Additional approaches via the mastoid fontanelle and foramen magnum may provide better views of the cerebellum. With the advent of the faster (rapid) MRI techniques, which can be conducted without sedation, MRI is commonly used in the evaluation of congenital malformation of the brain. Besides routine T1 and T2 weighted images, DWI and SWI are added to diagnose any associated anoxic/hypoxic damage and bleed.

CLASSIFICATION OF POSTERIOR CRANIAL FOSSA MALFORMATIONS

There is no clear consensus or guideline regarding the best way to classify malformations of the Posterior Cranial Fossa. Several classifications of congenital posterior fossa malformation based on neuroimaging, molecular genetic, and developmental biologic criteria have been proposed. Classifications are based on anatomic features which can be readily appreciated on imaging. One classic categorization is to divide malformations into cystic or noncystic. Additional anatomic-based classifications exist to further differentiate the cystic lesions, which may be described in terms of abnormal retrocerebellar fluid space and abnormal posterior fossa size.[7] Noncystic malformations are a more diverse group of conditions that share abnormalities related to varying degrees of cerebellar agenesis or dysgenesis.[9]

A more comprehensive approach to Posterior Cranial Fossa malformations can be made by classifying these lesions based on the features of embryonic development and neurogenetics, as proposed by Barkovich and colleagues in 2009[10] (**Box 1**). This particular classification system divides disorders by defects in steps of development as well as into groups that are components of identified genetic syndromes. This detailed categorization includes grouping by malformations that are due to mesenchymal-neuroepithelial signaling defects, abnormal neuronal and glial proliferation, defects in neuronal migration, or abnormal functioning ciliary proteins.[10] The disadvantage to such classification is that the Posterior Cranial Fossa malformations are multifactorial and often share significant overlap in genetic defects. Furthermore, genetic syndromes may manifest the same phenotype of malformation due to different mechanisms.

Great progress has been made in understanding the mechanisms underlying normal and abnormal development of the midbrain and hindbrain from various animal models. Doherty D, Millen K, and Barkovich J,[11] have redefined the midbrain and hindbrain malformations based on neuroimaging pattern (**Box 2**). They classified these malformations into 4 main categories: (a) predominantly cerebellar, (b) cerebellar and brainstem, (c) predominantly brainstem, and (d) predominantly midbrain malformations. In this article, we focus mainly on cerebellar-related malformations (8,11).

Box 1
Developmental and genetic classification of mid-hindbrain malformations as proposed by Barkovich and colleagues

a. Malformations secondary to early anteroposterior and dorsoventral patterning defects or to the misspecification of mid-hindbrain germinal zones.

Anteroposterior patterning defects
- Gain, loss, or transformation of the diencephalon and midbrain
- Gain, loss, or transformation of the midbrain and rhombomere 1
- Gain, loss, or transformation of lower hindbrain structures

Dorsoventral patterning defects
- Defects of alar and basal ventricular zones
- Defects of alar ventricular zones only
- Defects of basal ventricular zones only

b. Malformations associated with later generalized developmental disorders that significantly affect the brainstem and cerebellum (and have pathogenesis at least partly understood)
- Developmental encephalopathies associated with mid-hindbrain malformations
- Mesenchymal-neuroepithelial signaling defects associated with mid-hindbrain malformations
- Malformations of neuronal and glial proliferation that prominently affect the brainstem and cerebellum
- Malformation of neuronal migration that prominently affects the brainstem and cerebellum
  ○ Lissencephaly with cerebellar hypoplasia
  ○ Neuronal heterotopia with prominent brainstem and cerebellar hypoplasia
  ○ Polymicrogyria with cerebellar hypoplasia
  ○ Malformations with basement membrane and neuronal migration deficits
- Diffuse molar tooth type dysplasias associated with defects in ciliary proteins
  ○ Syndromes affecting the brain with low-frequency involvement of the retina and kidney
  ○ Syndromes affecting the brain, eyes, kidneys, liver, and variable other systems

c. Localized brain malformations that significantly affect the brainstem and cerebellum (pathogenesis partly or largely understood, includes local proliferation, cell specification, migration, and axonal guidance)
- Multiple levels of mid-hindbrain
- Midbrain malformations
- Malformations of rhombomere 1 including cerebellar malformations
- Pons malformations
- Medulla malformations

d. Combined hypoplasia and atrophy in putative prenatal onset degenerative disorders
- Pontocerebellar hypoplasia
- Mid-hindbrain malformations with congenital disorders of glycosylation
- Other metabolic disorders with cerebellar or brainstem hypoplasia or disruption
- Cerebellar hemisphere hypoplasia (rare, more commonly acquired than genetic, often associated with clefts or cortical malformation)

Adapted from Barkovich AJ, Millen KJ, Dobyns WB. A developmental and genetic classification for midbrain-hindbrain malformations. Brain. 2009 Dec;132(Pt 12):3199-230.

PREDOMINANTLY CEREBELLAR MALFORMATIONS

Cerebellar malformation may be caused by chromosomal disorders, specific genetic syndromes, or due to prenatal disruptions such as infection and ischemia.[8] Most commonly encountered posterior fossa malformation related to mesenchymal-neuroepithelial signaling defects include Dandy–Walker malformation (DWM),

---

Box 2
Midbrain and hindbrain malformations

Predominantly cerebellar involvement
- Predominantly vermian
  - Dandy–Walker malformation
  - Blake pouch cyst,
  - Mega cisterna magna,
  - Arachnoid cysts;
  - Isolated vermian hypoplasia
  - Rhombencephalosynapsis
- Global cerebellar
  - Cerebellar dysplasia
  - Malformations of cortical development
    - Lissencephaly
    - Polymicrogyria
    - Periventricular nodular heterotopia
  - Primary microcephaly
  - Macrocerebellum
  - Global cerebellar hypoplasia
  - Congenital CMV infection
- Unilateral cerebellar
  - Isolated unilateral cerebellar hypoplasia
  - PHACES syndrome
  - Cerebellar cleft

Cerebellar and brainstem involvement
- Pontocerebellar hypoplasia (PCH type 1–10)
- Joubert syndrome;
- Congenital muscular dystrophies
- Vanishing cerebellum in Chiari 2 malformation
- Cerebellar disruption secondary to prematurity

Predominantly brainstem involvement
- Pontine tegmental cap dysplasia
- Horizontal gaze palsy and progressive scoliosis (ROBO3 mutations)
- Duane retraction syndrome, Duane radial ray syndrome
- Athabaskan brainstem dysgenesis syndrome and Bosley–Salih Alorainy syndrome
- Moebius syndrome
- Diencephalic–mesencephalic junction dysplasia

Predominantly midbrain involvement
- Dysplasia of the diencephalic–mesencephalic junction

---

cerebellar vermis hypoplasia (CVH), mega-cisterna magna (MCM) with cerebellum vermis hypoplasia, isolated mega-cisterna magna, and arachnoid cysts of posterior fossa.

Dandy–Walker Malformation

The Dandy–Walker malformation occurs when the anterior membranous area (AMA) of the plica choroidalis does not involute, and continues to fill with cerebrospinal fluid to form an enlarged 4th ventricle that does not communicate with subarachnoid space.[2] As the AMA enlarges, the embryonic vermis is displaced, hypoplastic, and rotated.[12] The cerebellar hemispheres are also displaced by the expanded fourth ventricle, and therefore global cerebellar hypoplasia (with normal morphology) is an additional feature.[8] It should be noted that the entity Dandy–Walker *Variant* is a part of the continuum of the same mechanism of malformation, which may be differentiated in that these cases do not lead to enough expansion of the fourth ventricle to cause significant enlargement of the posterior cranial fossa.[5]

The etiology of Dandy–Walker malformation is genetically multifactorial and the abnormality can be seen as both an isolated defect or as a component of a syndrome. In many cases, Dandy–Walker Malformation is closely associated with FOXC1, which is expressed in the posterior fossa mesenchyme to promote cerebellar development. FOXC1 loss of function is closely associated with cerebellar hypoplasia.[10] Furthermore, a subset of patients with Dandy–Walker malformation are linked with mutations of ZIC1 and ZIC4. These genes are responsible for SHH dependent signaling as a component of posterior cranial fossa differentiation.[13] In more broad terms, the Dandy–Walker malformation can be seen as a presentation within many syndromes including Trisomy 13, Trisomy 18, PHACE, Walker–Warburg, Meckel–Grueber, and Ritscher–Schnizel cranio-cerebello-cardiac.[2]

The classic triad that represents the imaging features of Dandy–Walker malformation is described as vermian agenesis (or hypoplasia), cystic dilation of the fourth ventricle, and enlargement of the posterior cranial fossa[5,8] (Fig. 1). Typically, the cerebellar hemispheres are less affected than the vermis, and the brainstem is between normal and moderately hypoplastic. The elevation of the transverse sinuses, tentorium, and torcula together is a marker of enlarged posterior cranial fossa and can be identified in the midsagittal plane on both MRI and ultrasound.[14] Furthermore, the expansion of the fourth ventricle can lead to obstructive hydrocephalus, which is seen in 80% of cases in vivo,[15] and approximately 31% of cases identified prenatally.[9] Additional malformations, such as dysgenesis or agenesis of the corpus callosum, occipital encephalocele, polymicrogyria, and heterotopia, may be seen with Dandy–Walker malformation. Previously used terms such as "Dandy–Walker variant," "Dandy–Walker complex," or "Dandy–Walker spectrum" are avoided as they lack specificity and create clinical confusion.[8] Rather, the Radiologist needs to be more descriptive in detailing the findings when the definite criteria are not met for Dandy–Walker malformation.

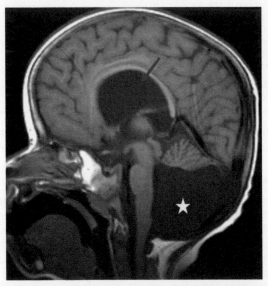

Fig. 1. Dandy–Walker malformation. Sagittal T1 WI shows a large Dandy–Walker Cyst (*yellow star*) with hypoplastic vermis with upward rotation and enlarged posterior fossa. Cystic dilated fourth ventricle is seen generously communicating with the cyst. Note supratentorial hydrocephalus (*red arrow*).

Arachnoid Cyst

An arachnoid cyst is a benign cerebrospinal fluid-containing lesion that can be found anywhere throughout the central nervous system. Intracranial Arachnoid cysts spontaneously form during development due to spontaneous duplication of the arachnoid membrane into inner and outer walls, which then fill with cerebrospinal fluid.[8] Their growth can be explained by active cerebrospinal fluid secretion from within the cyst as well osmotic gradient from the surrounding arachnoid space into the cyst.[16] A predisposition to intracranial arachnoid cyst development has been mapped to Chromosome 6p22.[17] Clinically, there is also documented association with Polycystic Kidney Disease, Glutaric aciduria type 1, mental retardation, pachygyria, and chromosome-12 trisomy.[17] They are often an incidental and asymptomatic finding. When large, they cause obstruction to the CSF flow and may clinically present with macrocephaly, signs of increased intracranial pressure, and developmental delay.

Posterior fossa arachnoid cyst may be located inferior or posterior to the vermis in a midsagittal location (retrocerebellar), cranial to the vermis in the tentorial hiatus (supravermian), anterior or lateral to the cerebellar hemispheres (**Fig. 2**), or anterior to the brainstem. Imaging features of arachnoid cysts include a well-circumscribed, space-occupying fluid collection that may exert mass effect on the adjacent structures.[2] The fluid composition should match that of cerebrospinal fluid in all imaging modalities and the cyst should not directly communicate with the fourth ventricle or surrounding arachnoid space.[5] While the entity can be seen on ultrasound, MRI is essential for differentiation from other cystic malformations by identifying this absence of communication.[8] Complications of growth can include obstructive hydrocephalus, osseous thinning, and direct mass effect.

Mega Cisterna Magna

Mega cisterna magna represents the expansion of the cisterna magna, with otherwise normal anatomy and morphology within the posterior cranial fossa. The malformation occurs due to a defect in the permeabilization of Blake's pouch, which is either

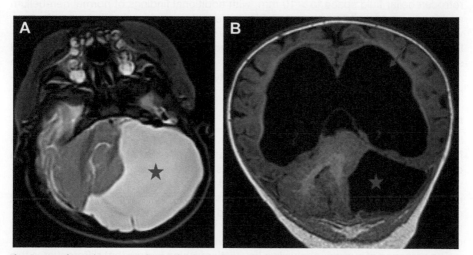

Fig. 2. Arachnoid cyst. Axial T2 (*A*) and coronal T1 (*B*) WIs show large left lateral cerebellar CSF intensity mass (*red star*), causing severe mass effect and rightward displacement of the cerebellum, severe compression of the fourth ventricle, and scalloping of the occipital bone. Compression of the fourth ventricle causes supratentorial hydrocephalus (*red arrow*).

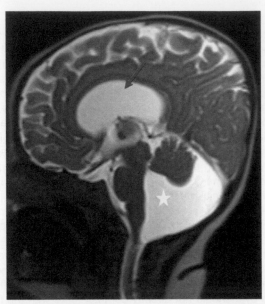

Fig. 3. Blake's pouch cyst. Sagittal image shows the prominence of the CSF space in the posterior fossa with the enlargement of the fourth ventricle communicating with the infravermian cystic compartment (*yellow star*) with supratentorial hydrocephalus (*red arrow*).

delayed or incomplete.[18] The pouch enlarges in size before it finally permeabilizes and involutes to form the connection to the subarachnoid space known as the Foramen of Magendi.[2] As an isolated finding, mega cisterna magna is considered a normal anatomic variant. However, it may be found in an association with vermian hypoplasia, in the context of FOXC1 loss of function mutations.

The imaging diagnosis of mega cisterna magna is made by the enlargement of the retrocerebellar fluid space to > 10 mm, with additional findings of normal cerebellum and fourth ventricle.[9] The absence of hydrocephalus is a key discriminating feature, which is prevented due to the delayed, however, eventually completes the permeabilization of Blake's pouch.[8] Additionally, the lack of any mass effect despite enlarged size differentiates it from space-occupying lesions such as Arachnoid cyst.[2] In many documented cases, if the abnormality is identified prenatally, it may self-resolve by the time the infant is born.[18]

Blake's Pouch Cyst

Blake's pouch Cyst is a malformation of a similar mechanism to Mega Cisterna Magna; however, in these patients, there is a complete absence of permeabilization of the anterior membranous area (AMA).[19] This leads to a Blake's Pouch that never involutes to form the Foramen of Magendie, and persists past 16 weeks of gestation. As result, the AMA becomes an enlarged cystic structure within the fourth ventricle that does not communicate with the subarachnoid space.[20] Blake's Pouch cyst is generally thought of as an anatomic variant rather than true pathology.[9] The only clinical concern is hydrocephalus, which can be alleviated by shunting.[5]

The presence of hydrocephalus is a key distinguishing feature that differentiates this malformation from Mega Cisterna Magna.[2] The characteristic appearance on MRI is a cystic collection in the posterior cranial fossa that is contiguous with the fourth ventricle and causes mass effect and obstructive hydrocephalus (**Fig. 3**). Furthermore, the Choroid plexus can be identified as an enhancing structure displaced beneath the cerebellar vermis and within the Blake's Pouch cyst.[8] Sonographically, the space occupied by the cyst can be represented by an increase in the tegmento-vermian angle.[9] Similar to mega cisterna magna, the remaining anatomic structures including the cerebellum are normal.

Macrocerebellum

Macrocerebellum is characterized by an abnormally large cerebellum with normal morphology. It may be seen in an isolated form (nonsyndromic) or part of syndromes such as Costello syndrome, Sotos syndrome or neurometabolic diseases (eg, fucosidosis, mucopolysaccharidosis type I and II).[21] Like most of the congenital cerebellar disorders child may present with ataxia, hypotonia, intellectual disability, and ocular movement disorders.

Sagittal and axial images on MRI demonstrate disproportionate enlargement of the cerebellar hemispheres in comparison to the cerebellar vermis with preserved architecture and shape.[21] This cerebellar hyperplasia may cause significant mass effect on the subjacent brainstem or cause upward or downward herniation. Supratentorial findings such as ventriculomegaly or white matter signal abnormalities may be present depending on the underlying disease.

Rhombencephalosynapsis

Rhombencephalosynapsis represents aplasia (partial or complete) of the cerebellar vermis with concomitant fusion of the cerebellar hemispheres, dentate nuclei, and superior cerebellar peduncles.[22] This is thought to occur due to extrinsic insult between 4 weeks and 6 weeks of gestation, following the initial formation of the cerebellar hemispheres from the rhomboid lips and before the initial formation of the cerebellar vermis.[23] Consequently, without proper vermian development the cerebellar hemispheres continue to grow until there is midline fusion.[2]

While there is a documented familial pattern of inheritance, there is no identified genetic mechanism for the embryonic development of Rhombencephalosynapsis. It is a hypothesized to be a consequence of abnormal vermian differentiation with defect dorsal and patterning, and as such is also associated with other midline abnormalities including fused tectum, dysgenesis of corpus callosum, and absent septum pellucidum.[8,24] Additional genetic associations include VACTERL and Gomez–Lopez–Hernandez syndrome.[2] The most common clinical presentation include truncal and/or limb ataxia, abnormal eye movements, head stereotypies, and delayed motor development. More severe neurodevelopmental impairment is seen with associated supratentorial anomalies.

Findings of Rhombencephalosynapsis can be identified on ultrasound, including absent cerebellar vermis as well as continuous hyperechoic white matter, representing the cerebellar hemispheres extending across the midline. On Sagittal view ultrasound, the distortion of the fourth ventricle can be identified,[14] however, is better appreciated on MRI. The absence of the vermis and fusion across midline cerebellum result in what is referred to as a diamond-shaped[2] or keyhole-shaped[5] fourth ventricle. In addition, axial/coronal MRI can identify continuity of the cerebellar folia and sulci to confirm their fusion[19] (**Fig. 4**). MR is very sensitive in identifying associated midbrain abnormalities such as aqueductal stenosis and midline fusion of the colliculi and supratentorial abnormalities such as absent septum pellucidum, absent olfactory bulbs, and corpus callosum dysmorphisms.[9]

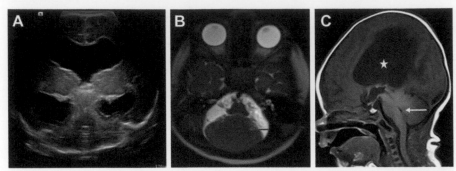

Fig. 4. Rhombencephalosynapsis. Coronal ultrasound image (*A*) and Axial T2 WI (*B*) show continuity of the cerebellar hemispheres with an abnormal transverse orientation of the cerebellar foliae (*red arrow*). Sagittal T1 WI (*C*) show severe effacement of the fourth ventricle (*yellow arrow*) and gross supratentorial hydrocephalus with interhemispheric cyst (*yellow star*).

GLOBAL AND UNILATERAL CEREBELLAR DISRUPTIONS

The long duration of cerebellar development, from 1st trimester to 2 years of age places the developing cerebellum at high risk for developmental and acquired injury. The cerebellum is particularly vulnerable to metabolic and toxic insults as well as prenatal infections and hemorrhages, whereas it is less vulnerable to prenatal, perinatal, and postnatal hypoxic-ischemic events.[8] Dysgenesis of the neocerebellum includes the developmental defects of aplasia, hypoplasia, and dysplasia of either one or both cerebellar hemispheres while the neocerebellar dysplasia include abnormalities such as heterotopias, microgyria polygyria, and agyria.[8]

Cerebellar Agenesis

Cerebellar agenesis represents the complete or near-complete absence of the cerebellum. While the presentation is the same in imaging, the etiology can be genetic or secondary to disruption, such as hemorrhage during perinatal development.[8]

Genetic etiology is associated with loss of function mutations in the PTF1A gene in chromosome 10, which has been linked to cerebellar malformation and therefore agenesis. PTF1A encodes for a transcription factor that is responsible for maintaining differentiation to cerebellar fate cells. Its loss of function disrupts the normal dorsal patterning of the cerebellum and therefore leads to abnormal ventral-only morphology. The cells intended for dorsal differentiation either become part of the brainstem or undergo apoptosis, leading to subsequent cerebellar agenesis.[25]

As expected, cerebellar agenesis is identified on both MRI and ultrasound as the absence of all or a majority of the cerebellum. MRI shows near-complete absence of cerebellar structures with remnants of the anterior vermis, floccules, and middle cerebellar peduncles (**Fig. 5**). Secondary pontine hypoplasia may be an additional associated finding.[8] The remaining posterior cranial fossa is normal in size and occupied by increased cerebrospinal fluid.[9]

Global Cerebellar Hypoplasia

Global cerebellar hypoplasia is a malformation that is distinct in etiology and presentation from cerebellar agenesis or vermian hypoplasia and represents a normal-appearing cerebellum that is reduced in size.[26] Like cerebellar agenesis, it can result from both genetic and acquired defects.

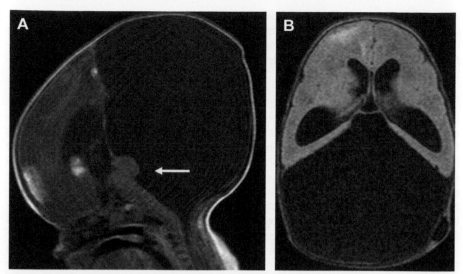

Fig. 5. Cerebellar agenesis. Sagittal T1 (*A*) and axial FLAIR (*B*) images show a complete absence of the cerebellum (*yellow arrow*), gross enlargement of the posterior fossa, and hypoplasia of the brainstem.

The malformation of cerebellar hypoplasia is multifactorial in origin and may occur due to defects at multiple possible steps in neurodevelopment. For example, Autosomal Recessive Lissencephaly with Cerebellar Hypoplasia occurs due to the defect of RELN, which is normally responsible for creating an extracellular matrix protein that binds to very low-density lipoprotein receptor (VLDR) in the pathway of cell migration. Mutation in RELN leads to the disruption of normal migration of neurons along the pathway of cerebellar development, leading to cerebellar hypoplasia.[27] The mutation of VLDR results in VLDR cerebellar hypoplasia due to the same defect of cerebellar neuromigration.[28] Additional associations of cerebellar hypoplasia include Trisomy 13 and 18, metabolic disorders such Adenylosuccinase deficiency, Smith–Lemli–Opitz syndrome, Zellweger syndrome, mitochondrial disorders (Leigh disease, pyruvate dehydrogenase deficiency), and Mucopolysaccharidoses (types I and II) as well as genetic syndromes such as CHARGE syndrome, oculocerebrocutaneous (Delleman) syndrome, and Neurofibromatosis type I.[29]

As previously noted, the cerebellum seems normal in shape and morphology on both ultrasound and MRI, with size smaller than expected for gestational age. In place of a normal-sized cerebellum, there is an increased volume of cerebrospinal fluid occupying the retrocerebellar space.[26] Notably, the diagnosis should be made after 6th months of gestation, as the still growing cerebellum may seem small if imaged too early (leading to false positives), and in some cases onset of the condition may be late (leading to false negatives).[9]

Unilateral Cerebellar Hypoplasia

As the name suggests, with Unilateral Cerebellar Hypoplasia there is mild asymmetry to congenital complete aplasia in the size of the cerebellar hemispheres. The most common cause of this anomaly is hemorrhage, leading to the developmental disruption of part or the entire cerebellar hemisphere.[8] The most common clinical presentations include delayed development and speech, hypotonia, ataxia, and abnormal ocular movements.

Prenatal ultrasound or MR demonstrates unilateral cerebellar hypoplasia and volume loss of the cerebellar hemisphere with a normal size (**Fig. 6**). GRE or SWI images may show the presence of hemosiderin deposition on the hypoplastic cerebellar surface. These findings along with porencephalic cysts or clefts may be seen in the supratentorial cerebral parenchyma.

Cerebellar Cleft

Unilateral cerebellar cleft is defined as a disruptive lesion affecting principally the cortical gray matter of one cerebellar hemisphere, extending from the hemisphere's surface into the parenchyma and reaching the fourth ventricle in some cases, but not involving the vermis.[30] This disruptive lesion is thought to be secondary to fetal cerebellar hemorrhages. Clinical presentation of the isolated cases of the cerebellar cleft is variable. Child may present with truncal ataxia, muscular hypotonia, oculomotor disorders, language and speech disorder, and behavioral abnormalities. Neurologic impairments and poor prognosis is seen when there is an associated supratentorial lesion such as schizencephaly.

Neuroimaging shows a cleft extending from the surface of the cerebellum toward the fourth ventricle with the malorientation of the cerebellar foliation, an irregular gray/white matter junction, and lack of normal architecture of the white matter in the region adjacent to the cleft.[8,30] Because of the adjacent loss of cerebellar tissue, the affected cerebellar hemispheres are usually reduced in volume, resulting in the asymmetric sizes of the cerebellar hemispheres.

Cerebral Dysplasia

Like cerebral dysplasia, cerebellar dysplasia may be either focal involve a small portion of a single hemisphere (focal dysplasia) or large portion of the cerebellar hemispheres (global dysplasia).[31,32] The etiology of these conditions could be due to inherited (developmental) or acquired (disruptive). Focal findings suggest a disruptive lesion, whereas global findings suggest inherited malformation. The clinical

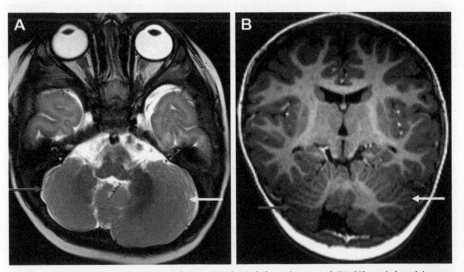

Fig. 6. Unilateral cerebellar hypoplasia. Axial T2 (*A*) and coronal T1 (*B*) weighted images show smaller right cerebellar hemisphere (*red arrows*) in comparison to the left hemisphere (*yellow arrows*).

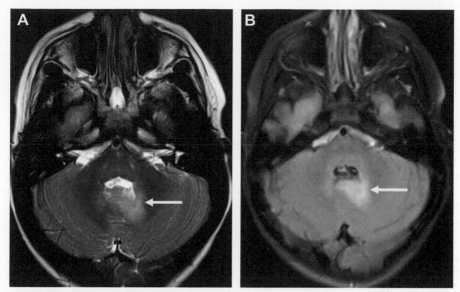

Fig. 7. Focal cerebellar dysplasia. Focal cerebellar dysplasia. Axial T2 (*A*) and FLAIR (*B*) images show irregular focal hyperintensity (*yellow arrow*) involving the dentate nucleus and periventricular region of the left cerebellar hemisphere. Lesion remained stable for 4 years in morphology and signal intensity.

manifestations of cerebellar dysplasia are highly variable, ranging from incidental finding to severe neurologic impairment and largely depend on the extent of the dysplasia. Most of the time, focal dysplasia is identified as an incidental finding, whereas global dysplasia is often associated with severe neurologic impairment.

On histopathology, cerebellar dysplasia may show various findings such as compact groups of mature neurons, focal or perivascular immature granular cell collections, mixed cell rests containing both mature neurons and immature granule cells, and heterotopias.[33] On imaging, focal cerebellar dysplasia is commonly found in the white matter and nodulus of the vermis (**Fig. 7**). Other findings may include asymmetry or focal disruption of cerebellar folial and sulcal morphology, disorganized and disordered foliation, enlarged and vertically oriented fissures, cerebellar gray-white matter heterotopia, bumpy gray-white matter interface in the cerebellum, lack of normal arborization of white matter, abnormal hyperintense signal in subcortical white matter[31–33] (**Fig. 8**). There may be associated supratentorial findings such as corpus callosal agenesis/dysgenesis, macro-/microscopic heterotopia, cerebral cortical dysplasia.

Injury Secondary to Prematurity/Cerebellum of the Premature Infant.

Similar to the supratentorial cerebral parenchyma, cerebellar parenchyma to a lesser extent is also vulnerable to destructive hemorrhage, infarction, or primarily under development in premature infants. Cerebellar injury occurs in up to 20% of preterm infants before 32 weeks gestation.[34] The surface area of the cerebellar cortex increases more than 30-fold, in the last trimester of the pregnancy. Any insult or injury, particularly during this period causes arrest of the cerebellar development thus reducing the final cerebellar volume. In preterm newborns this could be due to primary causes such as hemorrhage and/or ischemia or cerebellar underdevelopment could be due to hemosiderin–blood products deposition, glucocorticoid exposure, undernutrition.

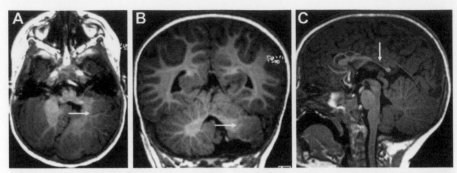

Fig. 8. Diffuse cerebellar dysplasia. Axial (A) and coronal thin T1WI (MPRAGE) (B), shows abnormal cerebellar foliation and sulcal morphology (*yellow arrow*). Sagittal T1 WI (C) shows associated corpus callosum dysgenesis (*white arrow*).

Neuroimaging shows a reduction in the cerebellar volume, with or without hemosiderin deposition, predominantly involving the cerebellar hemispheres.[8,34] In addition, there may be atrophy of the pons, with ex vacuo dilatation of the fourth ventricle (**Fig. 9**).

CEREBELLAR AND BRAINSTEM MALFORMATIONS
Joubert Syndrome

Joubert Syndrome is diverse in its developmental, imaging, and clinical presentations. There are 6 known subtypes based on the variable multisystem involvement.[8,35] As a posterior cranial fossa malformation, the abnormalities of Joubert Syndrome are centered on the agenesis or dysgenesis of the cerebellar vermis; additional components involving the brainstem and the pontomesencephalic junction are variable in extent and morphology.[2]

The genes NPHP1, AHI1, CEP290, RPGRIP1L, MKS3/TMEM67, CC2D2A, and ARL13 B[36] as well as additional loci, most notably 9q34, and 11p12-q13 have been associated with the development of Joubert syndrome.[18] Mutations in the several of these proteins are associated with defective cilia development and function. Additional defects are related to the disruption of the SHH signaling and dorsal-ventral patterning of the neural tube. Additionally, the genes affected in Joubert syndrome have correlated proteins located in other parts of the body, and therefore additional involvement in the liver (congenital hepatic fibrosis), kidney (cystic renal disease), and eyes (retinal dystrophy) is noted in the various subtypes of Joubert Syndrome.[36] Neonate with Joubert syndrome usually presents with neonatal hypotonia, abnormal eye movements, and alternating apnea and tachypnea.

The absence of the normally echogenic cerebellar vermis can be identified sonographically, best noted in the midsagittal plane.[14] Additionally, ultrasound in the axial plane may identify an elevated and horizontally oriented fourth ventricle with abnormally increased anterior–posterior diameter.[18] Findings better delineated on MRI include the cerebellar peduncles, which may be elongated and positioned perpendicular to the brainstem on Sagittal views[19] (**Fig. 10**). Notably, there is defective decussation in the presence of these abnormally configured cerebellar peduncles, as well as in the medullary pyramid, pontine tracts, and corticospinal tracts. The absence of decussation between the superior cerebellar peduncles and the brainstem leads to a thin, atrophic brainstem isthmus and therefore enlarged interpeduncular fossa.[5] While Joubert Syndrome may have a diverse imaging and clinical presentation, the

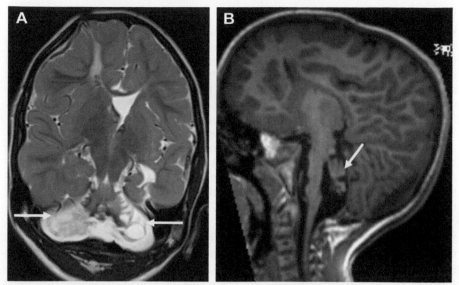

Fig. 9. Cerebellum of the Premature Infant. Coronal T2 (*A*) and Sagittal T1 (*B*) WIs show changes in periventricular leukomalacia in the cerebrum (*red arrow*). Posterior fossa is smaller in size, shows changes in pontine hypoplasia, severe loss of volume of the cerebellar parenchyma (*yellow arrows*).

criteria for its diagnosis are vermian agenesis/dysgenesis and the classic "molar tooth sign."[8,35] It is the combination of the malformations in the posterior cranial fossa described above that creates the classic "molar tooth sign" on axial MRI. More recently, diffusion tensor imaging (DTI) has been used to document the laterally displaced and dysmorphic deep cerebellar nuclei, hypoplastic medial lemnisci, and absent transverse fibers in the central vermis and deficient crossing of the superior cerebellar peduncles.[8,35] In addition, other brain malformations such as polymicrogyria, brainstem, and cortical heterotopia, and agenesis of the corpus callosum or cephalocele may be identified.

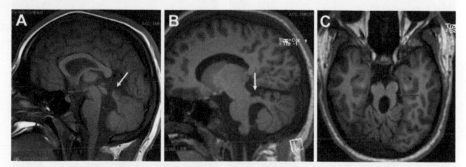

Fig. 10. Joubert syndrome. Sagittal T1-weighted images (*A, B*) show hypoplasia and dysplasia of the vermis (*arrow*), enlargement of the fourth ventricle with upward and posterior displacement of the fastigium. There is elongation and perpendicular positioning of the cerebellar peduncle to the brainstem (*white arrow*). Axial T1 image (*C*) shows elongated, thickened, and horizontally oriented superior cerebellar peduncles (*red arrow*) giving a characteristic appearance of the molar tooth sign.

Pontocerebellar Hypoplasia

Pontocerebellar hypoplasia is a group of autosomal recessive neurodegenerative disorders with prenatal onset, and is characterized by hypoplasia and variable atrophy of the cerebellum and pons.[8] Neurodegeneration predominantly affects the growth and survival of neurons in the cerebellar cortex, the dentate, inferior olivary and ventral pontine nuclei. To date, 10 types (PCH 1–11) and numerous subtypes have been defined depending on the gene defect. PCH1, PCH2, PCH4, and PCH6 are the most frequently reported types.[37,38] Common clinical presentation to most types and subtypes include progressive microcephaly and severe motor and cognitive impairments.

Neuroimaging shows hypoplasia and variable atrophy of the cerebellum and pons on sagittal images. Coronal images through the posterior fossa show a "dragonfly" appearance due to flattened cerebellar hemispheres ("the wings") and a relatively preserved vermis ("the body"). Additional imaging findings include ventriculomegaly, neocortical atrophy, and microcephaly[37] (**Fig. 11**).

Cobblestone Complex/Congenital Muscular Dystrophies

Cobble stone complex is classified based on the specific type of mutation into: (a) POMT mutation—Walker–Warburg syndrome, (b) FKRP mutation, (c) POMGnT1 mutation—muscle–eye–brain disease, (d) Fukuyama congenital muscular dystrophy (FCMD) mutation, and (e) LARGE mutation—muscle–eye–brain disease.[5,8,39] Pathologically, the cobblestone pattern is caused by the overmigration of neurons from the germinal matrix region that is thought to be the result of disrupted glycosylation.

Imaging shows irregular brain surface because of the presence of heterotopic tissue which results from over migration of glioneural elements, cobblestone cortex, dilated ventricles, abnormal white matter. Posterior fossa imaging shows cerebellar hypoplasia or dysplasia, cerebellar cysts, pontine hypoplasia, ventral pontine cleft, and pontomesencephalic kinking, a small brainstem, a hypoplastic vermis, and cerebellar polymicrogyria.[39] Cerebellar cysts are said to be a specific finding for this entity. In addition, it also shows a mild-to-severe eye malformation as well as congenital muscular dystrophy.

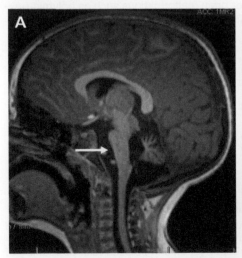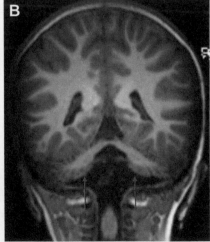

Fig. 11. Pontocerebellar hypoplasia sagittal (*A*) and coronal T1 (*B*) WIs show hypoplasia of the pons (*yellow arrow*) and cerebellar vermis. Coronal images show a dragonfly appearance due to severe reduction of the cerebellar hemispheres (*red arrows*).

The clinical presentation largely depends on the type and severity of mutation. The Walker–Warburg phenotype represents the severe end of the spectrum with profoundly small and dysmorphic cerebellar hemispheres, often with cysts, absent vermis, and very small brainstem. Clinically patients frequently presents with hydrocephalus, various eye abnormalities, seizures, hypotonia, and/or muscular dystrophy with creatine kinase levels 2- to 15-folds normal. Final diagnosis is confirmed by identifying the gene mutations (POMT1 MIM 607423, POMT2 MIM 607439, POMGNT1 MIM 606822, FKTN MIM 607440, FKRP MIM 606596, LARGE MIM 603590, ISPD MIM 614631, and GTDC2 MIM 614830).[40]

SUMMARY

The workup of a congenital cerebellar malformation is a multidisciplinary approach, most successful if all clinicians involved have an understanding of the anatomic, embryologic, genetic, and imaging features of the most common etiologies. While the phenotypic presentation is diverse, ultrasound and MRI can provide essential data that can provide context for both diagnosis and treatment.

CLINICS CARE POINTS

- Correct diagnosis of congenital malformations of the brain in regards to morphology, embryology, and molecular neurogenetics is of paramount importance to inform the parents or the caregiver of the prognosis, inheritance pattern and risk of recurrence, as well as genetic counseling.
- Prenatal imaging plays a vital role in diagnosing and understanding the pathogenesis.

DISCLOSURE

The authors have nothing to disclose.

REFERENCES

1. Shoja MM, Ramdhan R, Jensen CJ, et al. Embryology of the craniocervical junction and posterior cranial fossa, part II: embryogenesis of the hindbrain. Clin Anat 2018;31(4):488–500.
2. Nunes RH, Littig IA, da Rocha AJ, et al. Basic genetic principles applied to posterior fossa malformations. Top Magn Reson Imaging 2011;22(6):261–70.
3. Pertl B, Eder S, Stern C, et al. The fetal posterior fossa on prenatal ultrasound imaging: normal longitudinal development and posterior fossa anomalies. Eur J Ultrasound 2019;40(06):692–721.
4. Cotes C, Bonfante E, Lazor J, et al. Congenital basis of posterior fossa anomalies. Neuroradiology J 2015;28(3):238–53.
5. Shekdar K. Posterior fossa malformations. Semin Ultrasound CT MR 2011;32(3): 228–41.
6. Leibovitz Z, Shkolnik C, Haratz KK, et al. Assessment of fetal midbrain and hindbrain in mid-sagittal cranial plane by three-dimensional multiplanar sonography. part 1: comparison of new and established nomograms. Ultrasound Obstet Gynecol 2014;44(5):575–80.
7. Chapman T, Mahalingam S, Ishak GE, et al. Diagnostic imaging of posterior fossa anomalies in the fetus and neonate: Part 1, normal anatomy and classification of anomalies. Clin Imaging 2015;39(1):1–8.

8. Bosemani T, Orman G, Boltshauser E, et al. Congenital abnormalities of the posterior fossa. RadioGraphics 2015;35(1):200–20.
9. Massoud M, Guibaud L. Prenatal imaging of posterior fossa disorders. a review. Eur J Paediatric Neurol 2018;22(6):972–88.
10. Barkovich AJ, Millen KJ, Dobyns WB. A developmental and genetic classification for midbrain-hindbrain malformations. Brain 2009;132(12):3199–230.
11. Doherty D, Millen KJ, Barkovich AJ. Midbrain and hindbrain malformations: advances in clinical diagnosis, imaging, and genetics. Lancet Neurol 2013;12(4):381–93.
12. Poretti A, Boltshauser E, Huisman TA. Pre- and postnatal neuroimaging of congenital cerebellar abnormalities. Cerebellum 2015;15(1):5–9.
13. Blank MC, Grinberg I, Aryee E, et al. Multiple developmental programs are altered by loss of zic1 and ZIC4 to cause Dandy-Walker malformation cerebellar pathogenesis. Development 2011;138(6):1207–16.
14. Snyder E, Hwang M, Soares BP, et al. Ultrasound and CT of the posterior fossa in neonates. Cerebellum: From Embryology to Diagnostic Investigations; 2018. p. 205–17.
15. Spennato P, Mirone G, Nastro A, et al. Hydrocephalus in Dandy-Walker malformation. Childs Nerv Syst 2011;27(10):1665–81. Epub 2011 Sep 17.
16. Hellwig D, Bauer BL, List-Hellwig E. Stereotactic endoscopic interventions in cystic brain lesions. Adv Stereotactic Funct Neurosurg 1995;11:59–63.
17. Bayrakli F, Okten AI, Kartal U, et al. Intracranial arachnoid cyst family with autosomal recessive trait mapped to chromosome 6q22.31-23.2. Acta Neurochir 2012;154(7):1287–92.
18. Robinson AJ, Ederies MA. Diagnostic imaging of posterior fossa anomalies in the fetus. Semin Fetal Neonatal Med 2016;21(5):312–20.
19. Tortori-Donati P, Rossi A. Congenital malformations of the posterior cranial fossa. Rivista Di Neuroradiologia 2000;13(1_suppl):41–4.
20. Calabrò F, Arcuri T, Jinkins JR. Blake's pouch cyst: an entity within the Dandy-Walker Continuum. Neuroradiology 2000;42(4):290–5.
21. Poretti A, Mall V, Smitka M, et al. Macrocerebellum: significance and pathogenic considerations. Cerebellum 2012;11(4):1026–36.
22. Aldinger KA, Dempsey JC, Tully HM, et al. Rhombencephalosynapsis: fused cerebellum, confused geneticists. Am J Med Genet C: Semin Med Genet 2018;178(4):432–9.
23. Demaerel P, Morel C, Lagae L. Partial rhombencephalosynapsis. Am J Neuroradiol 2004;25(1):29–31.
24. Ishak GE, Dempsey JC, Shaw DW, et al. Rhombencephalosynapsis: a hindbrain malformation associated with incomplete separation of midbrain and forebrain, hydrocephalus and a broad spectrum of severity. Brain 2012;135(5):1370–86.
25. Millen KJ, Steshina EY, Iskusnykh IY, et al. Transformation of the cerebellum into more ventral brainstem fates causes cerebellar agenesis in the absence of ptf1a function. Proc Natl Acad Sci 2014;111(17):E1777–86.
26. Abdel Razek AA, Castillo M. Magnetic resonance imaging of malformations of midbrain-hindbrain. J Computer Assisted Tomography 2016;40(1):14–25.
27. Guerrini R, Parrini E. Neuronal migration disorders. Neurobiol Dis 2010;38(2):154–66.
28. Boycott KM, Bonnemann C, Herz J, et al. Mutations in VLDLR as a cause for autosomal recessive cerebellar ataxia with mental retardation (DYSEQUILIBRIUM syndrome). J Child Neurol 2009;24(10):1310–5.

29. Poretti A, Boltshauser E, Doherty D. Cerebellar hypoplasia: Differential diagnosis and diagnostic approach. Am J Med Genet C: Semin Med Genet 2014;166(2): 211–26.
30. Poretti A, Huisman TA, Cowan FM, et al. Cerebellar cleft: confirmation of the neuroimaging pattern. Neuropediatrics 2009;40(5):228–33.
31. Poretti A, Boltshauser E. Cerebellar dysplasia. In: Boltshauser E, Schmahmann JD, editors. Cerebellar disorders in children. London, England: Mac Keith; 2012. p. 172–6.
32. Demaerel P. Abnormalities of cerebellar foliation and fissuration: classification, neurogenetics and clinicoradiological correlations. Neuroradiology 2002;44(8): 639–46.
33. Soto-Ares G, Delmaire C, Deries B. Louis vallee, and jean pierre pruvo cerebellar cortical dysplasia: MR findings in a complex entity. AJNR Am J Neuroradiol 2000; 21:1511–9.
34. Volpe JJ. Cerebellum of the premature infant: rapidly developing, vulnerable, clinically important. J Child Neurol 2009;24(9):1085–104.
35. Poretti A, Huisman TAGM, Scheer I, et al. Joubert syndrome and related disorders: spectrum of neuroimaging findings in 75 patients. Neuropediatrics 2011; 42(S 01). https://doi.org/10.1055/s-0031-1274082.
36. Doherty D. Joubert syndrome: Insights into Brain Development, cilium biology, and complex disease. Semin Pediatr Neurol 2009;16(3):143–54.
37. Namavar Y, Barth PG, Poll-The BT, et al. Classification, diagnosis and potential mechanisms in pontocerebellar hypoplasia. Orphanet J Rare Dis 2011;6:50.
38. Schaffer AE, Eggens VR, Caglayan AO, et al. CLP1 founder mutation links tRNA splicing and maturation to cerebellar development and neurodegeneration. Cell 2014;157(3):651–63.
39. Clement E, Mercuri E, Godfrey C, et al. Brain involvement in muscular dystrophies with defective dystroglycan glycosylation. Ann Neurol 2008;64(5):573–82.
40. Devisme L, Bouchet C, Gonzalès M, et al. Cobblestone lissencephaly: neuropathological subtypes and correlations with genes of dystroglycanopathies. Brain 2012;135(Pt 2):469–82. Epub 2012 Feb 9.

Imaging of Congenital Spine Malformations

Christina White, DO*, Sarah Sarvis Milla, MD, John A. Maloney, MD,
Ilana Neuberger, MD

KEYWORDS

- Congenital malformations • Spinal dysraphisms • Zipper-like fusion
- Congenital abnormalities

KEY POINTS

- Congenital malformations of the spine and spinal cord are a large and diverse group of diagnoses that result from any number of disruptions in normal embryologic development.
- Knowledge of spinal cord embryology is helpful in understanding the imaging appearance of congenital spine anomalies.
- Open spinal dysraphisms, 98% of which are myelomeningocele, should be surgically managed prior to postnatal imaging due to high rates of placode infection and ulceration.
- Closed spinal dysraphisms may be diagnosed in the neonatal period or into later childhood/adolescence, depending on their complexity and association with a palpable subcutaneous mass. MRI is preferred for definitive assessment.

INTRODUCTION

Congenital malformations of the spine and spinal cord are a large and diverse group of diagnoses, which are often broadly referred to as spinal dysraphisms (SDs). Derived from the Greek words *dys* (bad) and *raphe* (suture), the term *dysraphism* describes missteps in the process of forming a midline seam during the zipper-like fusion of the neural folds in primary neurulation. As such, the term "spinal dysraphism" is a designation that should technically be reserved for malformations resulting from aberrations in primary neurulation. In medical practice, however, it is a catch-all designation regularly used to describe any of the numerous abnormalities demonstrating incomplete midline closure of mesenchymal, osseous, and nervous tissue, occurring at any point during embryologic development.[1] For the sake of clarity and completeness, this article will also include that breadth in the discussion of congenital abnormalities of the spine.

Neural tube defects are second only to congenital heart disease in the prevalence of birth anomalies.[2] Several of these entities are diagnosed in the prenatal period and require immediate postnatal management or are candidates for intra-utero repair, including the most common open SD, myelomeningocele (MMC). Therefore, it is

Department of Radiology, Children's Hospital Colorado, 13123 East 16th Avenue, Box 125, Aurora, CO 80045, USA
* Corresponding author.
E-mail address: christina.white@childrenscolorado.org

Clin Perinatol 49 (2022) 623–640
https://doi.org/10.1016/j.clp.2022.05.003
0095-5108/22/© 2022 Elsevier Inc. All rights reserved.

imperative that the neonatologist be aware of the various congenital abnormalities of the spine, the preferred imaging modalities, and current treatment standards of practice.

SPINAL CORD EMBRYOLOGY

To fully comprehend the imaging and physical examination findings in those patients with congenital spine abnormalities, it can be helpful to revisit the pertinent embryology of the spinal column, spinal cord, and surrounding mesenchymal structures.

Gastrulation

Gastrulation occurs around the second to third weeks of gestation and results in the formation of a trilaminar disk composed of endoderm, mesoderm, and ectoderm.[3] Before gastrulation, the developing fetus consists of a bilaminar sheet of cells composed of endoderm and ectoderm, without polarity or cell differentiation. During this phase of development, the intervening mesoderm is formed, to include a distinct column of mesodermal cells termed the notochord. This primitive notochord extends from anterior to posterior and will play a role in cell signaling during later stages of central nervous system development, eventually directing the formation of the neural tube.[4] Surrounding the notochord is paraxial mesoderm, which will form the osseous vertebral elements, skeletal muscle, and connective tissue.[3] The end product of gastrulation is a trilaminar disk with a defined midline and anterior–posterior axis.

Primary Neurulation

Once the trilaminar disk is fully formed and the notochord exists, primary neurulation can then take place around weeks 3 to 4.[4] The mesodermal notochord interacts with the overlying ectoderm and encourages a cascade of events that ultimately leads to the formation of the neural tube. Namely, on either side of midline along the long axis of the disk there is focal thickening and uplifting of the neural plate, resulting in the formation of distinct neural folds. These folds then continue to raise and fold inward, until they contact one another at midline and fuse to form a complete cylinder, the neural tube.[4] Historically, this process was understood to occur in a zipper-like fashion, originating at the cervicothoracic junction and extending in both directions.[5,6] However, a small minority of patients are born with defects affecting more than one spinal region and, as a result, additional theories have arisen that support several synchronous regions of ongoing fusion occurring at different spinal levels as a way to explain the existence of these multiple-site neural tube defects.[7]

Regardless of the timing or directionality of midline fusion, once the folds forming the neural tube are wholly in opposition with one another, the superficial and deep layers of the fold disconnect from one another in a process called dysjunction.[4] This allows the superficial ectodermal layer of the fold to fuse across midline, forming an intact contiguous skin surface (cutaneous ectoderm), while the deeper layers form the intact neural tube (neural ectoderm). Ultimately, the neural tube will give rise to the spinal cord and brain. Once dysjunction is complete, mesodermal cells are free to insinuate between the separated ectodermal layers and differentiate into various supporting elements adjacent to the spine, including subcutaneous fat and posterior spinal elements.[3]

Secondary Neurulation

Finally, secondary neurulation occurs at weeks 5 to 6.[4] During secondary neurulation, a caudal cell mass forms at the behest of the notochord and subsequently undergoes central cavitation and retrogressive differentiation.[4] This process transforms the solid cell mass into the conus medullaris and filum terminale, with a central lumen that reflects the terminal central canal. This separate caudal spinal cord segment then fuses with the primary neural tube to form one complete and continuous spinal cord, with fusion and continuity of the central canal also.[4,8] Transient expansion of the central canal within the lumbar spinal cord is evident during secondary neurulation, called the terminal ventricle or ventriculus terminalis, but subsequently regresses and is not detectable on postnatal MRI in most individuals.[5]

In reviewing the many steps involved in the formation of the spinal cord and surrounding osseous and soft tissue structures, it becomes clear how any misstep in this very complicated, multi-step process can result in a distinct malformation, thereby explaining the broad continuum of congenital spine malformations to be discussed in this article.

CLASSIFICATION

The most commonly used classification system for SDs is based on the work of Tortori-Donati and Rossi, and colleagues,[4] in the early 2000s, and relies on a combination of clinical and radiographic features for stratification (Fig. 1). This approach first broadly categorizes the defects as either having an intact skin covering or not (closed vs open), before further stratifying closed spinal dysraphisms (CSDs) depending on whether a subcutaneous mass is present or not (CSD with subcutaneous mass vs CSD without subcutaneous mass). Finally, those CSDs without a subcutaneous mass are subdivided into simple or complex dysraphic states.

An alternative approach to the classification of SDs is based on the embryologic stage during which the failure occurs, that is, MMC, intraspinal lipoma, and dermal sinus would all be lumped together as aberrations of primary neurulation.[3,4] Unfortunately, this method can be onerous and demands a mastery of the nuances of embryologic spine development, which many practitioners have not recently revisited

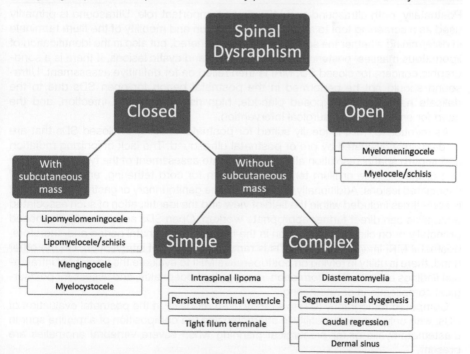

Fig. 1. Classification based on the clinical and radiographic features.

or reviewed. Instead, most clinicians and radiologists alike find the former method of classification more practical, particularly as it often belies the clinical severity of each entity and is therefore more useful.

ROLE OF IMAGING
Prenatal Imaging

Obstetric ultrasound provides fast and accessible prenatal screening of all developing fetuses and is a great initial tool in the evaluation of congenital spine abnormalities. Ultrasound is able to diagnose the vast majority of open SDs, via direct visualization of a CSF-filled sac herniating through a dorsal spinal defect or through the identification of associated findings of Chiari II malformation, such as a small posterior fossa with cerebellar crowding or marked bifrontal calvarial concavity with reduced biparietal diameter. The ultrasound diagnosis of closed SDs is somewhat less predictable. Obvious malformations featuring large lipomatous masses or cystic lesions are fairly reliably identified, but more subtle closed SDs may be missed.

Due to the challenges inherent to ultrasound, including variability in maternal body habitus, dependence on technologist experience, and less robust spatial resolution, fetal MRI has become the preferred choice for definitive prenatal characterization of SDs that are initially identified on screening ultrasound. Fetal MRI is not without its own limitations, which include cost, extended scan times, possible discomfort or anxiety experienced by the mother, difficulty obtaining images due to fetal motion, and lack of accessibility in more rural regions. In addition, fetal MRI requires specialized training and experience on the part of the MRI technologist and interpreting radiologist.

Postnatal Imaging

Postnatally, both ultrasound and MRI play an important role. Ultrasound is primarily used as a screening tool to assess for the position and mobility of the filum terminale in determining whether the spinal cord seems tethered, but also in the identification of lipomatous masses, posterior osseous defects, and cystic lesions. If there is a sonographic concern for closed SD, MRI is then relied on for definitive assessment. Ultrasound should not be performed in the postnatal period for open SDs due to the delicate nature of the exposed placode, high risk of postnatal infection, and the need for emergent neurosurgical intervention.

As mentioned, MRI is ideally suited for postnatal imaging of closed SDs that are inadequately evaluated by pre or postnatal ultrasound. The lack of ionizing radiation and superb spatial resolution allows for accurate assessment of the type of SD, position of the placode or filum terminale, concern for cord tethering, and existence of associated lesions. Additionally, pathology of the genitourinary or gastrointestinal tract is sometimes included within the field of view and the identification of such associated anomalies can direct further appropriate workup. Open SDs are generally diagnosed prenatally or on clinical examination in the immediate postnatal period and, therefore, postnatal MRI imaging of open SDs is rare before surgical intervention. On the other hand, there is utility in relying on postoperative MRI to evaluate the severity of intracranial findings of Chiari II malformation, manage hydrocephalus, and assess for postsurgical complications or retethering.

Computed tomography (CT) is a rarely used modality in the postnatal evaluation of SDs, with only occasional utility in characterizing the composition of a midline spur in diastematomyelia or for presurgical planning when severe vertebral anomalies are present.

OPEN SPINAL DYSRAPHISMS

As mentioned previously, open SDs are characterized by disruption in the skin covering the osseous spinal defect, allowing contents of the spinal canal to protrude outward and receive direct exposure to amniotic fluid. This contact has a caustic effect on sensitive neural tissues, resulting in greater clinical severity than those with closed SDs.[1,5,6] Because the defects are obvious and visible to the naked eye, patients are invariably diagnosed at birth, if not previously diagnosed during the prenatal period. If appropriate prenatal care is received and imaging is, indeed, performed, there is typically little uncertainty in the diagnosis of open spinal dysraphisms.

Myelocele/Myelomeningocele

The most widely discussed and commonly encountered open SD, comprising more than 98% of open neural tube defects, is MMC.[1,9] Embryologically, this results from the failure of the primary neural tube to fully close and subsequently detach from the cutaneous ectoderm.[4] Because the cutaneous ectoderm remains attached to the open neural tube, it cannot fuse across midline to form the overlying skin surface and the characteristic midline skin defect ensues.[1,4] The result is a flayed terminal spinal cord, termed the *placode*, that is elevated above the skin surface due to expansion of the underlying subarachnoid space.[4,6] The placode is anchored by nerve roots emerging from the ventral margins and coursing into corresponding neural foramen.[1,5,6] The lumbosacral level is most commonly involved and the spinal cord is invariably low and tethered by definition.[6]

This entity is typically diagnosed on fetal ultrasound and/or MRI and is rarely imaged postnatally unless the patient has already undergone repair, given the need for urgent surgical management to circumvent the high incidence of postnatal placode ulceration and infection.[9] On prenatal imaging, there is a defect in the posterior osseous spinal elements, through which the meninges and neural placode bulge (**Fig. 2**), with nearly all patients demonstrating intracranial findings of Chiari II malformation (small posterior fossa with inferior hindbrain descent, ventriculomegaly, and so forth). Higher the level of involvement, the more severe the clinical presentation.[1,5,10]

Though considerably more rare, myeloceles are often lumped in with MMCs, as the only differentiating feature between the 2 is the position of the neural placode. As discussed, in MMC, the expansion of the subarachnoid space results in protrusion of the placode above the skin surface, while the placode is flush with the skin surface in myelocele. The distinction between these entities is somewhat esoteric and does not alter the clinical picture in any meaningful way, but is occasionally useful information for the surgeon to have before repair as it impacts the amount of surrounding soft tissue available for mobilization and closure.

When MMC or myelocele is associated with cord splitting and only one hemicord fails to neurulate appropriately, it is termed hemimyelomeningocele or hemimyelocele, respectively.[1,4–6] While it is useful to be aware that various malformations can occur in conjunction, these are exceedingly rare and should not be considered primarily.

Within the past decade, treatment focus has shifted from postnatal repair with ventricular shunting to in utero fetal repair. This shift came with the conclusion of the Management of Myelomeningocele Study (MOMS trial) in 2011, a prospective randomized multicenter study comparing outcomes for those fetuses that underwent in utero surgical repair of MMC with those that did not. The trial demonstrated decreased need for ventricular shunting, improved hindbrain herniation, and better neurologic outcomes with fetal repair.[10] Greater incidences of neonatal/maternal morbidity and premature delivery were also observed, though not frequently enough to detract from the

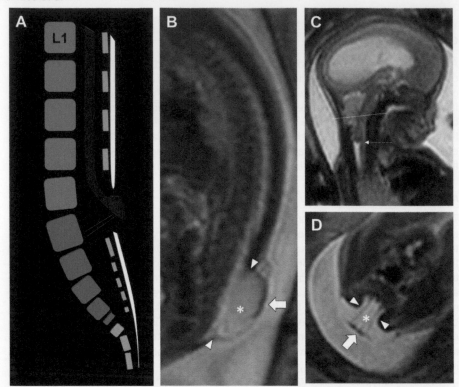

Fig. 2. Myelomeningocele with Chiari II malformation. (*A*) Digital rendition. (*B*) Sagittal and (*D*) axial oblique single-shot fast spine-echo T2-weighted MR images of the fetal spine demonstrate a focal defect in the dorsal skin and subcutaneous tissue of the thoracolumbar spine (*arrowheads*), with the expansion of the subarachnoid space (*asterisks*) through the dysraphic defect. The placode (*thick white arrows*) interfaces directly with amniotic fluid. (*C*) Sagittal single-shot fast spine-echo T2-weighted MR image of the cranio-cervical junction shows a small posterior fossa with inferior hindbrain herniation (*dashed arrow*) below the level of the foramen magnum (*thin white line*).

potential benefits of in utero repair.[10] As a result, fetal MMC repair is now the standard of care for cases diagnosed prenatally, if appropriate criteria are met.

CLOSED SPINAL DYSRAPHISMS WITH SUBCUTANEOUS MASS

In contradistinction to open neural tube defects, CSDs are covered with an intact layer of skin. Because the neural placode is not exposed to amniotic fluid and there is no CSF leakage, comparative preservation of neurologic function is seen.[9,11] Closed neural tube defects can be further subdivided by the presence or absence of an associated subcutaneous mass. Entities that demonstrate a palpable or visible mass on physical examination include lipomyelomeningocele, meningocele, and myelocystocele.

LIPOMAS WITH DURAL DEFECT

Lipomas with dural defects (LDDs) are a group of abnormalities that result from the premature separation of the cutaneous and neural ectodermal layers, allowing meso-dermal fat to insinuate into the still unfused neural tube.[4–6] The entities represented differ from one another based on the position of the cord-lipoma interface and include lipomyelomeningocele, lipomyelocele, and lipomyeloschisis.

Lipomyelomeningocele

Similar to MMC, lipomyelomeningocele also features the expansion of the subarachnoid space (with the lipoma-placode interface located outside of the spinal canal), but is distinguished by the presence of a fatty subcutaneous mass located at midline or just off midline with an intact overlying skin covering.[4–6,8] When occurring in the lumbosacral region, the subcutaneous fatty mass may be palpable above the gluteal crease, allowing for early clinical diagnosis. Because the mass is often apparent on clinical examination, the majority of patients present before the development of neurologic symptoms. Overlying skin lesions may occur in conjunction, including hairy nevus, skin dimple, and cutaneous hemangioma.[6]

On imaging, there is a posterior spinal defect and the low-lying spinal cord adheres to a fatty posterior subcutaneous mass (**Fig. 3**). Both ultrasound and MRI may be used to confirm the existence of lipomyelomeningocele, though MRI offers a more definitive evaluation of the cord position and extent of the lipomatous mass. Regardless, diagnosis is generally made within the first few months of life and treatment is the surgical resection of the lipoma with cord detethering.

Lipomyelocele/Lipomyeloschisis

Lipomyelocele and lipomyeloschisis reflect the same embryologic failing, also featuring a posterior spinal defect through which a lipomatous mass adheres to the tethered spinal cord. In contrast to lipomyelomeningocele, the cord-lipoma interface is located either within (lipomyeloschisis) or flush with (lipomyelocele) the neural arches (**Fig. 4**), a distinction that is again important for the surgeon when considering a repair.

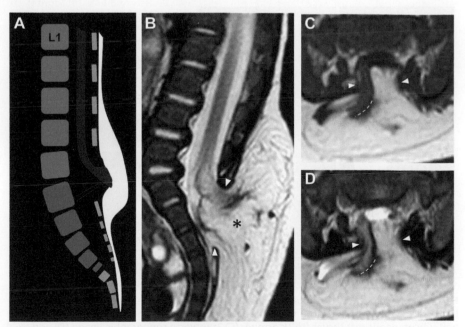

Fig. 3. Lipomyelomeningocele. (*A*) Digital rendition. (*B*) Sagittal (*D*) and axial oblique T2-weighted MR images and (*C*) axial oblique T1-weighted MR images of the lumbosacral spine demonstrate a posterior sacral dysraphic defect (*arrowheads*) through which a subcutaneous fatty mass (*asterisk*) communicates with the spinal canal. The placode-lipoma interface (*dashed line*) is positioned outside of the spinal canal.

Meningocele

Meningocele refers to the herniation of a CSF-filled sac that is lined by dura and arachnoid mater through a posterior dysraphic defect; the expanded subarachnoid space protrudes outward into the potential space left by the bony defect (**Fig. 5**). The exact embryologic underpinnings are uncertain, but currently, the most accepted theory is that this outward bulging of the meninges is a result of pronounced CSF pulsation expanding the sac.[5,6] By definition, the cord does not extend into the herniated sac, but may be tethered along the superior margin of its neck.[8] Nerve roots and filum terminale, on the other hand, may be contained in the sac.

When located posteriorly, meningocele most often occurs at the lumbosacral level, but can occur anywhere in the spine.[8] Overlying skin manifestations may be present, to include cutaneous dystrophy, hemangioma, or rudimentary tail-like structure.[5,6] Anterior meningoceles are commonly presacral in location and may be seen in conjunction with anorectal malformation and sacrococcygeal osseous defect (Currarino's triad).

Myelocystocele

In myelocystocele, there is ballooning of the central canal of the spinal cord through a posterior osseous dysraphic defect into a skin-covered meningocele (**Fig. 6**). This may occur within a low-lying, tethered distal spinal cord (terminal myelocystocele), or higher up in the spinal canal (nonterminal myelocystocele). Myelocystocele may occur in conjunction with Chiari II malformation or other CNS anomalies, and the nonterminal form is specifically associated with OEIS complex (omphalocele, exstrophy of the cloaca, imperforate anus, SD).[9,12] Occasionally, expansion of the central canal is

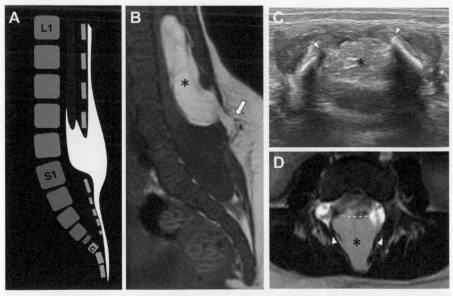

Fig. 4. Lipomyelocele. (*A*) Digital rendition. (*B*) Sagittal T1-weighted MR images of the lumbosacral spine show a large fatty mass contiguous between the spinal canal (*asterisk*) and subcutaneous soft tissues (*thick arrow*). (*C*) Transverse sonographic image (*D*) and axial oblique fat-saturated T2-weighted MR image confirm the dysraphic defect (*arrowheads*) and again highlights the intraspinal portion of the large fatty mass (*black asterisks*). As opposed to lipomyelomeningocele, the expansion of the subarachnoid space is absent and the lipoma-placode interface (*dashed white line*) is located within the spinal canal.

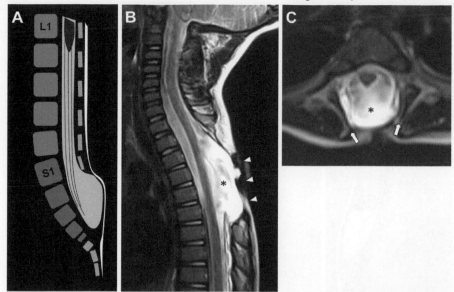

Fig. 5. Meningocele. (*A*) Digital rendition. (*B*) Sagittal and (*C*) axial oblique T2-weighted MR images of the cervicothoracic spine demonstrate a posterior dysraphic defect (*white arrows*) through which a CSF-filled sac bulges (*asterisk*). The overlying skin surface (*arrowheads*) is intact.

conspicuously absent in cases of nonterminal myelocystocele and only a thin fibrovascular stalk is seen extending from the dorsal surface of the cord into the meningocele, termed *abortive form nonterminal myelocystocele*.[5,9] In either form of nonterminal myelocystocele, as with terminal myelocystocele, the spinal cord is effectively tethered. Treatment is surgical, aimed at cord detethering and decreasing the size of the CSF-filled mass, in an effort to deter further enlargement.[13]

CLOSED SPINAL DYSRAPHISMS WITHOUT SUBCUTANEOUS MASS, SIMPLE

CSDs without subcutaneous masses can be further subdivided into complex and simple dysraphic states, based on their embryologic development.[4] Those deemed simple occur secondary to failures in dysjunction between cutaneous and neural ectoderm, and include intraspinal lipoma, persistence of the terminal ventricle, and tight filum terminale.[4,5] This is the category of dysraphisms that is most commonly diagnosed in older children, as the neurologic deficits are often more subtle and clinical examination findings may be absent.[14] As such, discussion of these entities will be limited to those that are more likely to be diagnosed with postnatal ultrasound, such as intraspinal lipoma.

Intradural Lipoma

Premature dysjunction of cutaneous ectoderm from neuroectoderm during primary neurulation allows fat to insinuate into the open neural tube.[4] The cutaneous ectoderm proceeds to fuse normally, meaning the skin surface is intact, but the mesenchymal elements that differentiate into fat are integrated into the open placode, preventing normal closure of the neural tube. The result is a fatty mass intimately associated with the spinal cord (**Fig. 7**), which is incompletely closed at the level of the integrated midline lipoma, and an intact overlying dura.[5] This latter feature allows the differentiation of an intradural lipoma from lipomyelocele or lipomyelomeningocele, whose dura is interrupted and accompanied by incomplete closure of the bony posterior elements.[9] Intraspinal lipomas occur most frequently in the lumbosacral spine and are associated with clinical symptoms of cord tethering, which are unlikely to manifest

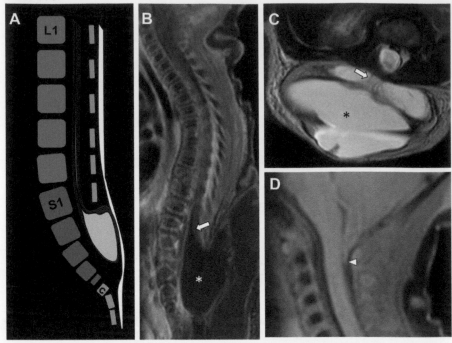

Fig. 6. Large terminal myelocystocele with Chiari I malformation. (*A*) Digital rendition. (*B*) Sagittal fat-saturated T1-weighted and (*C*) axial oblique fat-saturated T2-weighted MR images of the lumbosacral spine demonstrate the typical "trumpet" appearance of the low-lying distal spinal cord (*white arrow*) around a markedly dilated terminal central canal (*asterisk*). (*D*) Sagittal fat-saturated T1-weighted MR images of the cranio-cervical junction demonstrate inferior herniation of pointed cerebellar tonsils (*arrowhead*) below the foramen magnum.

in the neonatal period.[8] Therefore, if diagnosed neonatally, it is often because a screening ultrasound of the spine was performed.

Persistence of the Terminal Ventricle

An entity historically termed the "fifth ventricle," the persistent terminal ventricle reflects incomplete regression during secondary neurulation, leaving a small fluid-filled cavity in the conus medullaris.[4,5] On imaging, differentiating a persistent terminal ventricle from syrinx or arachnoid cyst may be challenging, but is generally accomplished based on the location.[8] Though a gratuitous distinction, a truly definitive diagnosis can only be made on postmortem examination by confirming the presence of ependymal cells lining the cyst walls, as opposed to arachnoid cells in arachnoid cyst, or neuronal cells in syrinx.[9] If large, it can be visualized by postnatal spinal ultrasound. As with any symptomatic cyst, the treatment includes excision or fenestration, though this is exceedingly rare as the majority are incidental and asymptomatic.[8]

The embryologic sequence of events leading to persistence of the terminal ventricle and terminal myelocystocele is notably similar; the only difference between the 2 being that persistent terminal ventricle preserves continuity with the central canal of the spinal cord, whereas terminal myelocystocele does not.[4,6]

CLOSED SPINAL DYSRAPHISMS WITHOUT SUBCUTANEOUS MASS, COMPLEX
Dermal Sinus Tract

Dermal sinus tract or dorsal dermal sinus is a fistulous tract leading inward from the skin surface, connecting the skin and underlying central nervous system or meninges,

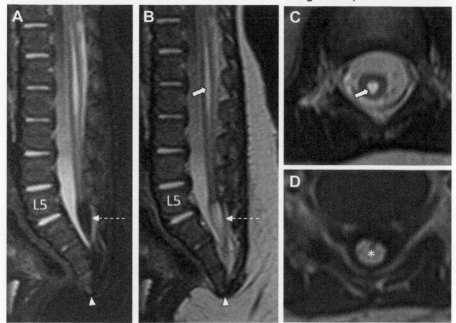

Fig. 7. Caudal agenesis type II with intraspinal lipoma and tethered cord. Sagittal (*A*) fat-saturated and (*B*) nonfat-saturated MR images of the thoracolumbar spine show only mild sacrococcygeal agenesis (*arrowheads*). The spinal cord is low-lying, effectively tethered to an intraspinal lipoma (*dashed arrows*) in the distal spinal canal. Axial (*C*) T2-weighted and (*D*) T1-weighted images of the same region again demonstrate a bulky intraspinal lipoma (*asterisk*), as well as a syrinx located slightly higher in the distal cord (*thick white arrow*).

and is lined by epithelium.[6] Embryologically, it occurs secondary to focal failure in dysjunction between cutaneous and neural ectoderm.[5] While it can occur anywhere, dermal sinus is most commonly observed in the lumbosacral region, whereby it may be associated with a spinal dermoid.[8]

A thin band is visible coursing obliquely through the midline dorsal subcutaneous fat on MRI, often most conspicuous on sagittal images (**Fig. 8**). On physical examination, a small ostium on the skin surface is visible at the midline and may be associated with a hairy nevus or hyperpigmentation.[6,8] Due to the potential for the tract to serve as a pathway for infectious organisms and subsequently result in meningitis, early surgical intervention is necessary.[8,9]

Diastematomyelia

This entity, also termed split cord malformation, reflects the formation of 2 separate, variably elongated hemicords that may be separated by a bony, cartilaginous, or fibrous septum. During the formation of the notochord, failure of midline integration results in the creation of 2 distinct paramedian notochordal procursors soparated by primitive streak cells.[4,5] The differentiation of those primitive streak cells determines which type of septum will develop, if at all.[6] For example, if they develop toward bone or cartilage, the hemicords will be contained in separate dural sacs separated by an osseocartilaginous division. Similarly, if there is complete or near-complete regression of the primitive streak, the cord halves will be housed within a single dural sac without intervening septum. The fate of those primitive streak cells is used to classify diastematomyelia into type I or II.[5]

In type I split cord malformation, each cord is confined within its own dural sac (**Fig. 9**A), most often separated by a bony or cartilaginous septum.[6] These patients will typically present with symptoms of cord tethering and scoliosis, and may exhibit cutaneous lesions caudal to the involved segment on physical examination, such as hairy nevus.[5] Associated vertebral anomalies are common and may include hemivertebrae, butterfly vertebrae, or spina bifida, among others. Dilation of the central canal, or hydromyelia, is also frequently encountered.

Type II split cord malformation tends to be less severe clinically, potentially asymptomatic, but can also be associated with symptoms of cord tethering.[4] By definition, both hemicords are contained within a single dural sac with either a thin fibrous septum or no intervening septum (**Fig. 9**B). The mildest end of the spectrum is a partial or incomplete division of the spinal cord. Vertebral anomalies are still encountered, but are also less severe, often consisting of spina bifida.[8] Hydromyelia may also be present, as in type I anomalies.

Caudal Regression

Also known as caudal agenesis or sacral agenesis, caudal regression syndrome (CRS) reflects a disruption in the normal development of the tail bud, occurring before the 4th

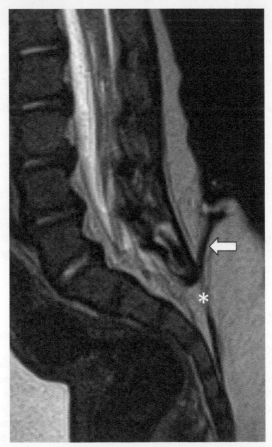

Fig. 8. Dorsal dermal sinus. Sagittal T2-weighted MR image of the lumbosacral spine demonstrates a fistula (*thick white arrow*) between the skin surface and spinal canal (*asterisk*), coursing obliquely through the subcutaneous soft tissues of the back.

gestational week at the crossover between primary and secondary neurulation.[4,5] This abnormal tail bud development has subsequent deleterious effects on the migration of mesodermal cells, resulting in associated abnormalities of the genitourinary, gastrointestinal, skeletal, and nervous systems.[4,5]

The constellation of anomalies varies, depending on the severity of the disorder, and may include anal atresia, neurogenic bladder, absent or hydronephrotic kidneys, clubfoot or limb contractures, and pulmonary hypoplasia, among others. An association with maternal diabetes mellitus is commonly described, with an estimated risk 170 to 400 times greater in infants of diabetic mothers as compared with the general population.[15] In general, the fetal karyotype is normal.[16]

If the insult takes place earlier and impacts both primary and secondary neurulation, the entity is classified as type I CRS.[4,6] These patients will have pronounced vertebral abnormalities, with the absence of the bony caudal spine at and below the affected level, occurring as high as the thoracic region. The corresponding caudal spinal cord metameres are also absent, resulting in high and abrupt termination of the blunted cauda equina (**Fig. 10**), often ending at T12.[5]

Type II, on the other hand, is related to aberrations in secondary neurulation only and is typified by less severe vertebral malformations, possibly involving only the sacrococcygeal segments or coccyx.[4,6] Rather than being blunted and foreshortened, as with type I, the spinal cord is often elongated and tethered to a thickened filum terminale or intraspinal lipoma (see **Fig. 7**).[6,9] While type I is characterized by major vertebral abnormalities, type II typically presents later with symptoms of cord tethering.[5]

Segmental Spinal Dysgenesis

Segmental spinal dysgenesis is a rare entity with similar pathophysiology to CRS,[4,5] characterized by segmental agenesis/dysgenesis of the lumbar or thoracolumbar spine, segmental abnormality of the corresponding spinal nerve roots and spinal cord, and congenital limb malformations. Patients exhibit signs of congenital paraparesis or paraplegia. The spinal cord may seem to be "cut in 2," either markedly hypoplastic or entirely absent at the level of the corresponding vertebral anomalies, with an intact and bulky lower cord segment (**Fig. 11**). The imaging appearance and morphologic severity of the abnormality go hand-in-hand with the clinical severity; specifically,

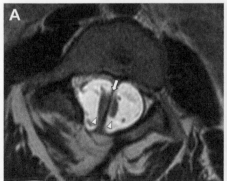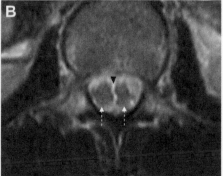

Fig. 9. Diastematomyelia, types I and II. (*A*) Axial T2-weighted MR image of the thoracic spine demonstrates a split spinal cord (*white arrowheads*), with each half contained in its own thecal sac separated by a osseocartilaginous spur (*thick white arrow*), consistent with type I. (*B*) Axial T2-weighted MR image of the thoracic spine in a different patient shows a split spinal cord (*dashed arrows*) contained within a single thecal sac separated only by CSF (*black arrowhead*), reflecting type II.

the amount of residual neural tissue present in the affected region correlates with neurologic outcomes.[4]

Inherent instability of the spinal column and the tendency toward the progression of neurologic defects necessitates careful assessment to determine whether immediate surgical evaluation and management are necessary.[17] Current treatment approaches are aimed at early fusion and decompression in patients with severe defects or evidence of neurologic decompensation, or bracing with a staged approach to fusion, when symptoms are less severe and stable.[18] Both approaches are challenging due to patient age and lack of vertebral body ossification. And unfortunately, while a small

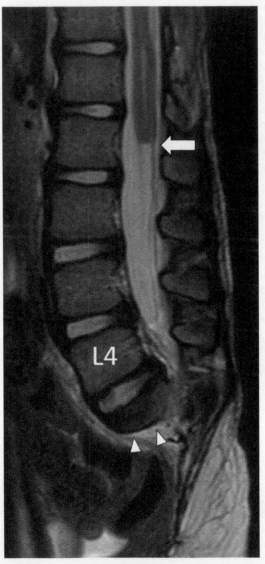

Fig. 10. Caudal agenesis type I. Abrupt termination of the bony spinal elements at the level of L5 (*white arrowheads*) with absent caudal spine below and associated high and blunt termination of the cauda equina (*thick white arrow*).

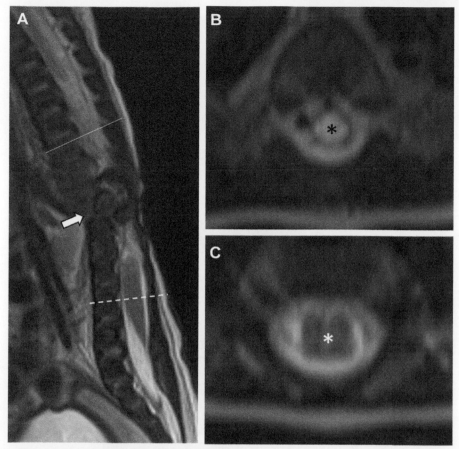

Fig. 11. Segmental spinal dysgenesis. (*A*) Sagittal T2-weighted MR image of the thoracolumbar spine shows focal marked dysgenesis (*thick white arrow*) of the spinal column at the thoracolumbar junction resulting in characteristic kyphotic deformity. Axial oblique T2-weighted MR images corresponding with the levels demarcated by the (*B*) solid and (*C*) dashed white lines on the sagittal image demonstrate a complete or near-complete absence of the spinal cord (*black asterisk*) just above the involved vertebral segment, with a bulky low-lying cord (*white asterisk*) inferior to the defect.

percent of patients improve the following surgery, many fail to show improvement and a few may deteriorate.[17]

Sacrococcygeal Teratoma

Though not a congenital malformation in the strictest sense, sacrococcygeal teratoma is a tumor that results from failed induction of totipotent somatic cells during spinal development and, therefore, is worth discussing alongside other congenital abnormalities of the spine.[19] Teratomas are the most common solid tumor in neonates, with a reported incidence of 1 in every 35,000 to 40,000 births, and are more common in women than men with a 3:1 female predominance.[19,20] Though the majority are histologically benign with good prognosis, early surgical resection is the standard of care due to the risk of malignant degeneration with increased age or in cases of incomplete surgical resection.[19]

Diagnosis with prenatal ultrasound is most often possible, particularly in cases whereby a large extra-pelvic component is present or when there is a mass effect

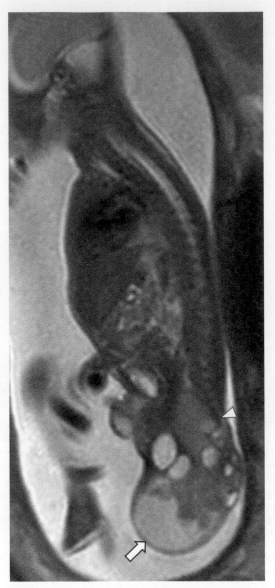

Fig. 12. Sacrococcygeal teratoma. Sagittal single-shot fast spine-echo T2-weighted MR image of the fetus shows a large cystic and solid mass (*thick arrow*) arising from the sacrococcygeal spine (*arrowhead*).

on the rectum or bladder outlet, resulting in ascites, hydronephrosis, and/or oligohydramnios.[19] Teratomas that are undiagnosed before birth are invariably identified on physical examination as a palpable mass in the sacrococcygeal region, if an extrapelvic component exits. A few cases are entirely intrapelvic/presacral (type 4) and may present only with gastrointestinal or genitourinary obstruction.

Most tumors are composed of both cystic and solid components (**Fig. 12**), though an entirely cystic composition is seen in 15% of cases. If widening of the lumbosacral spinal canal is identified on imaging, intraspinal extension is presumed.[19] Imaging with MRI is an important adjunct to ultrasound and is especially useful for evaluating the

Intrapelvic and intraabdominal extent, tumor composition, and involvement of nearby structures.[21]

SUMMARY

Congenital malformations of the spinal cord and associated osseous, mesenchymal, and nervous tissues encompass a broad group of abnormalities that occur secondary to missteps in a complex embryologic sequence of events. Based on the clinical and radiographic features, SDs are divided into open and closed SDs, with further stratification of closed SDs based on whether or not they are associated with a palpable subcutaneous mass. Because many spinal cord malformations are diagnosed and managed in the prenatal or immediate postnatal period, neonatologists should be aware of these entities, take care to conduct a thorough physical examination, and have familiarity with the preferred imaging modalities and treatment options.

Best practices

- The most commonly used classification system relies on a clinical and radiographic features for stratification and broadly categorizes the defects as either open or closed, before further stratifying closed spinal dysraphisms (CSDs) depending on whether a subcutaneous mass is present or not. CSDs without a subcutaneous mass are subdivided into simple or complex dysraphic states.

- Open spinal dysraphism: typically diagnosed (and often treated) prenatally. Requires emergent neurosurgical intervention prior to postnatal imaging.

- Closed spinal dysraphism with subcutaneous mass: ultrasound is useful as a screening entity in the neonatal period to assess for the position and mobility of the filum terminale, the identification of lipomatous masses, posterior osseous defects, and cystic lesions. MRI is valuable for definitive assessment.

- Closed spinal dysraphisms without subcutaneous mass: evaluate with MRI. If extensive osseous vertebral anomalies are present, CT may be useful for presurgical planning.

CLINICS CARE POINTS

- Open spinal dysraphisms are either diagnosed prenatally or, in cases of inadequate prenatal care, easily visible at birth. Imaging should be deferred until after appropriate surgical intervention, due to the high incidence of postnatal placode ulceration and infection.

- Closed spinal dysraphisms are further subdivided based on the presence or absence of an associated palpable subcutaneous mass. Closed dyraphisms with a subcutaneous mass are generally also diagnosed in the neonatal period and should be worked up with ultrasound and MRI.

- Closed sacral dysraphisms without an associated mass are often diagnosed in older children, as the neurologic deficits are more subtle and clinical examination findings may be absent. If there is concern for a closed spinal dysraphisms, MRI is preferred for definitive assessment.

DISCLOSURE

The authors have nothing to disclose.

REFERENCES

1. Schwartz EC, Barkovich AJ. Congenital anomalies of the spine. In: ZinnerS PecarichL, editor. Pediatric neuroimaging. 6th edition. Philadelphia: Wolters Kluwer; 2018. p. 1311–77.
2. Neural tube defects, susceptibility to; NTD. OMIM: online mendelian inheritance in man. Available at: https://www.omim.org/entry/182940. Accessed September 19, 2021.
3. Kaplan KM, Spivak JM, Bendo JA. Embryology of the spine and associated congenital abnormalities. Spine J 2005;5(5):564–76.
4. Tortori-Donati P, Rossi A, Cama A. Spinal dysraphism: a review of neuroradiological features with embryological correlations and proposal for a new classification. Neuroradiology 2000;42(7):471–91.
5. Rossi A, Biancheri R, Cama A, et al. Imaging in spine and spinal cord malformations. Eur J Radiol 2004;50(2):177–200.
6. Trapp B, de Andrade Lourencao Freddi T, de Oliveira Morais Hans M, et al. A practical approach to diagnosis of spinal dysraphism. Radiographics 2021; 41(2):559–75.
7. Van Allen MI, Kalousek DK, Chernoff GF, et al. Evidence for multi-site closure of the neural tube in humans. Am J Med Genet 1993;47(5):723–43.
8. Rufener SL, Ibrahim M, Raybaud CA, et al. Congenital spine and spinal cord malformations–pictorial review. AJR Am J Roentgenol 2010;194(3 Suppl):S26–37.
9. Reghunath A, Ghasi RG, Aggarwal A. Unveiling the tale of the tail: an illustration of spinal dysraphisms. Neurosurg Rev 2021;44(1):97–114.
10. Adzick NS, Thom EA, Spong CY, et al. A randomized trial of prenatal versus postnatal repair of myelomeningocele. N Engl J Med 2011;364(11):993–1004.
11. Grimme JD, Castillo M. Congenital anomalies of the spine. Neuroimaging Clin N Am 2007;17(1):1–16.
12. Wang LL, Bierbrauer KS. Congenital and hereditary diseases of the spinal cord. Semin Ultrasound CT MRI 2017;38:105–25.
13. Choi S, McComb JG. Long-term outcome of terminal myelocystocele patients. Pediatr Neurosurg 2000;32(2):86–91.
14. Kumar J, Afsal M, Garg A. Imaging spectrum of spinal dysraphism on magnetic resonance: a pictorial review. World J Radiol 2017;9(4):178–90.
15. Bell R, Glinianaia SV, Tennant PW, et al. Peri-conception hyperglycaemia and nephropathy are associated with risk of congenital anomaly in women with pre-existing diabetes: a population-based cohort study. Diabetologia 2012;55(4):936–47.
16. Heuser CC, Hulinky RS, Jackson GM. Caudal regression syndrome. In: Copel JA, D'Alton ME, Feltovich H, et al, editors. Obstetric imaging: fetal diagnosis and care. 2nd edition. Philadelphia: Elsevier; 2018. p. 291–4.
17. Remondino RG, Tello CA, Bersusky ES, et al. Surgical treatment of segmental spinal dysgenesis: a report of 19 cases. Spine Deform 2020;9:539–47.
18. Bristol RE, Theodore N, Rekate HL. Segmental spinal dysgenesis: report of four cases and proposed management strategy. Childs Nerv Syst 2007;23:359–64.
19. Wells RG, Sty JR. Imaging of sacrococcygeal germ cell tumors. RadioGraphics 1990;10(4):701–13.
20. Swamy R, Embleton N, Hale J. Sacrococcygeal teratoma over two decades: birth prevalence, prenatal diagnosis and clinical outcomes. Prenat Diagn 2008;28:1048–51.
21. Danzer E, Hubbard AM, Hedrick HL, et al. Diagnosis and characterization of fetal sacrococcygeal teratoma with prenatal MRI. Am J Roentgenol 2006;187(4): W350–6.

Imaging of Premature Infants

Abigail Locke, Sangam Kanekar, MD*

KEYWORDS

- Germinal matrix hemorrhage • Periventricular leukomalacia (PVL)
- Posthemorrhagic hydrocephalus of prematurity (PHHP)

KEY POINTS

- Preterm infants are those born at less than 37 weeks, while extremely and very preterm neonates include those born at 22 to <32 weeks gestational age.
- Neuroimaging, Brain MRI and cranial ultrasound (CUS), plays a key role in detecting and assessing the neurologic injuries that preterm infants are at risk.
- The very low birth weight (VLBW) infant, an infant 1500 g or less, have an increased risk for both GM and IVH, in addition to ischemic white matter injury.

INTRODUCTION

According to the World Health Organization (WHO), 15 million babies are born preterm each year. Preterm infants are those born at less than 37 weeks, while extremely and very preterm neonates include those born at 22 to less than 32 weeks gestational age.[1] Infants that fail to make it to term are missing a key part in neurodevelopment, as weeks 24 to 40 are a critical period of brain development.[2] Neonatal brain injury is a crucial predictor for mortality and morbidity in premature and low birth weight (<1500 g) infants.[3] Although the complications associated with preterm birth continue to be the number one cause of death in children under 5, the survival rates are increasing (Volpe, 2019). Despite this, the incidence of comorbidities, such as learning disabilities and visual and hearing problems, is still high.[4] The functional deficits seen in these infants can be contributed to the white matter abnormalities (WMA) that have been found in 50% to 80% of extremely and very preterm neonates.[1,2] While numerous, the etiology of the neonatal brain injury is essential for determining the mortality and morbidities of the infant,[3] as there is an increased risk for both intraventricular hemorrhage (IVH) and periventricular leukomalacia (PVL), which can be attributed to their lack of cerebrovascular autoregulation[5] and hypoxic events.[3] Neuroimaging plays a key role in detecting and assessing these neurologic injuries that preterm infants are at risk for.[6] It is essential to diagnose these events early on to assess neurologic damage, minimize disease progression, and provide supportive care.[5,6] Brain

The authors have nothing to disclose.
Radiology Research, Division of Neuroradiology, Penn State Health, Penn State College of Medicine, Mail Code H066 500 University Drive, Hershey, PA 17033, USA
* Corresponding author.
E-mail address: skanekar@pennstatehealth.psu.edu

Clin Perinatol 49 (2022) 641–655
https://doi.org/10.1016/j.clp.2022.06.001
0095-5108/22/© 2022 Elsevier Inc. All rights reserved.
perinatology.theclinics.com

MRI and cranial ultrasound (CUS) are both extensively used neuroimaging techniques to assess WMA,[7] and it has become ever more important to determine the best imaging techniques and modalities with the increasing survival rates and high incidence of comorbidities among these infants.[1,7]

Techniques

As of now, CUS is the primary modality used for imaging premature infants, as it serves as both an early diagnostic tool to minimize adverse outcomes and as a marker for long-term neurodevelopment.[5,7] To visualize the brain, CUS uses the anterior, posterior, and mastoid fontanelle as acoustic windows.[6] It is necessary to perform all views, as they each provide crucial information that may not be seen in the other windows. The posterior fontanelle view provides a more detailed assessment of the periventricular white matter, as well as the occipital lobes.[6] The mastoid fontanelle window is important for the visualization of the cerebellum, which is whereby most cases of cerebellar hypoplasia associated with cerebral white matter injury (WMI) occur.[6] Additionally, the cerebellum is a common site for significant hemorrhage due to injury, and the mastoid fontanelle window has a higher sensitivity at detecting this than any of the other views.[6] When performing the ultrasound, the images should be taken in the coronal plane with both anterior and posterior views, along with the sagittal plane using angulation on the left and right.[6] When serial CUS is performed within the first 2 week of life, it is able to detect 80% of germinal matrix (GM)/IVH.[2] Aside from the detection of brain injuries, CUS is widely available, inexpensive, and noninvasive.[2] Despite these advantages, there are several limitations and challenges to using CUS. Although mastoid views are able to detect hemorrhaging, they are unable to detect cerebellar microhemorrhages, which therefore need to be visualized using MRI.[2,6] Additionally, some white matter lesions including hyperechoic lesions, hypoechoic lesions, and ventricular enlargement, as well as the brain periphery and posterior fossa are not detected well on CUS.[2] Finally, interobserver variability is present, which must be taken into account.[2]

Aside from CUS, magnetic resonance imaging (MRI) is another modality used to visualize the brain of premature infants. MRI provides the most detailed imaging without ionizing radiation, unlike the CT.[6] Additionally, it provides more detailed images of lesions than CUS, which ultimately aids in determining the site, extent, and pathology of the lesion.[2] It is important to note that the MR sequences used for adults must be changed for neonates due to the higher water content and lower protein and lipid contents.[8] Specifically, the repetition time in T1- and T2-weighted images should be increased to increase the signal-to-noise ratio, as well as the contrast between white and gray matter.[8] When using MRI, the range for specific absorption rates, a measure of power of radiofrequency magnetic fields, is within an acceptable range.[6] Furthermore, with feeding 20 to 30 minutes before the scan, followed by swaddling to limit movement, there is no sedation needed.[6] Therefore, MRI is safe for the infant.[6] Despite these advantages, it is unclear if there is any predictive value of adverse neurodevelopmental outcomes when an abnormal MRI is obtained.[6] Finally, CT is no longer a standard modality used for routine imaging of premature infants due to the radiation risks that it imposes.[6]

Infants who are born at less than 30 weeks, along with those born at greater than 30 weeks with an increased risk for brain injury, should be imaged using CUS to check for IVH.[6] These risk factors include, but are not limited to, placental abruption, vigorous resuscitation, hypotension with pressor support, severe acidosis, prolonged mechanical ventilation, sepsis, and pneumothorax.[6] These infants should be imaged between 7 and 10 days of age.[6] However, if clinical signs and symptoms suggest brain injury, they should be imaged earlier.[6] Imaging should then be repeated at both 4 and 6 weeks of age and term equivalent age or when discharged from the hospital.[6] Additionally, if the initial CUS is abnormal, serial CUS should be obtained based on their chronologic and gestational age.[6] Although MRI has the ability to predict adverse neurodevelopmental outcomes, it is not currently indicated as a routine procedure, as there is not enough evidence that it is beneficial, unless the infant is < 29 weeks or less than 1000 g [2,6] For those preterm infants who do not meet the indicated criteria, MRI does not improve the prediction of early and late CUS that are already preformed.[6] Additionally, it does not improve maternal anxiety or quality of life for the infants and can increase health care costs, as well.[6] When offered to high risk infants as mentioned above, the limitations of long-term prognosis estimation should be discussed, and contrast should not be used.[6]

Pathophysiology of Preterm White Matter Injury

Despite the increasing rates of survival of preterm births, the rate of neurodevelopmental disability that results from the initial brain injury is high, as well.[4] During the premature period, there are a number of developmental events that are actively occurring. Consequently, these events are disturbed by WMI. WMI is the initiating event that results in a cascade of dysmaturational events to follow within the white matter, as well as in axonal structures.[4]

As mentioned above,[4] during the premature period of 20 to 40 weeks gestation, there are a variety of complex developmental events taking place in the cerebrum that are extremely vulnerable to disruptions.[4] The components of these processes include the oligodendroglia (OL) lineage, cerebral white matter axons, subplate neurons, cerebral cortex, thalamus, and basal ganglia. Within the cerebral white matter, the OL lineage of cells produce myelin, once they are mature.[4] It is not until postterm that most of these cells continue to develop and mature from preoligodendrocytes (pre-OLs), which arise from oligodendrocyte progenitors.[4] The pre-OLs are the driving force for the development of the cerebral cortex.[4] These highly vulnerable cells start ensheathing the axons at roughly 30 weeks' gestation.[4] Without this process occurring, the axons are not able to differentiate or function.[4] Additionally, cerebral matter white axons are rapidly developing during the premature period, especially in the cerebral white matter.[4] These too are vulnerable to insult, as they are very active during the premature period in the cerebrum.[4] Subplate neurons play an organizational role, in which they provide a transient synaptic site for afferents that are ascending from the thalamus toward other cortical sites.[4] The subplate reaches its max size between 24 and 32 weeks, which again is the most prevalent period for cerebral WMI to occur.[4] If these subplate neurons are not present as a transient target, the afferents will degenerate.[4] The cerebral cortex undergoes dramatic changes during the premature period that include the attainment of proper alignment, orientation and layering of cortical neurons, elaboration of dendritic and axonal ramifications (correlated with the development of cortical activity), onset of synaptogenesis, a marked increase in cortical surface area with gyral development, and arrival of late migrating GABAergic neurons, primarily to the upper cortical layer.[4] The arrival of these neurons does not actually peak until term.[4]

Microglia and astrocytes not only play a crucial role in development, but they are also mediators in the dysmaturation of the principal components discussed above.[4] Microglia aid in the development of axons, differentiation and myelination of OLs, vascularization, synaptogenesis, and synaptic pruning and neural circuit formation.[4] Astrocytes are important for axonal guidance, angiogenesis, formation of the BBB, synaptogenesis, neuronal survival, and axonal and synaptic pruning.[4] Despite the crucial role in development that these cells play, they also have the potential to cause harm.[4] Microglia are the principle neuroimmune cells that are involved in the neuroinflammatory response.[4] The M1 subtype is proinflammatory, while M2 is antiinflammatory.[4] The cerebral white matter of the premature infant brain has a large population of microglia present through the maturational process.[4] If a proinflammatory insult occurs during this time, the M1 phenotype is activated, resulting in WMI.[4] Furthermore, astrocytes also have the potential to become reactive and cause deleterious effects in white matter components, such as pre-OLs.[4]

One of the main cellular targets of WMI in premature infants is pre-OLs.[4] These cells are the main target as 90% of the OL lineage is in the pre-OL phase in premature infants when the highest period of WMI occurs.[4] The acute period of WMI includes the death of pre-OLs, which can result from a number of insults including hypoxia, ischemia, and inflammation.[4] The mechanisms for their death includes both excitotoxic and free-radical mediated.[4] The subacute period follows in which the proliferation of pre-OLs occurs to restore the population.[4] Despite this attempt, differentiation of these newly proliferated cells to the further phase of the OL lineage fails, which ultimately results is the hallmark of this disease: hypomyelination.[4]

Cerebral WMI has a range from PVL to diffuse white matter gliosis (DWMG).[4] It is this injury that then leads to the dysmaturational events that occur.[4] The WMI in addition to the neuronal and axonal disturbances encompass encephalopathy of prematurity.[4] PVL has two characteristics. The first being focal necroses that are a result of decreased cerebral blood flow due to a perinatal or neonatal event.[1,4] These necroses have a loss of cellular elements in the periventricular white matter, which are the infarcts.[4] The second is a diffuse lesion in cerebral white matter, which ultimately results in the death of early differentiating pre-OLs, which is then followed by astrogliosis and microgliosis.[1,4] Acutely, the pre-OL disturbance consists of cell death. This death results from acute insults or accompanying disturbances that have the potential to predispose the pre-OLs to injury, such as intrauterine growth retardation, systemic infection, or impaired nutrition.[4] This is subacutely and chronically followed by the proliferation of the pre-OLs.[4] Critically, there is failure of the maturation of these newly proliferated pre-OLs, which results in the hallmark of this disease mentioned above, hypomyelination.[4] This is likely related to the deleterious effects that microglia have that have been activated in addition to the reactive astrocytes.[4] In fact, it has been shown that the proinflammatory microglia have the ability to induce the formation of the reactive astrocytes, leading to the pre-OL maturational failure.[4] These astrocytes produce a large amount of IFN-gamma, for which the pre-OLs express a receptor for.[4] IFN-gamma activates these receptors, resulting in the inhibition of pre-OL differentiation.[4] The failure of the pre-OLs to ensheath axons results in impaired development.[4] There are diminished volumes of cerebral cortex and thalamus or basal ganglia, secondary to retrograde and anterograde effects.[4]

Neuroimaging

The likelihood of intracranial hemorrhage is increased in premature infants due to the difference in cerebral circulation.[3] Fetal blood supply is constantly changing, but the major modifications occur during the third trimester when the centrally located supply shifts to become predominantly peripheral, resulting in increased supply to the surface of the brain.[3] Furthermore, the deep white matter of the fetal brain is only supplied by a single artery making this area especially vulnerable to injury.[3] Finally, in contrast with term infants, premature infants have a marked presence of GM, which increases the risk of hemorrhage for these patients.[3]

In the event of intracranial hemorrhage, there is decreased oxygen delivered to the brain, resulting in injury.[3] This injury typically results due to fetal subjection to asphyxiation.[3] The degree of injury is determined by fetal compensation, in addition to the extent of the asphyxia.[3] In instances that the fetus is unable to compensate, or endures prolonged asphyxiation, there will ultimately be brain injury due to ischemia from the disruption in blood flow and gas exchange at the neuronal level.[3] There are typically 3 stages of injury: primary injury during asphyxiation, reperfusion injury during reperfusion or reoxygenation, and delayed and secondary neuronal loss, which typically occurs 6 to 12 hours after the primary injury and can last for several days.[3] Ultimately, the damage that results in intracranial hemorrhage is believed to be a result of the reperfusion injury.[3] A series of biochemical events occurs that results in free radical accumulation leading to tissue damage.[3] As this process is ever-changing, a series of cranial US must be performed both in utero and neonatally to monitor the condition.[3]

There are 2 different grading systems for which the severity of neonatal injury can be determined based on the results and findings of cranial US.[3] These systems convey the severity of injury, which is predictive of future outcomes for the infant.[3] Older grading system for Hemorrhage had four different grades of intracranial hemorrhage: Grade I is classified as slight in degree of severity, as the hemorrhage is restricted to the GM.[3] The GM is an area of brain tissue within the basal ganglia that receives a large amount of blood in premature infants.[3] It undergoes involution around 35 to 36 weeks gestation making term infants lower risk for GM hemorrhage.[5] On CUS coronal images, GM hemorrhages are seen as an area of increased echogenicity inferolateral to the floor of the frontal horns and medial to the head of the caudate nucleus.[5] (Fig. 1) On the parasagittal view, it is seen between the head of the caudate and the thalamus, also known as the caudothalamic groove.[5] In instances for which the hemorrhage is large, there is effacement of the frontal horn or body due to the elevation of the floor of the lateral ventricles.[5] A hemorrhage that occurs in the GM has the ability to extend to the ventricular system.[5] Grade II hemorrhages are still classified as slight in degree of severity, but are defined as IVH without ventricular enlargement.[3] With IVH, blood can fill the third and fourth ventricles.[5] On imaging, this will appear as homogeneously echogenic due to the clot forming.[5] (Fig. 2) However, it will start to look more heterogeneous as the hemorrhage evolves due to the retraction and lysis of the clot.[5] These hemorrhages result from rupture of a GM hemorrhage through the lateral

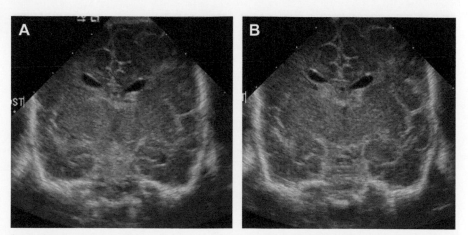

Fig. 1. Grade 1 intracranial hemorrhage: Coronal images of cranial US shows subependymal hemorrhage (*pink arrows*) located in the groove between the thalamus (*A*) and the nucleus caudate (*B*).

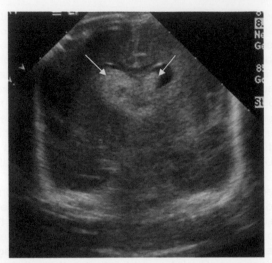

Fig. 2. Grade 2 intracranial hemorrhage: Coronal images of cranial US shows mild to moderate hemorrhage in the region of germinal matrix with the intraventricular extension of the bleed (yellow arrows). There is no hydrocephalus.

ependymal wall that results in filling of the ventricular system but does not dilate it more than 50%.[5] The severity increases to moderate when the IVH results in ventricular enlargement, and this is considered a Grade III hemorrhage.[3] (**Fig. 3**) Finally, Grade IV hemorrhages are classified as a severe degree of severity and are defined as IVH with parenchymal hemorrhage, and these can be associated with venous infarction.[3,5] (**Fig. 4**) On imaging, these will look brightly echogenic in the periventricular white matter found ipsilaterally to the IVH.[5] Despite this, the abnormality cannot always be seen on cranial US due to gliosis.[5]

The second system is Volpe's (2001b) Grading System for Hemorrhage, and the description for each of the severities is determined by the US findings.[3] Severity I is an isolated GM hemorrhage or one with less than 10% IVH.[3] Severity II is an IVH

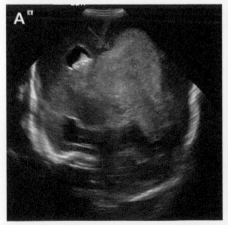
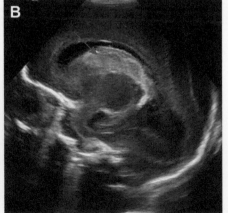

Fig. 3. Grade 3 intracranial hemorrhage: Coronal (*A*) and sagittal (*B*) images of cranial US shows large intraventricular hemorrhage (pink arrows) with the dilatation of the ventricular system– hydrocephalus..

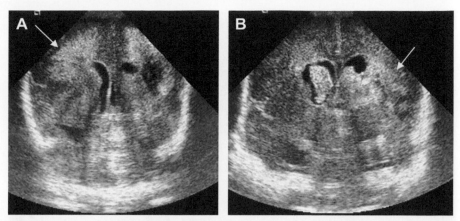

Fig. 4. Grade 4 intracranial hemorrhage: Coronal image of cranial US shows large parenchymal (*A*) and interventricular hematoma (*B*). There is extensive periventricular increased echogenicity of the brain parenchyma (*yellow arrows*).

constituting 10% to 50% of the ventricular area.[3] Finally, severity III is an IVH that is greater than 50% of the ventricular area and has a tendency to distend into the lateral ventricle.[3]

Additionally, premature infants can hemorrhage into the cerebellum.[5] This injury is typically due to prolonged labor and a traumatic delivery, and it tends to be seen more in delivery of infants with extremely low birth weight.[5] It is thought that this hemorrhage is a result of the GM zones within the subependymal layer of the fourth ventricle bleeding, which can be present without IVH.[5] However, this is not seen as well on cranial US.[5] To aid in visualization and detection, the mastoid view is used.[5] This view places the vermis, cerebellar hemisphere, and fourth ventricle closer to the transducer, which improves the visualization, especially compared with the standard fontanelle window.[5] When seen on cranial US, the hemorrhage is originally homogenously echogenic but will become heterogenous and then hyperechoic as the clot undergoes lysis.[5] (**Fig. 5**).

IVH has the potential to result in ventricular dilation, resulting in posthemorrhagic hydrocephalus, which will present with rapidly increasing head circumference, a tense anterior fontanelle, apnea, vomiting, and abnormal posture.[5] (**Fig. 6**) The resulting

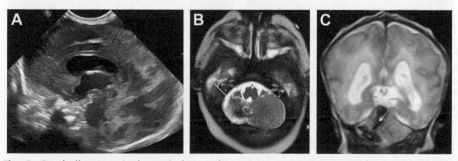

Fig. 5. Cerebellar germinal matrix hemorrhage in a preterm neonate born at 24 weeks gestation. Sagittal view (*A*) of the cranial US demonstrates an area of echogenicity (*pink arrow*) in the left cerebellar hemisphere, a finding that is compatible with hemorrhage. Axial T2 (*B*) and coronal GRE (*C*) Large right cerebellar hemisphere Hg (*yellow arrows*), with severe loss of volume.

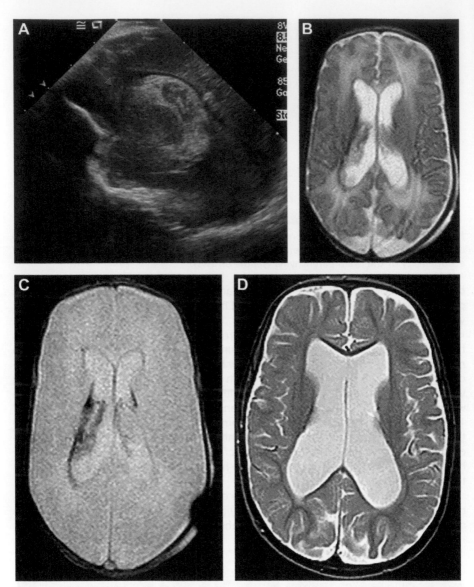

Fig. 6. Posthemorrhagic hydrocephalus of prematurity (PHHP). Coronal image (*A*) of cranial US shows intraventricular hemorrhage with possible areas of ischemia or hemorrhage (*pink arrow*) in the periventricular white matter. T2 (*B*) and GRE (*C*) MRI images show bled in the body and occipital horn of the right lateral ventricle. Two years follow-up MRI scan (*D*) of the brain shows moderate dilatation of the lateral ventricles with the paucity of the white matter.

obstruction is either classified as noncommunicating or communicating, although posthemorrhagic are typically communicating.[5] Communicating obstructions occur outside the ventricular system, while noncommunicating are obstructions within the ventricular system.[5] In communicating, the absorption of CSF is impaired due to chemical arachnoiditis that developed from blood products, which eventually leads to both arachnoid granulation fibrosis and meningeal fibrosis.[5] Inflammatory factor

TGF-beta also plays a role in posthemorrhagic hydrocephalus, due to its stimulation and production of extracellular matrix leading to blockage of the arachnoid villi.[5] To monitor infants and determine those who require the placement of a shunt, serial cranial US can be used.[5] Following shunt placement, cranial US can continued to be used to determine ventricular decompression.[5]

Hypoxic-Ischemic Injury in Preterm Neonates

Hypoxic-ischemic injury (HII) occurs in both preterm and term neonates and primarily damages the deep gray matter, which ultimately leads to death or long-term neurologic disability.[9] Not only can imaging be useful for the diagnosis of HII, but it can also be used for managing the injury and predicting the prognosis of the infant based on the degree of injury.[9] However, HII imaging findings can vary based on the maturity of brain, severity, and duration of insult, and the type and timing of the imaging study.[9] This puts an emphasis as to why it is crucial to understand and know the various patterns and locations of HII when it is suspected.[9]

When infants experience asphyxiation, they suffer from hypoxemia, which leads to brain hypoxia.[9] Hypoxemia, when prolonged, results in cardiac hypoxia and decreased cardiac output.[9] This drop in cardiac output decreases blood flow to the brain, resulting in brain ischemia, as well.[9] Although the origin of insult can vary, the pathophysiologic process remains the same in all cases: ischemia from diminished cerebral blood flow and reduced blood oxygenation, or hypoxemia.[9] With HII, there is selective vulnerability, meaning that there are specific regions of the brain that are more readily injured.[9] When the brain undergoes ischemia, the lack of oxygen results in anerobic metabolism predominating over oxidative phosphorylation, which is not competent.[9] This switch results in the depletion of adenosine triphosphate (ATP), lactate accumulation within cells, and loss of normal cellular membrane function.[9] The depolarization of the presynaptic neuronal membrane results in a substantial release of various excitatory neurotransmitters.[9] Glutamate is one of the major neurotransmitters released, and it primarily binds to N-methyl-D-aspartate (NMDA) receptor-mediated calcium (Ca2+) channels in the immature brain.[9] When these channels are activated, Ca^{2+} rushes into the postsynaptic cell causing membrane phospholipases to be activated and oxygen free radical production that damage the cell membrane.[9] Additionally, mitochondrial damage can follow and cause a greater depletion of ATP production.[9] The overall result of this reduction in energy is rapid cell death from necrosis.[9] If ATP is not depleted to as severe of a degree, there is a chance that the neurons may survive.[9] However, this is short lived as it is followed by apoptosis, which is a major component of injury in the premature brain.[9] The previously stated phenomena[9] conveys the 3 characteristics seen in infants with HII[9]: the areas of the brain most likely to be damaged from excitotoxic injury from hypoxia-ischemia are those with the highest concentration of excitatory amino acids, the most energy demanding locations of the brain will lose ATP the fastest resulting in earlier injury due to loss of energy, and finally, injury can show up days after the initial insult due to the delay of apoptosis.[9] HII varies between term and preterm neonates, as the maturity of the brain is different and this is a major determining factor of areas that are most susceptible to hypoxic injury.[9] Therefore, the imaging of HII will not be the same for these 2 different neonatal age groups, and this emphasizes why it is important to keep the 3 key characteristics of HII in mind when analyzing imaging.[9]

In term infants, severe asphyxia and partial asphyxia have different pathophysiologic processes, which result in different imaging findings, as well as outcomes. In severe asphyxia events, the deep gray matter is the primary target of injury.[9] This includes the putamina, ventrolateral thalami, hippocampi, dorsal brainstem, and lateral geniculate nuclei.[9] Additionally, the periolandic cortex can be affected.[9] These structures are the most vulnerable due to the active myelination that occurs, in addition to the high NMDA receptor concentrations.[9] In instances that the asphyxia is chronic, the injury can spread beyond these areas to the cortex, which is correlated with a worsened neurologic outcome.[9] Both cranial US and MR imaging are used to visualize HII. When the possibility of HII is being considered, transcranial US is the first study to be performed.[9] Although US can detect abnormalities, within the first week of life it only has a sensitivity of ∼50% for detecting abnormalities for HII.[9] After the 7 day mark, the sensitivity begins to rise.[9] When performing cranial US for HII suspicion, there are several early findings to look for. The first of these includes a global increase in cerebral echogenicity and obliteration of the cerebrospinal fluid (CSF)-containing spaces, which suggests diffuse cerebral edema.[9] There will also be increased echogenicity in the basal ganglia, thalami, and brainstem, and this is especially apparent after the 7 day mark.[9] If a thalamic echogenicity is found, it is suggestive of a more severe injury, which indicates a worse outcome.[9] Findings found on later studies can include prominence of the ventricles and extra-axial CSF-containing spaces, which is likely due to atrophy.[9] As the sensitivity is low, a cranial US study that is interpreted as negative should not be used to rule out HII.[9] MR imaging may be used to identify injury and determine the severity of it.[9] To obtain the most sensitive images within the first 24 hours, diffusion-weighted imaging should be used as conventional T1- and T2-weighted images can be seemingly normal.[9] On these images, there will be increased signal intensity of the ventrolateral thalami and basal ganglia in the periolandic regions, as well as the corticospinal tracts.[9] (**Fig. 7**) Despite this benefit of diffusion-weighted MR imaging, there are also drawbacks. When injury is detected via this modality, the extent is often underestimated due to the role of apoptosis in HII.[9] Additionally, there is the possibility of normal findings being reported.[9] When using diffusion-weighted imaging, it is important to remember that abnormalities are seen best when they peak at three to 5 days before they begin to pseudonormalize.[8,9] Once they pseudonormalize, the images will seem to be normal, but this does not mean there was any resolution of the HII.[8,9] Although it is unclear why, after pseudonormalization occurs around the 1 week mark, T1- and T2-weighted images begin to hold the most diagnostic value as they display hyperintensity in injured areas, as well as changes in the intensity of signal in both the dorsal brainstem and hippocampi.[9] Both T1 and T2 shortening are observed in imaging.[9] T2 is expected to be seen by week two after insult in the thalami and posterior putamina, while T1 will be seen in the thalami, basal ganglia, and periolandic cortex and has the potential to persist for much longer.[9] T1 shortening has several potential causes including calcification, lipid release from myelin breakdown, and free radical paramagnetic effects.[9] In T2 weighted images, it is difficult to appreciate signal intensity changes before the 7 to 10 day time period, which may be attributed to the high water content of the neonatal brain.[9] However, when there is chronic injury, T2 hyperintensity can be appreciated along with atrophy of the structures affected.[9]

Term neonates with partial HII do not follow the same pattern of injury.[9] The autoregulatory mechanisms present provide blood flow to the vital brain structures, such as the brainstem, cerebellum, and deep gray matter structures, during mild-moderate hypoxic ischemic insults.[9] In fact, if these insults are of short duration, there is usually not any injury to the brain.[9] Once these start to become prolonged, the intervascular boundary, also known as watershed, zones begin to become hypoperfused due to the shunting of blood to the vital structures mentioned above.[9] When detecting injuries in these zones, CUS has minimal use due to their area in relation to the calvaria.[9] Therefore, for partial asphyxia HII, MR imaging has the superior detection capability.[9] Similarly to profound HII, diffusion-weighted imaging is able to detect change within the

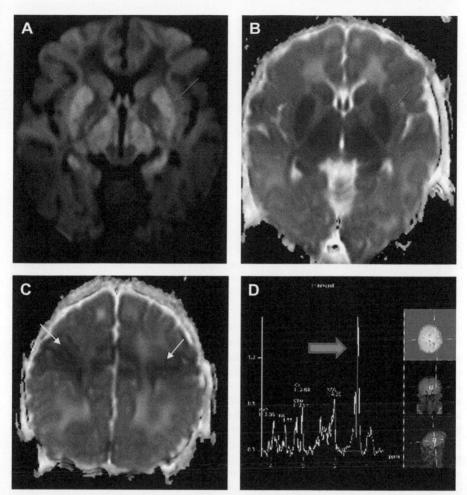

Fig. 7. Severe neonatal HII in a 3-day-old term infant. Diffusion weighted (*A*) and ADC (*B*) MR images show symmetric restricted diffusion in the deep gray matter nuclei (*pink arrows*) and perirolandic cortex (*yellow arrows*) (*C*). MRI spectroscopy demonstrates decreased NAA and a prominent lactate peak (*blue arrow*) (*D*), also supportive of the diagnosis of HIE.

first 24 hours after injury.[9] However, the abnormalities in these images can be extremely hard to see.[9] Most of the neonatal brain is unmyelinated, which causes high T2 values that essentially cover-up the areas of restricted diffusion.[9] With this in mind, diffusion-weighted images should be compared with the corresponding ADC maps or calculated ADC values.[9] T1- and T2-weighted images will not demonstrate changes until the second day after injury and will often display cortical swelling with loss of differentiation between gray and white matter, as well as hyperintensity in the cortex and subcortical white matter.[9] This will be predominantly seen in the parasagittal watershed zones.[9] In instances whereby HII persists and becomes chronic, these images will begin to show atrophy with cortical thinning, in addition to diminished white matter volume.[9] (**Fig. 8**).

Preterm neonates have a higher chance of being exposed to events that result in hypoperfusion, which results in HII being more common in preterm than term

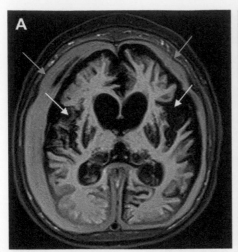
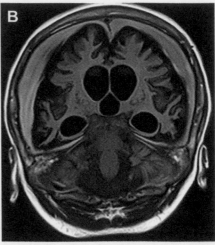

Fig. 8. Hypoxic-ischemic injury-sequela. Diffuse hypoxic damage to GM or WM may lead to severe cortical atrophy (*yellow arrows*) with large extra-axial collections (*pink arrows*) (*A, B*) or may cause postanoxic Leukoencephalopathy depending on the primary site of damage.

neonates.[9] In addition to these events, the preterm brain lacks the autoregulatory mechanisms that have developed in the term brain, so blood is not shunted to vital areas of the brain in instances of hypoperfusion as they are in term neonates.[9] Furthermore, HII can be extremely difficult to diagnose clinically, which is why imaging is crucial for the diagnosis of HII in preterm infants.[9] The pattern observed, however, varies from that seen in term neonates.[9] When preterm neonates undergo profound hypoxic-ischemic events, the damage is seen primarily in the deep gray matter structures and brainstem, while those that are more mild typically manifest as GM-IVH or PVL.[9] Although the pattern seen for severe asphyxia has similarities to that for profound HII in term neonates, there are key differences, as well.[9] In these patients, the structures involved in injury are most frequently the thalami, anterior vermis, and the dorsal brainstem, as these are the areas in which metabolic activity is the highest due to increased myelination taking place, which ultimately makes them more susceptible to oxygen deprivation.[9] The basal ganglia is less likely to be involved in the preterm brain due to its late myelination.[9] In instances that is involved in injury, it typically cavitates and shrinks without scarring.[9] Cranial US will start to show increased echogenicity in the thalami by 48 to 72 hours after insult.[9] However, in the first 2 days, it can seem normal.[9] Following cranial US, MR should be performed when HII is suspected in preterm neonates.[9] While the abnormalities seen on diffusion-weighted imaging will be seen best at 3 to 5 days, they will again start to become noticeable in the thalami in the first 24 hours following injury.[9] Similarly to the T1- and T2-weighted imaging performed in term neonates, T2 prolongation is apparent after 2 days in the thalami and basal ganglia, while T1 shortening is not seen until after the third day following injury and commonly continues into the chronic stages of injury.[9]

When premature infants endure WMI, it is referred to a PVL.[9] This common injury may be associated with the vulnerability of the oligodendrocyte lineage, especially to hypoxic-ischemia changes.[9] Compared with their mature counterparts, pre-OLs are much more vulnerable to both oxidative and excitotoxic injuries, which result from hypoxia, and it is these cells that are primarily populating the cerebral white matter before myelination onset.[9] This is why this is the period of highest risk of PVL for premature infants.[9] Aside from the pre-OLs, the cells that aid in normal fetal thalamo-cortical development, subplate neurons, may also have a part in PVL development.[9] The most common areas of PVL are seen adjacent to trigones of lateral ventricles and adjacent to the foramina of Monro, which is why motor and visual impairment are both the most common consequences of WMI in premature infants, as both these pathways travel through the injured area.[9] On cranial US, PVL is described in 4 stages.[9] Congestion is seen first as globular areas of increased echogenicity in the periventricular regions, and it can be observed within the first 48 hours.[9] However, this finding is neither sensitive nor predictive.[9] A transient period of normalization then occurs by the second to fourth week of life.[9] At 3 to 6 weeks of life, periventricular cysts develop.[9] The final stage occurs by 6 months of age, which is characterized by the resolution of the cysts and ventricular enlargement.[9] CUS is extremely useful in detecting cystic changes of PVL later in perinatal life, and is considered better when performed over the first 6 weeks of life to detect subsequent cystic changes.[9] Although CUS has its benefits, MR imaging is better at visualizing periventricular WMA and is also able to detect them at an earlier stage.[9] MR is considered especially useful when the neonate has noncystic areas of echogenicity on US.[8] On MR, the WMI will primarily be detected as periventricular foci of T1 shortening within larger areas of T2 prolongation, which can typically be detected by 3 to 4 days.[9] T2 weighted images will display abnormal periventricular white matter hyperintensity, especially in the per-trigonal regions.[9] (Figs. 9 and 10) Furthermore, hemorrhage is present in 64% of PVL cases, and it will have a much lower signal intensity on T2 images.[9] It is likely that the MR imaging abnormalities described above can be attributed to reactive astriogliosis.[9] Although head CT has the ability of confirming findings of end-stage PVL later in life, it should be avoided due to the ionizing radiation that the neonates would have to be exposed to.[9] Both MR and CT have a distinct end-stage PVL appearance of reduction in the volume of periventricular white matter and centra semiovale, ventriculomegaly with the dilation of the trigones, and an irregular ventricular outline.[9]

The very low birth weight (VLBW) infant, an infant 1500 g or less, is a progressively increasing population with roughly 63,000 infants falling into this category every

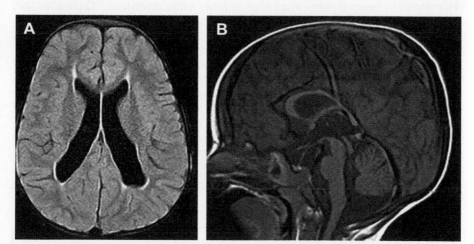

Fig. 9. Periventricular leukomalacia (PVL). Axial FLAIR (*A*) and sagittal T1 Wis (*B*) show classic features of PVL with gliosis and significant volume loss of the periventricular white matter with associated thinning of the corpus callosum and ex vacuo enlargement of the lateral ventricles as noted.

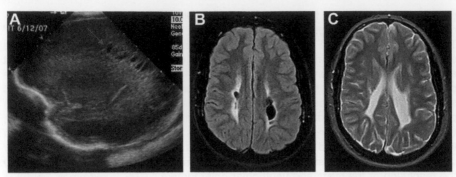

Fig. 10. Cystic periventricular leukomalacia. Sagittal image (*A*) of cranial US shows cystic PVL (pink arrow) along the periventricular white matter adjacent to the left lateral ventricle. Axial FLAIR (*B*) and T2 (*C*) WI show periventricular white matter volume loss with cystic white matter changes and gliosis. There is moderate paucity of white matter.

year.[6,10] These infants have an increased risk for both GM and IVH, in addition to ischemic WMI.[6] MRI imaging has shown the cerebral cortex to specifically be affected in VLBW infants, particularly in the instances in which they suffer from PVL, as well.[10] Other structures that seem to have abnormalities include the cerebellum.[10] In fact, it has been shown that 25% to 30% of VLBW infants suffer neuronal loss in both the dentate nucleus and the cerebellar cortex,[10] while 15% to 20% endured loss in the cerebellar relay nuclei, the basis pontis, and the inferior olive.[10] In addition to the increased risk for injury, they are also more likely to suffer from cognitive deficits.[10] When evaluating these infants for injury, it has been shown that CUS is the best modality for WM injury, particularly cystic lesions as it has a 75% sensitivity and a 100% specificity.[2]

Clinical Outcomes of Preterm Cerebral White Matter Injury

The neurodevelopmental outcomes that result from WMI include both motor and cognitive outcomes.[1] Abnormalities in the white matter due to injury have been shown to be related to cerebral palsy, in addition to other motor disabilities.[1] Qualitative MRI can be used to determine the prognostic likelihood of developing either of these outcomes. Cognitively, general intellectual ability, language development, executive functioning, and behavior were all affected based on the severity of injury.[1]

One of the largest predictors of clinical outcome in infants with IVH is the degree of PVL, if present.[3] When infants undergo preterm WMI, the treatment typically consists of supportive care as there is not much that can be conducted to prevent an injury that is occurring.[9] In the instances when treatment is administered, the early detection of WMI is emphasized as there is a very narrow window in which treatment can be effective.[9] Different treatment options include hypothermia and administration of excitatory amino acid antagonists, as they can potentially reduce the extent of lesions in the thalamus and basal ganglia.[8,9]

CLINICS CARE POINTS

- Neonatal brain injury is a crucial predictor for mortality and morbidity in premature and low birth weight (<1,500 g) infants. Neuroimaging plays a key role in detecting and assessing these neurologic injuries.

REFERENCES

1. Hinojosa-Rodríguez M, Harmony T, Carrillo-Prado C, et al. Clinical neuroimaging in the preterm infant: diagnosis and prognosis. Neuroimage Clin 2017;16:355–68.
2. Ibrahim J, Mir I, Chalak L. Brain imaging in preterm infants <32 weeks gestation: a clinical review and algorithm for the use of cranial ultrasound and qualitative brain MRI. Pediatr Res 2018;84(6):799–806.
3. Bloch JR. Antenatal events causing neonatal brain injury in premature infants. J Obstet Gynecol Neonatal Nurs 2005;34(3):358–66.
4. Volpe JJ. Dysmaturation of premature brain: importance, cellular mechanisms, and potential interventions. Pediatr Neurol 2019;95:42–66.
5. Maller VV, Cohen HL. Neurosonography: assessing the premature infant. Pediatr Radiol 2017;47(9):1031–45.
6. Hand IL, Shellhaas RA, Milla SS, Committee on fetus and newborn secon, S. E. C.TION on radiology. Routine neuroimaging of the preterm brain. Pediatrics 2020;146(5). e2020029082.
7. Hintz SR, Barnes PD, Bulas D, et al. Neuroimaging and neurodevelopmental outcome in extremely preterm infants. Pediatrics 2015;135(1):e32–42.
8. Shroff MM, Soares-Fernandes JP, Whyte H, et al. MR imaging for diagnostic evaluation of encephalopathy in the newborn. Radiographics 2010;30(3):763–80.
9. Huang BY, Castillo M. Hypoxic-ischemic brain injury: imaging findings from birth to adulthood. Radiographics 2008;28(2):417–39 [quiz: 617].
10. Volpe JJ. Brain injury in premature infants: a complex amalgam of destructive and developmental disturbances. Lancet Neurol 2009;8(1):110–24.

Imaging of Inherited Metabolic and Endocrine Disorders

Anna V. Trofimova, MD, PhD[a,b],*, Kartik M. Reddy, MD[a,b]

KEYWORDS

- Metabolic • Neurometabolic • Devastating • Encephalopathy
- Leukoencephalopathy • Endocrine • Newborn • Fetus

KEY POINTS

- Inherited metabolic disorders represent a large, heterogeneous and growing group of disorders, of which approximately 25% have neonatal onset.
- Neuroimaging findings are often nonspecific and overlap with other types of brain injury, such as hypoxic ischemic injury and infection, and need to be interpreted in conjunction with clinical, biochemical, and genetic information.
- Goals of imaging are multifold and include identification and characterization of the pattern of brain injury, suggesting a possibility of an inherited error of metabolism as a causative cause, differential diagnosis with other types of brain injury, identification of life-threatening complications, and treatment monitoring.
- Several metabolic disorders have characteristic neuroimaging findings that allow for narrowing of the differential diagnosis or to even suggest a specific diagnosis. Radiologists play a pivotal role in early diagnosis of this group of metabolic disorders, facilitating timely initiation of therapy to prevent severe brain damage and neurologic sequelae in affected neonates.

INTRODUCTION/HISTORY/DEFINITIONS/BACKGROUND

Inherited metabolic disorders represent a large, heterogeneous and growing group of inborn errors of metabolism,[1–8] which due to the rarity of individual disorders, often nonspecific clinical and imaging features as well as gravity of the clinical course, pose a difficult diagnostic challenge to clinicians and radiologists alike.[3,5] Approximately 25% of inborn error of metabolism have neonatal presentation.[5,9–12] Clinical presentation of inherited metabolic disorders in the neonatal period signifies the

---

[a] Children's Healthcare of Atlanta, Radiology Department, 1405 Clifton Road NE, Atlanta, GA 30322, USA; [b] Emory University, Department of Radiology and Imaging Sciences, 1364 Clifton Road NE, Atlanta, GA, 30322, USA
* Corresponding author.
E-mail address: atrofim@emory.edu
Twitter: @DrTrofimova (A.V.T.)

Clin Perinatol 49 (2022) 657–673
https://doi.org/10.1016/j.clp.2022.05.004
0095-5108/22/© 2022 Elsevier Inc. All rights reserved.
perinatology.theclinics.com

profound severity of the metabolic abnormality compared with cases presenting later in infancy and childhood[2,4,13,14] and necessitates rapid diagnosis and urgent therapeutic measures in an attempt to decrease the extent of brain injury and prevent grave neurologic sequela or even death.[9,15] Revolutionary achievements in molecular diagnosis with advancements in genomics, metabolomics, and transcriptomics,[3,16,17] have resulted in an increased ability to detect impairment of specific enzymes or biochemical pathways.[3] Despite these advances, in approximately 40% to 50% of cases a specific diagnosis is never established. Neuroimaging plays pivotal role in diagnosis, treatment, and prognostication of this group of disorders in neonates.[3] The goals of imaging are multifold and include characterization of the imaging patterns of brain injury, establishing differential diagnoses including more common neonatal pathologies such as hypoxic-ischemic brain injury or infection; alerting clinical providers to a possibility of inherited error of metabolism as a causative cause; potential narrowing of the biochemical and genetic workup by suggesting a specific diagnosis or a group of potential diagnoses; identification of life-threatening complications such as brain edema, intracranial hemorrhage, and herniation; and treatment response monitoring.[2,3]

Clinical Presentation

Clinical presentation of neurometabolic disorders in neonates is variable and broadly can be divided into 2 groups[13]:

- Type 1 presentation: affected neonates are healthy at birth and develop clinical deterioration after a short symptom-free interval.[2,13] In this group of inherited metabolic disorders, the placental circulation functions as a protective buffer allowing for elimination of endogenous toxic substances accumulating as a result of an inherited error of metabolism or by providing supply of biochemical substances that are missing due to a biochemical pathway abnormality.[2,13,18] However, within a few days after birth, the underlying metabolic disturbances start to manifest as acute encephalopathy and rapidly developing profound metabolic decompensation. Clinically, affected neonates refuse to feed, develop vomiting, followed by lethargy and coma.[2,13] Examples of metabolic disorders with type 1 presentation include maple syrup urine disorder (MSUD) and urea cycle disorders.[13]
- Type 2 presentation: affected neonates are profoundly symptomatic at birth with acute encephalopathy, seizures, hypotonia, and apnea.[13] Symptom-free interval is absent. Examples of metabolic disorders in these groups are nonketotic hyperglycinemia (NKH) and molybdenum cofactor deficiency among others.[13]

Seizures are a common but nonspecific complication of metabolic disorders, signifying involvement of the cerebral cortex.[4] Muscle tone changes are often present, for example, hypertonia seen in Krabbe disease and alternating muscle tonus in MSUD.[2] If not treated promptly, progressively worsening toxicity leads to irreversible brain damage or death. Some inherited metabolic disorders have unique clinical features that can be helpful in narrowing the differential diagnosis. For example, several metabolic disorders are known to have abnormal body odors, such as "burnt sugar" or "maple syrup" odor in MSUD, "sweaty feet" in glutaric aciduria type II and isovaleric acidemia, "cat urine" in 3-hydroxy-3-methylglutaric aciduria, and multiple carboxylase deficiency.[2] Peroxisomal disorders characteristically present with multiorgan involvement including skeletal dysplasia, cataract and optic nerve atrophy, hepatosplenomegaly, and cardiomyopathy.[13] Multiple inherited disorders of metabolism have associated malformations of central nervous system, for example, Zellweger syndrome (cerebellar dysgenesis, corpus callosum abnormalities, dentate nuclei, and inferior olivary nucleus abnormalities) and glutaric acidemia type 2 (posterior fossa abnormalities, cerebral dysgenesis, corpus callosum abnormalities, gray matter heterotopia, pachygyria).[2,3,15,18]

Imaging Techniques Considerations in Diagnosis of Inherited Metabolic and Endocrine Disorders

Ultrasound (US) is commonly used during the neonatal period as an initial screening tool.[2,14] US findings are nonspecific and may include echogenic white matter, ventriculomegaly, lenticulostriate vasculopathy, germinolytic cysts, calcifications, as well as cortical or corpus callosum abnormalities.[14,19] CT has limited role as well due to its low contrast resolution and associated radiation exposure.[2] CT is often used for expedited evaluation in a critically ill patient to evaluate for life-threatening hemorrhage or intracranial mass effect. MRI is the modality of choice for evaluating neurometabolic brain injuries.[2] However, structural MRI findings are often nonspecific and overlap with other causes. Advanced imaging modalities, including diffusion-weighted images (DWI) and MR spectroscopy (MRS), represent an important adjunct to structural MRI brain protocols in evaluation of inherited metabolic disorders in neonates,[2,5,18] providing additional diagnostic information and allowing to narrow the differential diagnosis or in rare cases even suggest a specific diagnosis, for example, by identifying an abnormal glycine peak at 3.56 ppm in NKH or by demonstrating an abnormal branched chain amino acids peak at 0.9 ppm in MSUD.[2]

Classification

Currently, no single unifying classification of inherited metabolic disorders exists.[4,6,8] Multiple different approaches have been described in an attempt to classify inherited errors of metabolism including clinical, pathophysiological, and imaging pattern recognition approach, pioneered by van der Knaap and Valk and Barkovich.[3,4,20,21] For the purpose of this discussion the authors will be using classification scheme initially proposed by Saudubray and colleagues[11] and further built on by Labarthe and colleagues[22] and Poretti and colleagues,[9,13] which categorizes inherited metabolic disorders with neonatal onset into 4 major groups: (1) disorders of intoxication, (2) disorders of energy production, (3) disorders of biosynthesis and catabolism of complex molecules, and (4) neurotransmitter disorders.[3,9,13]

Disorders of Intoxication

The unifying pathophysiologic characteristic of the disorders of intoxication is accumulation of toxic to the brain metabolites proximal to the biochemical pathway interruption.[5] This group includes organic acid and amino acid metabolism disorders.[2,5] Classically, disorders of intoxication do not interfere with embryo and fetal development and present in the neonatal period after a symptom-free period of a variable duration.[6,18] Overall, imaging findings are nonspecific; however, several disorders demonstrate distinct imaging characteristic allowing for more specific differential diagnosis.

MAPLE SYRUP URINE DISEASE

In MSUD, the genetic defect affects the catalytic proteins of the branched-chain alpha-ketoacid dehydrogenase complex, leading to impaired oxidative decarboxylation of the branched-chain amino acids leucine, isoleucine, and valine.[2,4,23,24] MSUD can be identified at newborn screening, which facilitates timely initiation of therapy. Treatment requires dietary restriction of branched-chain amino acids to avoid brain injury; however, commonly, children develop metabolic decompensations in the setting of nonspecific illnesses.[4] Several clinical phenotypes have been described, which correlate with the severity of the enzyme deficiency.[4,24]

In classic type, MSUD manifests in the neonatal period typically with poor feeding, dystonia, and/or seizures. Prompt diagnosis and onset of therapy with dietary restriction is crucial to avoid rapid progression to coma and death and to prevent a potentially grave neurologic prognosis.

Imaging plays an important role in timely diagnosis, as imaging findings can be quite characteristic. In particular, MSUD preferentially involves myelinating and myelinated white matter with development of intramyelinic edema, resulting in low density on CT, as well as T1 hypointense and T2 hyperintense signal on brain MRI. Corresponding to the myelination pattern in a neonatal brain, the following brain structures are characteristically involved: deep cerebellar white matter and corticospinal tracts from the brainstem to perirolandic white matter including the dorsal pons, cerebral peduncles, posterior limb of the internal capsule, and posterior centrum semiovale; thalami and globi pallidi can also be affected. In the brainstem, a characteristic "4 dots" imaging appearance have been described with 2 ventrally located "dots" representing involvement of the corticospinal tracts and 2 dorsally located "dots" representing affected central tegmental tracts.[3] Diffusion imaging is particularly helpful, as areas of intramyelinic edema show reduced diffusivity with low apparent diffusion coefficient (ADC) values consistent with reduced diffusivity, whereas vasogenic edema affecting nonmyelinated white matter manifests as increased ADC values (increased diffusivity). Diffusion abnormalities mostly resolve after the acute toxic phase of the disease with varying degrees of residual brain damage. Relapses occurring later during infancy or early childhood typically demonstrate imaging pattern reflective of child's current state of myelination. MR spectroscopy can demonstrate a characteristic broad peak at 0.9 ppm, thought to be reflective of accumulating branched-chain amino acids and branched-chain alpha ketoacids and seen on both short and long echo spectra; this finding is considered more specific for pathology when seen on long echo time (TE) spectra[3,4,24,25]; **Figs. 1, 2, and 3** illustrate cases of neonatal onset of MSUD.

Disorders of the Urea Cycle and Ammonia

Urea cycle disorders represent a subgroup of amino acid metabolism disorders that is characterized by impaired ability to remove the excess of nitrogen in the body[2,26] and include ornithine transcarbamylase deficiency (**Fig. 4**), carbonic anhydrase VA deficiency (**Fig. 5**), carbamoyl phosphate synthetase deficiency, argininosuccinic aciduria, citrullinemia, and hyperargininemia.[4] As a result of the metabolic defect, accumulating ammonia freely crosses the blood-brain barrier and promotes synthesis of glutamate, which in turn hypothesized to cause astrocytic swelling and brain edema.[2] Similar to other inherited metabolic disorders, neonatal presentation is seen in cases with the most severe metabolic abnormality.[26] Overall, imaging patterns of brain injury are similar for all disorders in this group. Characteristically in neonates, the insular cortex is affected earliest in the course of the disease, followed by perirolandic cortex and basal ganglia, in particular globi pallidi.[26] Predominant involvement of the basal ganglia helps to differentiate the pattern of injury from that seen in hypoxic-ischemic encephalopathy where predominant thalamic involvement is seen. Affected brain regions will demonstrate T2 and variable T1 hypointense as well as later in the course T1 hyperintense signal. The pattern of brain edema in older children is slightly different, with preferential involvement of the insula, however, with sparing of the perirolandic and occipital cortices. MR spectroscopy findings are

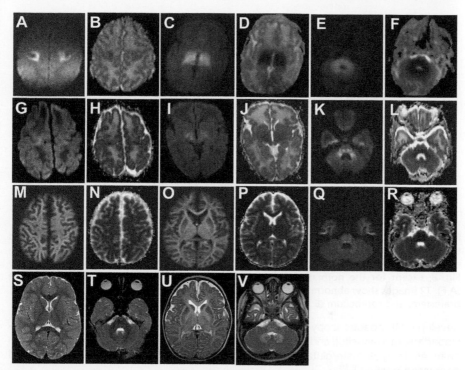

Fig. 1. Multiple MRIs of a man with maple syrup urine disease, obtained on DOL 12 (*A–F*) and at ages 1 month (*G–L*) and 18 months (*M–R, U, V*). MRI on DOL 12 shows robust diffusion restriction in the sensorimotor tracts (*A, B*), basal ganglia and thalami (*C, D*), and brainstem and cerebellum (*E, F*). Follow-up at 1 month of age shows persistent but decreased diffusion restriction in the same structures likely due to improvement in intramyelinic edema after initiation of therapy with dietary restrictions (*G–L*). DWI, ADC, and T2 images at 18 months during an acute exacerbation with metabolic acidosis show diffuse white matter diffusion restriction (*M–P*) and T2 hyperintense signal involving cerebral white matter, thalami, globi pallidi, dorsal putamen (*U*), brainstem, and cerebellar dentate nuclei (*V*). Normal pattern of white matter myelination in a neurologically normal 18 month old is shown for comparison (*S, T*). MSUD preferentially affects myelinated/myelinating tissue; thus the interval maturation of myelination in this child over 18 months has influenced the pattern of signal abnormality thought to represent intramyelinic edema.

nonspecific and demonstrate decreased N-acetylaspartate, elevation of lactate as well as a broad peak of glutamine and glutamate at 2.1 to 2.4 ppm as well as 3.75 ppm.[2,4]

Propionic Acidemia

Propionic acidemia (PA) is an autosomal recessive disorder characterized by a deficiency of propionyl coenzyme A carboxylase, which results in ketoacidosis, hypoglycemia, and hyperammonemia.[2,4,9] In neonatal onset PPA, main imaging finding is diffuse brain swelling.[14] Pathologically, white matter spongiosis has been demonstrated in PA.[9] Areas more commonly involved include midbrain, dentate nuclei, and cerebral cortex. Involvement of the basal ganglia in neonatal period is variable and may be absent.[9] With disease progression, atrophy and delayed myelination

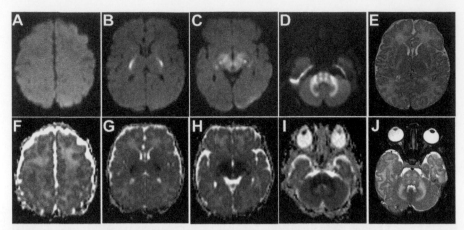

Fig. 2. MRI of a man with MSUD on DOL 19. DWI and ADC maps show diffusion restriction in the internal capsule posterior limbs (B,G), globi pallidi (C,H), brainstem (C,D,H,I), and dentate nuclei (D,I); the pattern of findings are nearly identical to that shown in case from **Fig. 8**, except for the normal appearance of the upper sensorimotor tracts in this case (A,F). T2 images show abnormal hyperintense signal in the internal capsule posterior limbs, brainstem, and cerebellum (E,J).

develops. MR spectroscopy findings are nonspecific as well with decreased N-acetylaspartate, myo-inositol, and increased lactate during acute metabolic crisis.[2] Variable changes in glutamate/glutamine have been reported with both increased and decreased peaks.[2,9,18]

Methylmalonic Acidemia

Methylmalonic acidemia (MMA) is an autosomal recessive disorder characterized by a deficiency of methylmalonyl coenzyme A mutase, which through inhibition of multiple metabolic pathways, results in ketoacidosis, hyperammonemia, and hyperglycinemia.[2,27] In the neonatal period imaging findings are nonspecific and in acute phase may include brain edema with T2 hyperintense signal primarily involving nonmyelinated white matter.[28] Involvement of the central tegmental tracks in the brainstem has been described in MMA with characteristic appearance of 2 "dots," which might be helpful in attempt to differentiate from brainstem involvement in MSUD, which has "4 dots" appearance.[3] With time, diffuse parenchymal brain atrophy develops. Symmetric involvement of globi pallidi has been also described in late-onset MMA.[3]

Disorders of Energy Metabolism

This heterogeneous group includes primary lactic acidosis, fatty acid oxidation disorders, sulfite oxidase deficiency, and molybdenum cofactor deficiency. Primary lactic acidosis in turn includes pyruvate dehydrogenase deficiency (PDH), pyruvate carboxylase deficiency, and mitochondrial respiratory chain defects (cytochrome oxidase deficiency, complex succinate dehydrogenase [type II] deficiency)[23]; **Figs. 6–8** illustrate neuroimaging findings in mitochondriopathies with neonatal presentation. Clinical symptoms are mutisystemic and primarily affect highly metabolically structures, including heart and brain. Central nervous system involvement can clinically and radiologically mimic moderate to severe hypoxic ischemic injury[3,5] (**Fig. 9**). Disproportionate lactic acidosis is a characteristic and mandatory for diagnosis[9] clinical laboratory marker of disorders of energy metabolism. Imaging findings at early stage are absent or, when present, are nonspecific and primarily include diffuse brain edema

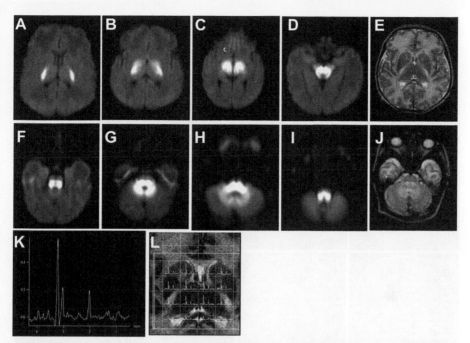

Fig. 3. MRI of a 2-week-old mane with MSUD. DWI at multiple levels show a similar pattern of diffusion restriction (A–D, F) to MSUD cases from **Figs. 8** and **9**. Abnormal T2 hyperintense signal in the internal capsule posterior limbs (E), brainstem, cerebellar dentate nuclei, and peridentate white matter (J). Single-voxel long TE MRS reveals abnormal peaks corresponding to branched chain amino acids and ketoacids at 0.9 ppm and lactate at 1.3 ppm (K). Multivoxel MRS, a technique used to evaluate multiple regions of the brain concurrently, shows small BCAA/BCKA and lactate peaks at several voxels including the basal ganglia and thalami (L). This case shows how MRS can be a useful tool to narrow the differential diagnosis and potentially expedite life- and brain-saving therapy. (*Courtesy of* Dr Goldman-Yassen, Atlanta, Georgia and Children's Hospital of Philadelphia.)

with predominant involvement of nonmyelinated white matter as well as basal ganglia, periaqueductal areas, and cerebellar peduncles.[2] MR spectroscopy demonstrates a lactate peak at 1.3 ppm; however, it is important to note that it is not specific for primary lactic acidosis and can be present in other metabolic disorders. Absence of the lactate peak does not exclude the disease as well.[2,3] Pyruvate dehydrogenase complex deficiency (PDHc) is an important cause of primary lactic acidosis. Cerebral dysgenesis is commonly seen in affected neonates with a large spectrum of developmental abnormalities including corpus callosum dysgenesis, subcortical heterotopia, and pachygyria. It is hypothesized that cerebral dysgenesis may be related to the critical role of PDHc in energy metabolism of proliferating and migrating neurons.[9] In addition, periventricular leukomalacia and germinolytic cysts are seen in cases of prenatal onset of PDHc deficiency.

Disorders of Biosynthesis and Catabolism of Complex Molecules

This group of disorders consists of peroxisomal and lysosomal disorders including Zellweger syndrome, neonatal adrenoleukodystrophy, peroxisomal bifunctional deficiency as well as Krabbe disease, among others.[3,9] Peroxisomal function is critical

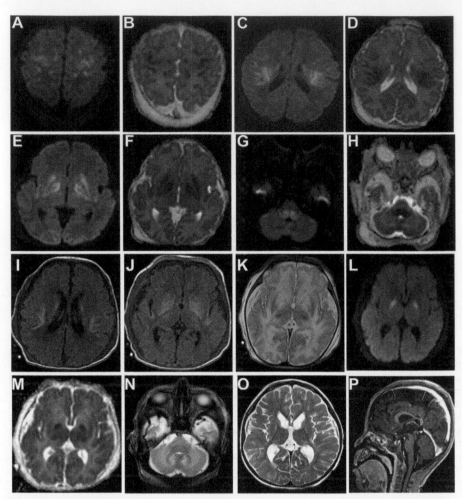

Fig. 4. Multiple MRIs of a man with ornithine transcarbamylase deficiency performed on DOL 6 (*A–H*), DOL 12 (*I–N*), and at 2 years of age (*O, P*). DWI and ADC maps show restricted diffusion in the sensorimotor and adjacent cortex (*A, B*), opercula (*C, D*), lentiform nuclei, internal capsules (*E, F*), and dorsal brainstem (*G, H*). MRI on DOL 12 shows abnormal T1 hyperintense signal in the basal ganglia and insula, a pattern commonly seen after hyper-ammonemic brain injuries (*I, J*). Injuries to the caudate nuclei and putamen are shown on T2 (*K*). DWI and ADC show persistent diffusion restriction in the globi pallidi and resolution elsewhere (*L, M*). T2 of the posterior fossa shows dorsal brainstem and dentate nuclei signal abnormality (*N*). Follow-up imaging performed at 2 years of age shows diffuse volume loss with white matter and deep nuclei shrinkage and ex-vacuo dilation of the ventricles (*O*). Enhanced sagittal T1 shows relative preservation of the supratentorial white matter (mild callosal thinning), brainstem, and cerebellar volume as well as an incidental pars intermedia cyst (*P*).

for neuronal migration, organization, and myelin formation[3]; as a result, these disorders commonly manifest prenatally with cerebral dysgenesis and dysmorphic features.[15]

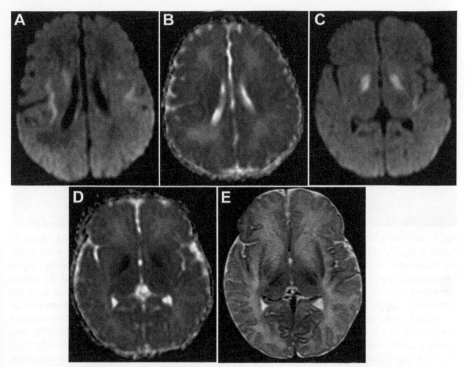

Fig. 5. MRI in a woman with carbonic anhydrase-VA deficiency on DOL 8. DWI and ADC maps show restricted diffusion in the right frontoparietal cortex (*A*, *B*) and bilateral globi pallidi (*C*, *D*). T2-weighted imaging demonstrates abnormal T2 hyperintense signal in the bilateral caudate nuclei, putamen and globi pallidi (*E*). Lack of diffusion restriction in the caudate and putamen suggests that these injuries are older, possibly occurring within the first few days of life.

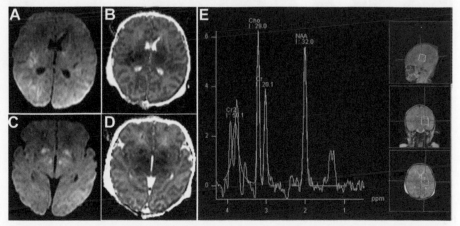

Fig. 6. MRI in a woman with MPV17-related hepatocerebral type mitochondrial DNA depletion syndrome on DOL 9 showing diffusion restriction in the right frontoparietal operculum (*A*, *B*), globi pallidi, internal capsules, and inferomedial thalami (*C*, *D*). Single-voxel long TE MRS shows a lactate doublet peak at 1.3 ppm (*E*). The patient died on DOL 55.

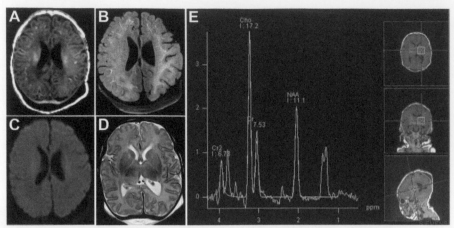

Fig. 7. MRI of a woman with mitochondrial DNA Mt-ATP6 mutation on DOL 11. Axial T1 shows diffusely scattered cortical and subcortical hyperintense foci, compatible with multiple subacute injuries (*A*). Axial FLAIR images show abnormal hyperintense signal throughout the white matter (*B*). DWI was within normal limits (*C*). Axial T2 shows decreased volume of the left thalamus with ex-vacuo dilation of the left lateral ventricle atrium (*D*). Single-voxel long TE spectroscopy at the left basal ganglia demonstrates an elevated lactate doublet peak at 1.3 ppm (*E*). This patient's mitochondrial DNAmutation was considered a variant of uncertain significance; however, a mitochondriopathy was strongly suspected, and the patient died on DOL 12 due to multiorgan failure despite therapy; this highlights the fact that many metabolic derangements are difficult to diagnose, likely in part due to extreme rarity, and in some cases even novelty of a genetic mutation. FLAIR, fluid-attenuated inversion recovery.

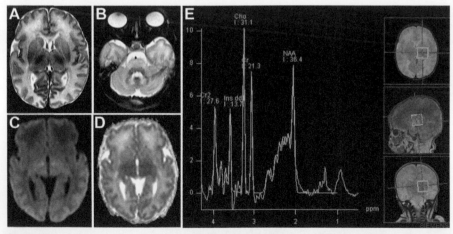

Fig. 8. MRI of a man with mitochondrial disease complex V deficiency on DOL 6. T2 images demonstrate diffusely hyperintense white matter, hyperintense thalami and basal ganglia (*A*), and hyperintense pons (*B*). DWI and ADC show restricted diffusion in the inferomedial thalami at the thalamopeduncular junction (*C*, *D*). Single-voxel long TE MRS demonstrates no definite lactate peak at 1.3 ppm (*E*).

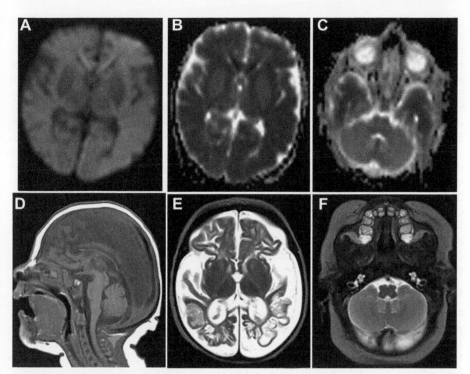

Fig. 9. MRI of a woman with anoxic brain injury on DOL 5 (*A–C*) and on DOL 35 (*D–F*). This case illustrates a differential diagnosis for diffuse, symmetric brain injury in a neonate. DWI and ADC maps on DOL 5 show global diffusion restriction throughout the supratentorial brain, with sparing of the lentiform nuclei, ventral thalami, brainstem, and cerebellum. The pattern of HIE in this neonate differs from that of a neonate with a devastating neurometabolic derangement primarily due to the former's ability to divert blood flow and thus oxygenation to critical brain structures in order to survive. Follow-up MRI on DOL 35 shows diffuse supratentorial volume loss (*E*), relative preservation of basal ganglia and thalami (*E*), and normal appearance of the cerebellum and brainstem (*F*). Sagittal T1 shows diffuse thinning of the corpus callosum (*C*), a common finding seen after diffuse cerebral volume loss. HIE, hypoxic-ischemic encephalopathy.

Zellweger Syndrome

Zellweger syndrome is a prototype of the peroxisomal biogenesis disorders.[15,29] It presents in early neonatal period with a multitude of clinical symptoms including hypotonia, failure to thrive, poor swallowing, irritability, and seizures, among others, due to multiorgan involvement secondary to ubiquitous nature of peroxisomes.[9] Characteristic neuroimaging features include cortical malformations, germinolytic cysts, hypomyelination, and brain atrophy.[29] Cortical malformations include polymicrogyria, pachygyria, and periventricular heterotopia.[2,9] MR spectroscopy shows increased lipid and decreased N-acetylaspartate levels.[2]

Krabbe Disease

Krabbe disease, also known as globoid cell leukodystrophy, is an autosomal recessive lysosomal disorder characterized by a deficiency in galactosylceramide beta-galactosidase, an enzyme involved in myelin turnover and breakdown[4,30]; this results in pathologic accumulation of galactosylsphingosine, which is toxic to neurons, oligodendrocytes, and Schwann cells.[4] Most commonly (90-95%), clinical manifestation is between 3 and 6 months of age, known as an infantile form of the disease.[4] Neonatal (early infantile) form is rare and associated with rapidly progressive clinical course and poor prognosis.[13,31,32] In particular, early in the course of disease CT demonstrates hyperdensity of thalami, caudate nuclei, corona radiata, and cerebellar dentate nuclei.[2,4,13,33] On MRI, hyperintense T1 and hypointense T2 signal can be seen in thalami,[13] with delayed appearance in expected hyperintensity of the internal capsules.[4] Central leukodystrophy with characteristic sparing of the subcortical U-fibers is present.[13] On T2, abnormal hyperintense signal is also seen within the splenium of the corpus callosum, corticospinal tracts, cerebellar white matter, and hila of cerebellar nuclei.[4,13,34] In addition, optic nerves enlargement and contrast enhancement of cranial and spinal nerves can be seen in some patients.[4,13,35–38] MR spectroscopy findings are nonspecific including increased choline, reduced N-acetylaspartate, and a prominent lactate peak.[25] When present, this constellation of imaging findings can be helpful in suggesting possible diagnosis of early infantile form of Krabbe disease.

Neurotransmitter Disorders

Neurotransmitter disorders encompass inherited disorders of neurotransmitter transport or metabolism.[39] Clinical presentation is variable and may include acute encephalopathy, developmental delay or regression, seizures, and movement disorders.[39] Major groups of inherited neurotransmitter disorders include disorders of monoamine biosynthesis, primary cerebral folate deficiency, disorders of pyridoxine and gammaaminobutyric acid metabolism, cerebral creatine deficiency, and disorders of serine biosynthesis.[39] Neurotransmitter disorders with neonatal presentation include nonketotic hyperglycinemia, pyridoxine deficiency, and disorders of biopterin metabolism.[3]

Nonketotic Hyperglycinemia

NKH, also known as glycine encephalopathy, is an autosomal recessive disorder caused by a genetic defect in mitochondrial glycine breakage system. As a result, large quantities of glycine accumulate in body fluids and cerebrospinal fluid (CSF). Up to 70% of cases have classic presentation in early neonatal period. Affected neonates develop myoclonic encephalopathy presenting with lethargy, hypotonia, and myoclonic jerks, which rapidly progress to apnea and even death. Hiccups maybe present. Infants that survive through this acute phase develop seizures and profound developmental delay. The diagnosis is established by an increased plasma glycine as well as an increased CSF glycine to plasma glycine levels.

On MRI, imaging findings in NKH can be similar to those seen in MSUD; however, there are a few additional findings that might assist in differentiating between these 2 causes[3] (**Figs. 10** and **11**). Similar to MSUD, there is involvement of the myelinated white matter in NKH, characterized by abnormal T2 hyperintense signal and restricted diffusion with low ADC values, reflective of vacuolating myelopathy, with involvement of the corticospinal tracts, central tegmental tracts, and internal capsule.[40,41] A distinctive imaging finding in NKH is presence of structural brain abnormalities, of which agenesis or dysgenesis of the corpus callosum being the most common.[40] With time, brain atrophy develops with accompanying increase in ADC, likely reflective of axonal degeneration.

MR spectroscopy plays a critical role in diagnosis, demonstrating a characteristic abnormal glycine peak at 3.56 ppm.[4,14,25] It is important to mention that myo-

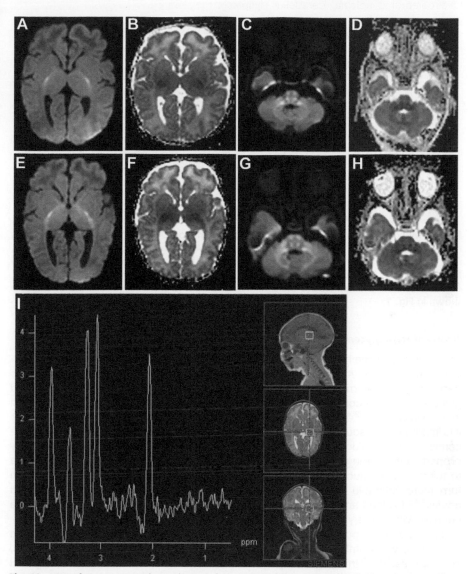

Fig. 10. MRI of a woman with nonketotic hyperglycinemia on DOL 7 (*A–D*) and DOL 23 (*E–I*). DWI and ADC maps show restricted diffusion in the bilateral internal capsule posterior limbs (*A, B*) and in the posterior fossa involving brainstem and cerebellum (*C, D*); these images also demonstrate focal involvement of the corticospinal tracts ventrally and the central tegmental tracts dorsally, the "4 dot sign" (*C, D, G, H*). Images obtained on DOL 23 show a similar pattern of brain injury (*E–H*). Single-voxel long TE spectroscopy at the left thalamus performed on DOL 23 shows a glycine peak at 3.6 ppm, characteristic of nonketotic hyperglycinemia (*I*). The patient died on DOL 33.

inositol has a similar chemical shift to glycine when a short echo time is used. For this reason, it is important to obtain MR spectra with a long echo time when NKH is suspected.[25] In addition to potentially providing a specific diagnosis, MR spectroscopy can also be used for treatment response monitoring in NKH.[14]

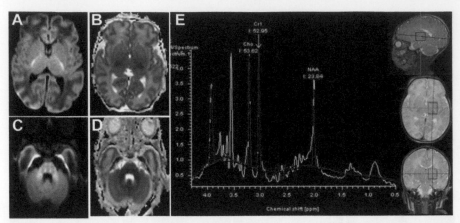

Fig. 11. MRI of a man with nonketotic hyperglycinemia on DOL 7. DWI and ADC map show restricted diffusion in the bilateral internal capsules (*A*, *B*) and cerebellum and brainstem (*C*, *D*). Within the brainstem, focal involvement of the corticospinal tracts and central tegmental tracts is shown (*C*). Single-voxel short TE MRS shows a glycine peak at 3.6 ppm, characteristic of NKH (*E*). Notice the similarity of findings in this case to those of the case shown in **Fig. 1**.

Neonatal Hypoglycemia

Hypoglycemia is the most common[42,43] and likely underrecognized[4] metabolic disturbance in neonates. It is important to note that the definition of hypoglycemia varies depending on the maturational state of a neonate.[4,42] Different suggested blood glucose threshold concentrations exist at which to consider therapeutic intervention in hypoglycemia,[4,42,44,45] review of which is beyond the scope of this article; however it is important to discuss several concepts related to the association between hypoglycemia and brain injury. The ability of a neonate to tolerate hypoglycemia is inversely proportionate to the degree of their maturity, with less mature neonates being able to tolerate lower glucose levels compared with more mature neonates, which are in turn more tolerable to lower glucose levels compared with older children and adults.[4,42] Prolong and severe hypoglycemia is required to result in brain injury in a neonate with primary predilection to parietal and occipital lobes, followed by hippocampi, caudates, putamen, brainstem, and cerebellum.[4] Clinical presentation is nonspecific with dominant features including altered mental status, irritability, tremors, and seizures.[4,42,45] Imaging findings in acute phase include brain edema, in a regional brain pattern described earlier, with the most severe injury to the parietal and occipital lobes.[21] The involved cortex and subjacent white matter demonstrate prolongation of T1 and T2 signal with reduced diffusivity.[4] Shortening of T1/T2 signal can be seen in acute phase in deep gray matter structures,[42] as well as in the cortex in subacute phase.[4] It is important to mention that when coinciding, mild neonatal hypoglycemia and mild hypoxic-ischemic injury tend to result in brain injury, whereas in isolation they do not. In these cases, the pattern of brain injury is similar to normoglycemic perinatal injury with additional involvement of the corticospinal tracts.[4]

SUMMARY

Inherited metabolic and endocrine disorders with neonatal presentation signify profound severity of the underlying metabolic abnormality and grave prognosis. Timely diagnosis and treatment initiation is a paramount prerequisite for successful mitigation of devastating brain injury and potentially improved short- and long-term outcome. Although clinical and imaging findings are commonly nonspecific, in a minority of cases, a specific diagnosis or a group of diagnoses can be suggested based on the constellation of imaging findings. Advanced imaging techniques provide valuable additional diagnostic information and should be routinely used in the diagnostic workup of a suspected inherited metabolic abnormality in a neonate.

Best practices

Major Recommendations:

- A multidisciplinary approach is needed when inherited metabolic disorders are suspected and require interpretation of neuroimaging findings in conjunction with clinical, biochemical and genetic information.

- Neuroimaging should be obtained as soon as possible in the acute phase of the disease as early imaging findings might provide more specific diagnostic information compared to later stages.

- MRI is the modality of choice for evaluation of suspected inherited metabolic disorders, and is superior to US and CT in evaluation of suspected inherited metabolic disorders.

- MRI protocol should include combination of structural images, DWI and MR spectroscopy.

DISCLOSURE

The authors have nothing to disclose.

REFERENCES

1. Tabarki B, Ortigoza-Escobar JD, Lee W-T, et al. Editorial: pediatric neurometabolic disorders. Editorial. Front Neurol 2021;12. https://doi.org/10.3389/fneur.2021.737398.

2. Yoon HJ, Kim JH, Jeon TY, et al. Devastating metabolic brain disorders of newborns and young infants. Radiographics 2014;34(5):1257–72.

3. Biswas A, Malhotra M, Mankad K, et al. Clinico-radiological phenotyping and diagnostic pathways in childhood neurometabolic disorders-a practical introductory guide. Transl Pediatr 2021;10(4):1201–30.

4. James A. Barkovich CR. Pediatric neuroimaging. Sixth edition. Wolters Kluwer: Philadelphia; 2019.

5. Patay Z, Blaser SI, Poretti A, et al. Neurometabolic diseases of childhood. Pediatr Radiol 2015;45(Suppl 3):S473–84.

6. Saudubray JM, Garcia-Cazorla A. Inborn errors of metabolism overview: pathophysiology, manifestations, evaluation, and management. Pediatr Clin North Am 2018;65(2):179–208.

7. Morava E, Rahman S, Peters V, et al. Quo vadis: the re-definition of "inborn metabolic diseases". J Inherit Metab Dis 2015;38(6):1003–6.

8. Saudubray JM, Mochel F, Lamari F, et al. Proposal for a simplified classification of IMD based on a pathophysiological approach: a practical guide for clinicians. J Inherit Metab Dis 2019;42(4):706–27.

9. Poretti A, Blaser SI, Lequin MH, et al. Neonatal neuroimaging findings in inborn errors of metabolism. J Magn Reson Imaging 2013;37(2):294–312.

10. Leonard JV, Morris AA. Diagnosis and early management of inborn errors of metabolism presenting around the time of birth. Acta Paediatr 2006;95(1):6–14.

11. Saudubray JM, Sedel F, Walter JH. Clinical approach to treatable inborn metabolic diseases: an introduction. J Inherit Metab Dis 2006;29(2–3):261–74.

12. El-Hattab AW. Inborn errors of metabolism. Clin Perinatol 2015;42(2):413–39, x.

13. Mankad K, Talenti G, Tan AP, et al. Neurometabolic disorders of the newborn. Top Magn Reson Imaging 2018;27(4):179–96.

14. Reddy N, Calloni SF, Vernon HJ, et al. Neuroimaging findings of organic acidemias and aminoacidopathies. Radiographics 2018;38(3):912–31.

15. Blaser S, Feigenbaum A. A neuroimaging approach to inborn errors of metabolism. Neuroimaging Clin N Am 2004;14(2):307–29, ix.

16. Mordaunt D, Cox D, Fuller M. Metabolomics to improve the diagnostic efficiency of inborn errors of metabolism. Int J Mol Sci 2020;21(4). https://doi.org/10.3390/ijms21041195.

17. Menezes MJ, Riley LG, Christodoulou J. Mitochondrial respiratory chain disorders in childhood: insights into diagnosis and management in the new era of genomic medicine. Biochim Biophys Acta 2014;1840(4):1368–79.

18. Patay Z. MR imaging workup of inborn errors of metabolism of early postnatal onset. Magn Reson Imaging Clin N Am 2011;19(4):733–59, vii.

19. Leijser LM, de Vries LS, Rutherford MA, et al. Cranial ultrasound in metabolic disorders presenting in the neonatal period: characteristic features and comparison with MR imaging. AJNR Am J Neuroradiol 2007;28(7):1223–31.

20. Barkovich AJ. An approach to MRI of metabolic disorders in children. J Neuroradiol 2007;34(2):75–88.

21. Schiffmann R, van der Knaap MS. Invited article: an MRI-based approach to the diagnosis of white matter disorders. Neurology 2009;72(8):750–9.

22. Labarthe F, Tardieu M, de Parscau L, et al. [Clinical presentation of inborn metabolic diseases in the neonatal period]. Arch Pediatr 2012;19(9):953–8. Signes néonatals des maladies héréditaires du métabolisme.

23. Kontzialis M, Huisman T. Toxic-metabolic neurologic disorders in children: a neuroimaging review. J Neuroimaging 2018;28(6):587–95.

24. Li Y, Liu X, Duan CF, et al. Brain magnetic resonance imaging findings and radiologic review of maple syrup urine disease: report of three cases. World J Clin Cases 2021;9(8):1844–52.

25. Rossi A, Biancheri R. Magnetic resonance spectroscopy in metabolic disorders. Neuroimaging Clin N Am 2013;23(3):425–48.

26. Ozturk K, McKinney AM, Nascene D. Urea cycle disorders: a neuroimaging pattern approach using diffusion and FLAIR MRI. J Neuroimaging 2021;31(1):144–50.

27. Zhou X, Cui Y, Han J. Methylmalonic acidemia: current status and research priorities. Intractable Rare Dis Res 2018;7(2):73–8.

28. Radmanesh A, Zaman T, Ghanaati H, et al. Methylmalonic acidemia: brain imaging findings in 52 children and a review of the literature. Pediatr Radiol 2008;38(10):1054–61.

29. Cheillan D. Zellweger syndrome disorders: from severe neonatal disease to atypical adult presentation. Adv Exp Med Biol 2020;1299:71–80.

30. Kwon JM, Matern D, Kurtzberg J, et al. Consensus guidelines for newborn screening, diagnosis and treatment of infantile Krabbe disease. Orphanet J Rare Dis 2018;13(1):30.

31. Beltran-Quintero ML, Bascou NA, Poe MD, et al. Early progression of Krabbe disease in patients with symptom onset between 0 and 5 months. Orphanet J Rare Dis 2019;14(1):46.
32. Duffner PK, Barczykowski A, Jalal K, et al. Early infantile Krabbe disease: results of the world-wide Krabbe registry. Pediatr Neurol 2011;45(3):141–8.
33. Sasaki M, Sakuragawa N, Takashima S, et al. MRI and CT findings in Krabbe disease. Pediatr Neurol 1991;7(4):283–8.
34. Muthusamy K, Sudhakar SV, Thomas M, et al. Revisiting magnetic resonance imaging pattern of Krabbe disease - lessons from an Indian cohort. J Clin Imaging Sci 2019;9:25.
35. Bernal OG, Lenn N. Multiple cranial nerve enhancement in early infantile Krabbe's disease. Neurology 2000;54(12):2348–9.
36. Ganesan K, Desai S, Hegde A. Multiple cranial nerve enhancement: uncommon imaging finding in early infantile Krabbe's disease. J Neuroimaging 2010;20(2):195–7.
37. Hwang M, Zuccoli G, Panigrahy A, et al. Thickening of the cauda equina roots: a common finding in Krabbe disease. Eur Radiol 2016;26(10):3377–82.
38. Beslow LA, Schwartz ES, Bönnemann CG. Thickening and enhancement of multiple cranial nerves in conjunction with cystic white matter lesions in early infantile Krabbe disease. Pediatr Radiol 2008;38(6):694–6.
39. Lim YT, Mankad K, Kinali M, et al. Neuroimaging spectrum of inherited neurotransmitter disorders. Neuropediatrics 2020;51(1):6–21.
40. Stence NV, Fenton LZ, Levek C, et al. Brain imaging in classic nonketotic hyperglycinemia: quantitative analysis and relation to phenotype. J Inherit Metab Dis 2019;42(3):438–50.
41. Butler CJ, Likeman M, Mallick AA. Distinctive magnetic resonance imaging findings in neonatal nonketotic hyperglycinemia. Pediatr Neurol 2017;72:90–1.
42. Filatov A, Milla S, Shekdar K, et al. Imaging features of acquired pediatric metabolic and toxic white matter disorders. Top Magn Reson Imaging 2011;22(5):239–50.
43. Abramowski A, Ward R, Hamdan AH. Neonatal hypoglycemia. StatPearls. StatPearls Publishing Copyright © 2021, Philadelphia: StatPearls Publishing LLC.; 2021.
44. Tin W. Defining neonatal hypoglycaemia: a continuing debate. Semin Fetal Neonatal Med 2014;19(1):27–32.
45. Adamkin DH. Neonatal hypoglycemia. Semin Fetal Neonatal Med 2017;22(1):36–41.

Perinatal Ischemic Stroke
Etiology and Imaging

Nicholas V. Stence, MD*, David M. Mirsky, MD,
Ilana Neuberger, MD

KEYWORDS

- Perinatal stroke • Neonatal arterial ischemic stroke
- Periventricular venous infarction • Presumed perinatal arterial ischemic stroke

KEY POINTS

- Perinatal ischemic stroke is a common cause of acute neonatal neurologic symptoms. It can be most effectively diagnosed in the acute period with imaging, preferably MRI if available.
- Perinatal ischemic stroke can cause lifelong morbidity, including hemiparesis, language impairment, and cognitive disability.
- The risk for poor outcome in perinatal stroke can be predicted early on acute imaging and managed with proactive referral to rehabilitation services.

INTRODUCTION

Perinatal ischemic stroke is common, exceeding the risk of childhood stroke 10-fold.[1] Most cases of unilateral hemiparesis are due to perinatal stroke.[2] Early identification of affected patients and prediction of their risk for future morbidity on acute imaging can aid in determining rehabilitation strategies and clinical follow-up. This review will provide an overview of perinatal ischemic stroke, including clinical features, imaging, and outcome.

DEFINITIONS

A workshop was convened in August 2006 by the National Institute of Child Health and Human Development (NICHD) and the National Institute of Neurologic Disorders and Stroke (NINDS) to review the topic of stroke in the perinatal period and create research goals. The proceedings noted that various terms have been used to define both stroke and the perinatal period, leading to numerous different labels for the condition. Thus, the workshop specifically chose the term ischemic perinatal stroke (IPS) and defined it

Department of Radiology, Children's Hospital Colorado, University of Colorado School of Medicine, 13123 East 16th Avenue, Box 125, Aurora, CO 80045, USA
* Corresponding author.
E-mail address: nicholas.stence@childrenscolorado.org

Clin Perinatol 49 (2022) 675–692
https://doi.org/10.1016/j.clp.2022.05.005
0095-5108/22/© 2022 Elsevier Inc. All rights reserved.
perinatology.theclinics.com

as "a group of heterogeneous conditions in which there is focal disruption of cerebral blood flow secondary to arterial or cerebral venous thrombosis or embolization, between 20 weeks of fetal life and the 28th-day postnatal day, confirmed by neuroimaging or neuropathologic studies."[3] They further defined various subsets of IPS based on the time of diagnosis, to include (1) fetal ischemic stroke diagnosed before birth, (2) neonatal ischemic stroke diagnosed in either term or preterm infants after birth and on or before the day of life 28, (3) presumed perinatal ischemic stroke (PPIS) diagnosed in patients greater than 28 days of age, in whom it is inferred that an ischemic event occurred sometime between 20th week of fetal life and the 28th postnatal day, with said inference typically made from the interpretation of imaging and clinical history.[3]

More recent publications have further refined the classification of perinatal stroke. The current standard is to categorize perinatal stroke based on whether it is arterial or venous in origin, whether it is purely ischemic or contains hemorrhage, and age at diagnosis.[4] This leads to 6 commonly used categories of perinatal stroke. In this review, we will focus on the ischemic stroke subtypes, which are currently typically termed neonatal arterial ischemic stroke (NAIS), synonymous with neonatal ischemic stroke as defined above, presumed perinatal arterial ischemic stroke (PPAIS), synonymous with PPIS as defined above, and periventricular venous infarction (PVI), another presumed perinatal ischemic stroke subtype.[4] Of note, NAIS is synonymous with perinatal arterial ischemic stroke (PAIS) as used in much of the literature on neonatal stroke, but for consistency in this review, the term NAIS will be used.

NEONATAL ARTERIAL ISCHEMIC STROKE
Epidemiology

Neonatal arterial ischemic stroke (NAIS) incidence estimates range from 17.8/100,000 to 35/100,000.[5–8] Incidence estimates have increased over time, and it is unclear whether this is due to a true increase in disease or improved detection. Perinatal stroke overall accounts for 25% of stroke in children,[9] and NAIS represents 71% of all perinatal strokes.[10] Most of the reported NAIS cases are male, ranging up to 70%.[11] NAIS was the etiology of 15% of neonatal seizures in one study.[12] Mortality is generally considered rare, with incidence estimates ranging from 2.67/100,000 to 3.49/100,000 live births,[5] although more recent case series have reported no deaths.[7]

Table 1 Risk Factors of NAIS		
Maternal	**Fetal/Intrapartum**	**Placental**
First pregnancy	Male sex	Maternal vascular malperfusion
Twin pregnancy	Congenital heart disease	Fetal vascular malperfusion
Prolonged second stage	Hypoglycemia	Amniotic fluid inflammation
Emergency caesarean section	Perinatal hypoxia	Chronic villitis
Preeclampsia	Infection/inflammation	Large placenta with chorangiosis
IUGR	Need for resuscitation	
Maternal Smoking	Apgar <7 at 5 min	
Maternal Fever	Arteriopathy	
PPROM	Presence of meconium	
Family history of seizures		

Data from Refs.[10,11,13–15,54]

Risk Factors

Most sources separate NAIS risk factors into maternal, fetal, and placental categories (**Table 1**). The most commonly reported risk factors include first pregnancy, perinatal infection/inflammation, prolonged second stage, need for resuscitation, male sex, and congenital heart disease.[10,11,13–15] In many cases, multiple risk factors are present and increase the likelihood of NAIS.[6]

Although global hypoxia is considered a risk factor for NAIS, it and HIE are typically considered separate entities. One study did identify an overlap of multiple risk factors for NAIS and neonatal hypoxic-ischemic encephalopathy (HIE), including male sex, premature rupture of membranes (PROM), presence of meconium, and need for resuscitation.[11] Intrapartum inflammatory complications such as PROM and maternal fever are still more common in NAIS, which further implicates inflammation as an important risk factor.[15]

Evidence regarding thrombophilia as a risk factor is mixed. Some reports have strongly implicated thrombophilia in infants and/or mothers in NAIS,[16,17] although more recent studies have not found an association.[18,19] Curtis and colleagues thus do not recommend routine testing for thrombophilia in patients with NAIS.

Causes

Regardless of the risk factor background, NAIS likely occurs due to some of the same underlying mechanisms as stroke at older ages. These include embolus (of either cardiac or aortic origin), arteriopathy, and thrombosis due to disordered hemostasis.[20] Emboli can result from either congenital heart disease or placental pathology (both known risk factors), arteriopathy can result from either genetic causes or neonatal meningitis causing nearby arteritis, and thrombosis can be caused from systemic perinatal infection and/or inflammation.[21]

Clinical Presentation

Patients with NAIS will present before 28 days of life in 58% to 68% of cases.[6,14] Seizures are the classic and most common presentation of NAIS, occurring in up to 88% of neonates, and they are most often focal although they can be generalized.[22] Focal motor seizure presenting after 12 hours of life in the neonate strongly favors NAIS over HIE.[23] Neonates can also present with other neurologic deficits, including encephalopathy, abnormal tone, and feeding and respiratory difficulties.[22]

Imaging

Cranial ultrasound

Cranial ultrasound (CUS) is frequently the first diagnostic imaging test undertaken on the neurologically compromised NICU patient. A study of CUS in term infants with NAIS found that the modality detected 68% of cases in scans performed between days 1 to 3 of life, and 87% of cases performed between days of life 4 to 14.[24] However, in a major series of childhood stroke patients from Canada, CUS was the first test to diagnose NAIS in only 7%.[22]

Infarcted tissue on neonatal CUS is typically abnormally echogenic relative to surrounding normal brain. CUS is superior at detecting areas of infarction that are within the view of the ultrasound probe, including the lenticulostriate territory, the medial anterior cerebral artery, and more lateral middle cerebral artery territories (**Fig. 1A, B**). Small infarctions, particularly over the more superior convexities outside of the probe range, can be missed (**Fig. 1C, D**). As alluded to above, CUS sensitivity increases in the earlier subacute period compared with the acute period (<3 days).[24]

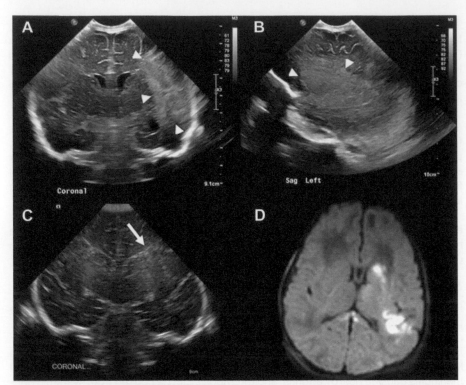

Fig. 1. Cranial US coronal (*A*) and sagittal (*B*) images were obtained in an infant at DOL 7 who was already diagnosed with stroke on MRI at DOL 1 after presenting with seizures. Images demonstrate a roughly wedge-shaped area of increased echogenicity in the left MCA territory compatible with infarction (*arrowheads*). Coronal cranial US (*C*) in a different patient at DOL 1 was called normal. In retrospect, there is a subtle area of increased echogenicity near the left caudate head (*arrow*). The areas of infarction are demonstrated on the follow-up DWI MRI performed at DOL 2 (*D*).

Head computed tomography

Head computed tomography (HCT) is often not the first-choice modality for imaging of neonatal neurologic symptoms for several reasons. CUS is more easily and quickly obtained as it can be performed at the bedside in critically ill neonates. HCT generally requires transport to the CT scanner, which entails extra risk for neonates in the NICU. Further, if transport is required, MRI (if available) is a more sensitive modality for most neurologic diseases, including NAIS. HCT is also less sensitive to parenchymal disease in the neonate due to its generally unmyelinated state.

However, HCT is still a reasonable alternative to MRI in those neonates who are so critically ill that they cannot undergo a (generally longer) MRI examination or in institutions whereby MRI is not available. In fact, HCT was the first test to diagnose NAIS in 87% of patients in a large national series of patients with stroke.[22]

The HCT findings of acute arterial ischemic stroke in the neonate are the same as in older children and adults—an area of hypodensity corresponding to an arterial territory (**Fig. 2**A, B). The characteristic hypodensity of acute infarction is more difficult to detect on HCT in neonates, because the relatively unmyelinated neonatal brain is more diffusely hypodense, creating less inherent contrast between normal and

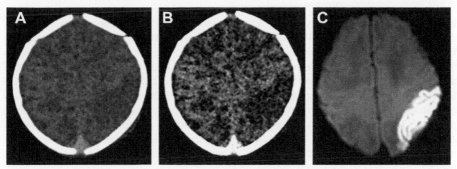

Fig. 2. Term newborn with focal seizures. Axial CT image at DOL 0 displayed with routine brain windowing (A) demonstrates a very subtle area of hypodensity in the left parietal lobe that is better seen on a narrower stroke window (B). DWI at DOL 1 (C) shows the area of restricted diffusion compatible with arterial ischemic stroke to much better advantage.

infarcted brain. Using a narrower "stroke" window setting increases the contrast between infarcted and normal brain (see **Fig. 2**B). Also, like older patients, HCT is less likely to show a stroke less than 12 to 24 hours old compared with DWI on MRI (see Fig. 2C).

Brain magnetic resonance imaging
General considerations. MRI is the gold standard for imaging of neurologic disease at any age. It is particularly valuable in imaging neonates with concern for central nervous system pathology for many reasons, including avoidance of ionizing radiation and superior depiction of tissue contrast. Furthermore, multiple different types of anatomic and physiologic imaging can be performed during a single MR examination, including multicontrast imaging of the brain parenchyma, luminal imaging of the intracranial arterial and venous systems, MR spectroscopy, and perfusion-weighted imaging (**Fig. 3**).

MRI does present specific challenges in neonatal imaging compared with other modalities. There are safety concerns with the high magnetic field strengths necessary for clinical MRI. Although these are routinely managed by MRI staff, additional MR safety

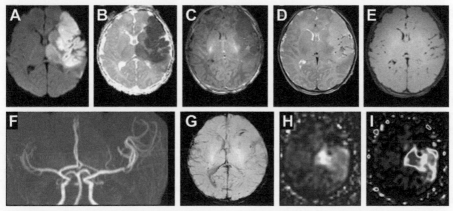

Fig. 3. This figure illustrates the different types of MRI sequences commonly used to image perinatal arterial ischemic stroke, including DWI (A), ADC (B), T1 (C), T2 (D), FLAIR (E), time of flight MRA (F), SWI minIP (G), grayscale (H) and color-coded (I) pCASL.

training is usually necessary for NICU staff transporting the patient. In most institutions, transport from the NICU to the MRI suite and a transition from the incubator to the MRI scanner table is required. Some institutions have acquired MRI scanners in the NICU, obviating the need for lengthy transport, and many other children's hospitals have used MRI compatible incubators to maintain neonatal life support without the need to move the patient to a separate table.[25] Finally, MRI requires a relatively motionless subject for diagnostic imaging. While general anesthesia is often used in pediatric MRI examinations to ensure patients remain motionless, most neonates can be imaged safely and easily without anesthesia using a feed and sleep technique.[26,27] Multiple new MRI techniques have also been developed to acquire images more quickly and to decrease motion artifacts.[28]

Diffusion-weighted imaging. While most routine MR sequences generate image contrast by varying parameters to accentuate differences in local proton magnetic environments (known as the T1 and T2 tissue times), diffusion-weighted imaging (DWI) uses a specific sequence of strong magnetic gradients to ensure that only relatively stationary protons will return signal. Protons in brain tissue tend to return the signal on DWI in several pathologies, but most often in cytotoxic edema, which is a state of intracellular swelling often brought about by metabolic derangements such as ischemia.[29]

DWI is thus extraordinarily sensitive to acute arterial ischemic stroke in both adults and children, and it can demonstrate changes in infarction earlier than most other imaging modalities. Areas of infarction are hyperintense on DWI. An apparent diffusion coefficient (ADC) map is routinely generated with DWI to show diffusion restriction in a quantifiable manner and to remove the effects of T2 hyperintensity. Thus, any areas of hyperintensity on DWI should be correlated with hypointensity on ADC maps to confirm true restricted diffusion indicative of infarction.[29]

Several publications have studied the time course of DWI and ADC changes after infarction (**Fig. 4**). While usually positive soon after symptom onset, DWI can underestimate the extent of infarction and the degree of associated network injuries if performed within 24 hours of presentation.[30] The time course of diffusion-weighted changes has also been studied on ADC maps, showing that the lowest ADC values are usually seen 3 to 4 days after presentation, with so-called pseudonormalization (apparent return to normal ADC values) at approximately 7 to 9 days.[31]

T1 and T2-weighted imaging. In general, T1-weighted images depict areas with higher lipid content (such as the myelin sheath) as hyperintense, and T2-weighted images depict areas with higher water content as hyperintense. In the unmyelinated neonatal brain, this results in the normal cortex being relatively T1 hyperintense and T2 hypointense, and normal white matter being T1 hypointense and T2 hyperintense.

Loss of gray/white differentiation is the first sign of infarction in the neonatal brain on T1 and T2-weighted images, manifesting as abnormal cortical T1 hypointensity and T2 hyperintensity. This occurs after findings are apparent on DWI/ADC, usually greater than 12 to 24 hours after presentation. This persists through approximately day 6 to 7, after which the cortex gradually becomes more T1 hyperintense and T2 hypointense through the first or second month after infarction[32] (see **Fig. 4**G, H). Tissue atrophy and cyst formation begin approximately 1 month after the initial insult, and the area of infarction will usually take on its chronic appearance within 2 to 3 months (see **Fig. 4**K, L).

Although a mainstay for diagnosis in older children and adults, FLAIR imaging (see **Fig. 3**E) is of limited utility for parenchymal evaluation and NAIS in neonates,

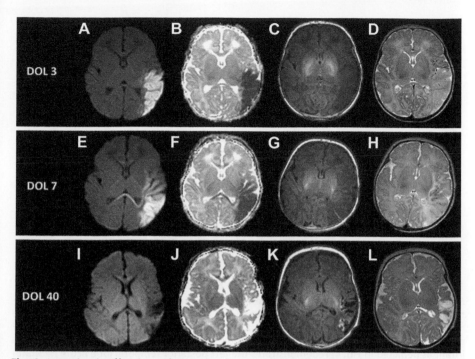

Fig. 4. Lettering is off. D is on their twice. Term neonate who presented at DOL 2 with seizures. Successive DWI, ADC, T1, and T2-weighted images demonstrate the maturation of signal changes in a perinatal arterial ischemic stroke single patient over time. On the patient's first examination performed at DOL 3, DWI image (*A*) depicts a circumscribed area of marked hyperintensity in the left posterior temporal lobe with corresponding decreased ADC values (*B*), compatible with restricted diffusion. In this context, the diffusion restriction indicates cytotoxic edema from acute arterial ischemic stroke. T1 (*C*) and T2 (*D*) images show the area of infarction as a homogeneous area of loss of gray/white differentiation. On DOL 7, the area of infarction is still hyperintense on DWI (*E*) and shows persistently decreased ADC values (*F*), although they have slightly increased since DOL 3. DWI image also demonstrates diffusion restriction in the corpus callosum splenium, compatible with an associated network injury. The involved white matter in the left posterior temporal lobe has become more T2 hyperintense, and the cortex has become slightly more T1 hyperintense (*G*) and T2 hypointense (*H*). By DOL 40, diffusion restriction on DWI (*I*) has resolved, and ADC values in the area of infarction have become diffusely increased relative to normal brain (*J*). Associated cortical T1 hyperintensity throughout this region has become even more conspicuous (*K*) and cystic changes and atrophy of the affected parenchyma have already developed on T2-weighted images (*L*).

secondary to their unmyelinated white matter. It is, therefore, not a routine part of many neonatal brain imaging protocols, although it can aid in the detection of extra-axial hemorrhage.

Magnetic resonance angiography. Most routine intracranial magnetic resonance angiography (MRA) techniques are designed to use the signal from fast-moving blood flowing into the area of interest to generate images of the arterial lumen; thus, no intravenous contrast is necessary.

MRA findings in NAIS can range from stenosis or occlusion of involved arterial segments (**Fig. 5**A, B, C), to paradoxic enlargement and hyperintensity of involved

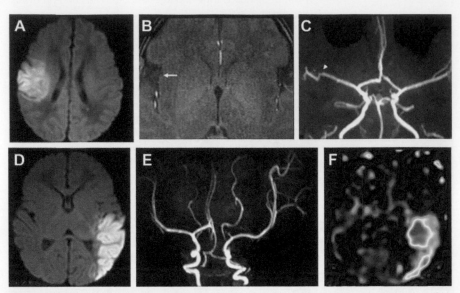

Fig. 5. DWI (*A*) of a 2-day-old woman presenting with seizures demonstrates acute infarction in the right posterior frontal lobe. MRA source image (*B*) shows the asymmetric absence of flow-related enhancement in right MCA M2 branches (*arrow*), also seen on a frontal MIP projection (*C, arrowhead*). DWI image (*D*) obtained at DOL 3 in a different patient (same infant as depicted in **Fig. 4**) redemonstrates the left posterior temporal lobe acute neonatal arterial ischemic stroke. Time of flight MR angiography from DOL 3 (*E*) shows increased caliber and intensity of flow-related enhancement in left MCA branches supplying the area of infarction. Color pCASL image (*F*) demonstrates that the area of infarction is correspondingly hyperperfused.

segments, a phenomenon sometimes referred to as reperfusion or luxury perfusion (**Fig. 5**D, E). In one study of 37 patients with NAIS, 23 had abnormalities on MRA, including occlusion in 6, thrombus formation in 9, and increased flow in 8.[33] Those patients with NAIS with MRA abnormalities also demonstrated worse outcomes, especially those with occlusion. These findings may provide additional evidence that embolism is a frequent cause of NAIS.

Arterial spin labeling. Arterial spin labeling (ASL) perfusion techniques are increasingly used in routine brain imaging to depict changes in cerebral blood flow without the need for intravenous contrast. Various ASL techniques are available that vary by manufacturer, including continuous, pulsed, and pseudocontinuous. Each technique has its own advantages, disadvantages, and availability, although pseudocontinuous ASL (pCASL) has been shown to be superior to pulsed ASL (PASL) in neonates.[34] Regardless of the available technique, ASL can be technically challenging in neonates due to their size and smaller volume of circulating blood. Modification of default parameters to optimize the detection of neonatal cerebral blood flow is often necessary and may require vendor support.

ASL in NAIS often depicts an area of increased blood flow corresponding to the area of infarction (**Fig. 5**F), corresponding to findings often seen on MRA. In one large series of neonatal stroke imaged with ASL, 8/11 NAIS cases demonstrated hyperperfusion, and a penumbra was seldom seen,[35] in contrast to older patients.

Network injury. Secondary neuronal degeneration in a part of the brain distant from an injury has been called diaschisis, Wallerian degeneration, or network injury by various authors. All these terms refer to the structural and/or functional changes that can occur in the central nodes of the various neuronal networks distant from a site of injury. This phenomenon is perhaps most famously recognized in crossed cerebellar diaschisis, whereby hypoperfusion or atrophy occurs in the cerebellar hemisphere contralateral to a large cerebral insult,[36,37] although it has also been described in the striatum and thalami of adults following surgery.[38]

The unmyelinated neonatal brain may be particularly vulnerable to this sort of secondary neuronal degeneration.[39,40] Network injuries in neonates most often manifest as areas of mild diffusion restriction (with higher ADC values than the area of infarction) in central areas of the brain not supplied directly by the middle cerebral artery, including the corpus callosum splenium, thalamus, and corticospinal tracts in the cerebral peduncle (**Fig. 6**). Recognition of these sites of diffusion restriction as network injury and not additional sites of infarction is important to accurately determine the extent of injury and to aid in the prognostication of outcome. Notably, network injuries on DWI are more likely to be demonstrated on imaging performed more than 48 hours after presentation, which has implications for outcome prediction (see **Fig. 4**A, E).[30]

Stroke evolution. Large territory AIS in adults and older children can result in malignant edema, causing significant midline shift and transfalcine herniation that can require decompressive hemicraniectomy.[41] In contrast, even very large territory arterial ischemic strokes in neonates do not swell to a significant degree (see **Fig. 6**A, C). As is often the case with any difference noted between neonatal and childhood stroke, this could be attributable to the lack of myelination in the neonatal brain. Open sutures in the neonate can also better accommodate degrees of brain swelling than older children and adults.

After several months, the infarcted tissue in NAIS takes on a chronic appearance of largely cystic volume loss,[32] in contrast to cortical infarctions in older children and adults that more often manifest at least partially as gliosis. As is the case with any injury occurring early during brain development, the affected hemisphere is often smaller, and the calvarium over it is also smaller to accommodate the difference in cerebral hemisphere size (see **Fig. 6**B, D). Atrophy of central structures such as the thalami that are involved in network injuries also often occurs. Recurrence risk of NAIS is very low outside of the context of congenital heart disease. Therefore, follow-up imaging is not indicated for stroke follow-up, although it is sometimes performed for secondary complications such as seizures or developmental delays.

PRESUMED PERINATAL ISCHEMIC STROKE

Some children with brain imaging compatible with a remote infarction only come to clinical attention after the neonatal period. These are typically categorized as either presumed perinatal arterial ischemic stroke (PPAIS) or periventricular venous infarction (PVI).

Presumed Perinatal Arterial Ischemic Stroke

PPAIS is diagnosed in patients older than 28 days of age who lack significant perinatal neurologic history and who usually require imaging for hemiparesis or seizures in infancy.[3] Imaging in these patients is indistinguishable from the chronic imaging of NAIS diagnosed symptomatically in the neonatal period. The injured areas of brain demonstrate cystic volume loss and contain thin membranes, central structures such as the thalamus are often correspondingly atrophied, and the affected

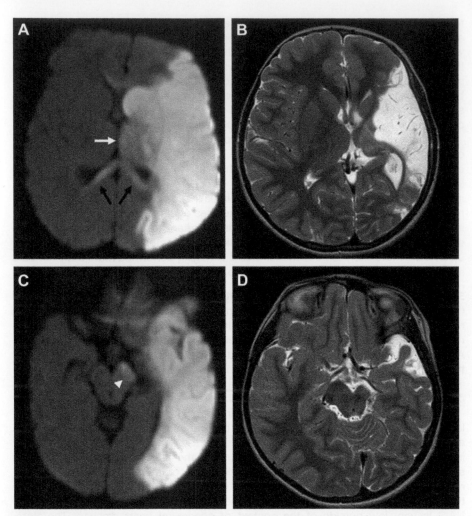

Fig. 6. Axial DWI images (*A*, *C*) obtained in a term neonate at DOL 3 demonstrate a large area of marked diffusion restriction in the left MCA territory, compatible with an acute neonatal arterial ischemic stroke. Areas of milder diffusion restriction not in the left MCA territory, including the thalamus (*A, white arrow*) corpus callosum splenium (*A, black arrow*) and cerebral peduncle (*C, white arrowhead*) indicate areas of network injury. Note that despite the large territory of infarction, there is no significant midline shift or swelling of the large area of infarcted tissue. Axial T2 images (*B, D*) from a follow-up MRI obtained at 7 years of age demonstrate marked cystic volume loss of the left MCA territory infarction, marked atrophy of the ipsilateral thalamus and cerebral peduncle as a result of the network injury. Further, the left cerebral hemisphere is much smaller than the left overall, and the calvarial vault accommodates this different size.

hemisphere is usually smaller with a correspondingly smaller cranial vault volume (**Fig. 7**). For these reasons, the putative etiology is NAIS which was simply not diagnosed in the neonatal period.

Debate exists over the reasons why NAIS presentation is sometimes delayed. Possible explanations include neonatal seizures that are missed clinically, an insult that occurred in utero with missed hemiparesis in the neonatal period, or a smaller

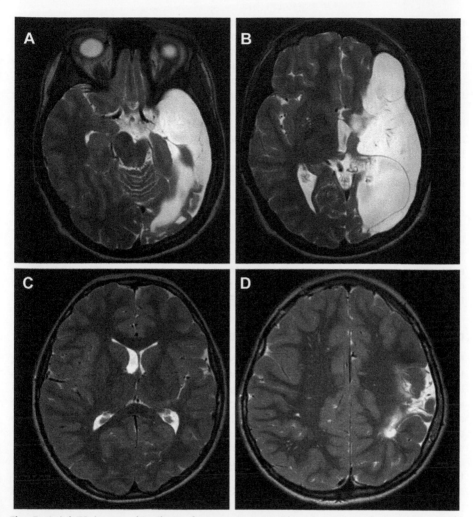

Fig. 7. Axial T2 images (*A, B*) are from a 15 year old with presumed perinatal arterial ischemic stroke. The extensive area of left MCA territory cystic infarction, associated atrophy of the thalamus and cerebral peduncle, and smaller left cerebral hemisphere size are nearly identical in appearance to the perinatal arterial ischemic stroke diagnosed in the neonatal period acutely in the patient in **Fig. 6**. Axial T2 images (*C, D*) from a patient with mild right hemiparesis first imaged at 7 years of age demonstrate a smaller area of chronic infarction in the left posterior MCA territory, with milder volume loss in the left thalamus and cerebral hemisphere. This was also diagnosed as a presumed perinatal arterial ischemic stroke as symptoms had been present as infancy but not imaged until later in life.

infarction that correspondingly lacked seizures.[42] However, most studies of PPAIS find that the risk factors are very similar to acute symptomatic cases of NAIS, which argues against many cases occurring in utero.[43]

Periventricular Venous Infarction

Some patients presenting during the first year of life with hemiparesis have a different pattern of abnormality on brain imaging, consisting of cystic periventricular white matter volume loss focally dilating the ventricular margin (porencephaly) and occasionally lined by chronic blood products indicating remote hemorrhage (**Fig. 8**). As the appearance is identical to the chronic evolution of periventricular white matter infarctions seen in preterm infants, it is presumed to represent a similar mechanism of infarction occurring in utero, and thus has been termed periventricular venous infarction (PVI).[44,45] In fact, with the growing use of fetal MRI for diagnosis of in utero brain abnormalities, more cases of PVI are diagnosed in the fetus that otherwise appears like what is seen in the preterm infant[46] (**Fig. 9**). In keeping with their proposed differing mechanisms, patients diagnosed with PVI are more likely to have antenatal or maternal risk factors such as preeclampsia, small for gestational age or primigravida, while those with PPAIS are more likely to have acute peripartum risk factors such as low Apgar and prolonged rupture of membranes.[2,42]

An important differential consideration for porencephaly diagnosed in infancy is a mutation in the COL4A1 gene that encodes type IV collagen. These mutations can cause weakening of the basement membranes whereby type IV collagen is located, including blood vessels of the brain, eyes, and muscles.[47] Thus, the clinical phenotypes are broad, but they can include intracerebral hemorrhages in infancy that present with a similar appearance as periventricular venous infarction (**Fig. 10**A). Some of these patients will also have a distinctive type of congenital cataract with a characteristic lens shape[47] (posterior lenticonus, **Fig. 10**B, C).

OUTCOME PREDICTION IN PERINATAL ISCHEMIC STROKE

Mortality and stroke recurrence are rare in NAIS.[42] Siblings are also at no greater risk than the general population.[42] The risk of epilepsy is high and likely varies with the location and size of the infarction, with rates ranging historically from 9% to 16%,[42] although a recent meta-analysis noted an overall epilepsy rate of 27.2%.[48] A recent study found the risk of infantile spasms in NAIS increases with larger infarct volume and involvement of deep cerebral structures.[49] Other studies have correlated larger stroke volumes with the development of cerebral palsy.[50]

The presence and location of network injuries have been used for outcome prediction on acute imaging of NAIS. One study quantifying the diffusion restriction in the cerebral peduncle on acute imaging of NAIS found that the percentage of cerebral peduncle involvement and length and volume of the abnormal corticospinal tracts

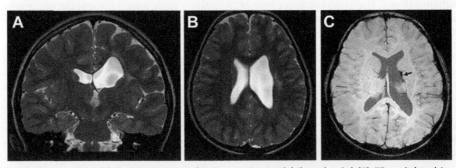

Fig. 8. 5-year-old with hemiparesis and seizures. Coronal (*A*) and axial (*B*) T2-weighted images demonstrate focal enlargement and outward scalloping of the left lateral ventricular surface, with small areas of nearby abnormal T2 hyperintensity. Axial SWI image (*C*) demonstrates a small area of hemosiderin along the ependymal surface near the caudothalamic notch (*black arrow*).

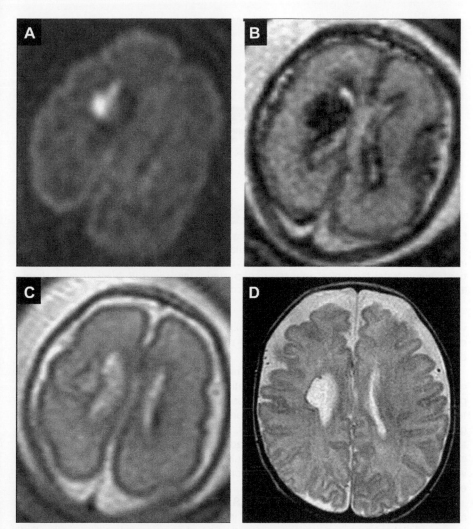

Fig. 9. Images from a fetal MRI performed at 26 weeks gestation (*A–C*) demonstrate a focal area of diffusion restriction in the right periventricular white matter on DWI (*A*), with corresponding susceptibility on an EPI T2*-weighted sequence compatible with internal hemorrhage (*B*), and faint T2 hyperintensity with a hypointense rim (*C*). An axial T2-weighted imagine (*D*) from a follow-up MRI performed at DOL 3 shows the typical appearance of a chronic periventricular venous infarction.

correlated with poor motor outcome.[39] Another study of diaschisis in NAIS measured thalamic volumes in patients with NAIS after 6 months of age and compared them to control patients. While the thalamic volume of patients with NAIS ipsilateral to the stroke did not correlate with motor deficits, an inverse correlation was found between their contralateral thalamic volume and motor function. This implies that the thalamus is involved in the mechanisms of plasticity that occur in the healthy cerebral hemisphere after a unilateral infarction.[51]

A recent study of cognitive outcomes in NAIS and PPAIS found that deficits in attention and executive function correlated with a diagnosis of PPAIS, larger infarct

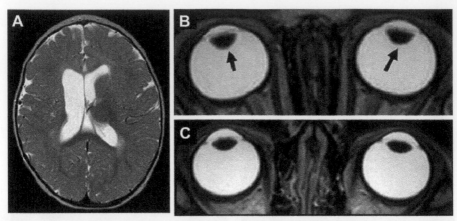

Fig. 10. An axial T2-weighted image (*A*) from a 9 month old with a COL4A1 mutation demonstrates a similar appearance of periventricular volume loss and T2 hyperintensity as seen in periventricular venous infarction. Axial T2-weighted image through the globes in this patient demonstrates the typical appearance of posterior lenticonus (B, *black arrows*). Normal appearance of the lenses in a control (*C*) for comparison.

volumes, and history of epilepsy.[52] The unexpectedly worse outcomes noted in PPAIS could be due either to referral biases, or the potential for earlier intervention in NAIS as diagnosed in the neonatal period.

Wagenaar and colleagues classified areas of infarction in NAIS on acute DWI into 1 of 8 territories (main MCA, anterior MCA, middle MCA, posterior MCA, cortical MCA, perforator, PCA, ACA), and included injuries in the thalamus, basal ganglia, and posterior limb internal capsule. Adverse outcomes were defined as cerebral palsy, language delay, epilepsy, behavioral issues, and visual deficits. Main MCA branch strokes were associated with universally adverse outcomes, basal ganglia/thalamic injuries were correlated with cognitive deficits and behavioral difficulties, and lesions in the cerebral peduncles and bilateral lesions were correlated with increased risk for epilepsy.[53]

Differences in outcomes between PPAIS and PVI have also been studied.[44] The amount of cortical involvement, as seen in PPAIS but not PVI, is correlated with increased risk of seizures, language disorders, and poor cognitive outcomes. Both presumed ischemic stroke subtypes carry a risk of poor motor outcomes, although PVI has a greater risk of spasticity than some patients with PPAIS.[44]

SUMMARY

Acute imaging in NAIS is preferentially performed with MRI, whereby it can be promptly diagnosed and managed. Patients who are diagnosed with perinatal stroke either in the neonatal period or later in childhood experience a range of morbidities, often hemiparesis and epilepsy. Both acute and chronic imaging can be used to estimate the risk of various long-term complications, and aid in the determination of rehabilitation strategies.

Best practices

What is the current practice for perinatal arterial ischemic stroke?

Acute imaging with MRI, DWI, MRA, and MR perfusion is recommended for the best assessment of stroke size and location, and to provide the optimal opportunity for outcome prediction.

Best Practice/Guideline/Care Path Objective:

What changes in current practice are likely to improve outcomes?
   Adoption of methods to predict poor neurodevelopmental and motor outcomes, such as the detection of network injuries and classification of stroke location and size, will enable improved patient surveillance and earlier rehabilitation referral.

Pearls/Pitfalls at point-of-care:

Do not mistake network injuries for new or additional sites of infarction.

CLINICS CARE POINTS

- CUS and CT have been used in acute diagnosis of NAIS, although both can miss acute infarction when performed within 1-2 days.
- MRI is the preferred modality for diagnosis of NAIS and PVI, due to it's superior contrast resolution, ability to diagnose stroke earlier, and multimodality capabilities such as MRA and ASL.
- Network injuries detected on MRI acutely can be used in outcome prediction.
- Risk of adverse outcomes can be also predicted based on arterial territory involvement and stroke subtype (NAIS vs PPAIS, PPAIS vs PVI).

DISCLOSURE

The author has nothing to disclose.

REFERENCES

1. Martinez-Biarge M, Ferriero DM, Cowan FM. Perinatal arterial ischemic stroke. Handb Clin Neurol 2019;162:239–66.
2. Vitagliano M, Dunbar M, Dyck Holzinger S, et al. Perinatal arterial ischemic stroke and periventricular venous infarction in infants with unilateral cerebral palsy. Dev Med Child Neurol 2022;64(1):56–62.
3. Raju TN, Nelson KB, Ferriero D, et al. Ischemic perinatal stroke: summary of a workshop sponsored by the national Institute of Child Health and human development and the national Institute of neurological disorders and stroke. Pediatrics 2007;120(3):609–16.
4. Dunbar M, Kirton A. Perinatal stroke: mechanisms, management, and outcomes of early cerebrovascular brain injury. Lancet Child Adolesc Health 2018;2(9):666–76.
5. Lynch JK, Nelson KB. Epidemiology of perinatal stroke. Curr Opin Pediatr 2001;13(6):499–505.
6. Lee J, Croen LA, Backstrand KH, et al. Maternal and infant characteristics associated with perinatal arterial stroke in the infant. Jama 2005;293(6):723–9.
7. Clive B, Vincer M, Ahmad T, et al. Epidemiology of neonatal stroke: a population-based study. Paediatr Child Health 2020;25(1):20–5.
8. Dunbar MJ, Kirton A. The incidence of perinatal stroke is 1: 1200 live births: a population-based study in Alberta Canada. Stroke 2020;51(Suppl_1):A51.

9. deVeber GA, MacGregor D, Curtis R, et al. Neurologic outcome in survivors of childhood arterial ischemic stroke and sinovenous thrombosis. J Child Neurol 2000;15(5):316–24.

10. Kirton A, Armstrong-Wells J, Chang T, et al. Symptomatic neonatal arterial ischemic stroke: the International pediatric stroke study. Pediatrics 2011;128(6): e1402–10.

11. Martinez-Biarge M, Cheong JL, Diez-Sebastian J, et al. Risk factors for neonatal arterial ischemic stroke: the importance of the intrapartum period. J Pediatr 2016; 173:62–8.e1.

12. Tekgul H, Gauvreau K, Soul J, et al. The current etiologic profile and neurodevelopmental outcome of seizures in term newborn infants. Pediatrics 2006;117(4): 1270–80.

13. Lynch JK. Epidemiology and classification of perinatal stroke. Semin Fetal Neonatal Med 2009;14(5):245–9.

14. Lehman LL, Rivkin MJ. Perinatal arterial ischemic stroke: presentation, risk factors, evaluation, and outcome. Pediatr Neurol 2014;51(6):760–8.

15. Giraud A, Guiraut C, Chevin M, et al. Role of perinatal inflammation in neonatal arterial ischemic stroke. Front Neurol 2017;8:612.

16. Lynch JK, Han CJ, Nee LE, et al. Prothrombotic factors in children with stroke or porencephaly. Pediatrics 2005;116(2):447–53.

17. Kenet G, Lutkhoff LK, Albisetti M, et al. Impact of thrombophilia on risk of arterial ischemic stroke or cerebral sinovenous thrombosis in neonates and children: a systematic review and meta-analysis of observational studies. Circulation 2010; 121(16):1838–47.

18. Curtis C, Mineyko A, Massicotte P, et al. Thrombophilia risk is not increased in children after perinatal stroke. Blood 2017;129(20):2793–800.

19. Arnaez J, Arca G, Martin-Ancel A, et al. Neonatal arterial ischemic stroke: risk related to family history, maternal diseases, and genetic thrombophilia. Clin Appl Thromb Hemost 2018;24(1):79–84.

20. Govaert P, Ramenghi L, Taal R, et al. Diagnosis of perinatal stroke I: definitions, differential diagnosis and registration. Acta Paediatr 2009;98(10):1556–67.

21. Govaert P, Ramenghi L, Taal R, et al. Diagnosis of perinatal stroke II: mechanisms and clinical phenotypes. Acta Paediatr 2009;98(11):1720–6.

22. deVeber GA, Kirton A, Booth FA, et al. Epidemiology and outcomes of arterial ischemic stroke in children: the Canadian pediatric ischemic stroke registry. Pediatr Neurol 2017;69:58–70.

23. Rafay MF, Cortez MA, de Veber GA, et al. Predictive value of clinical and EEG features in the diagnosis of stroke and hypoxic ischemic encephalopathy in neonates with seizures. Stroke 2009;40(7):2402–7.

24. Cowan F, Mercuri E, Groenendaal F, et al. Does cranial ultrasound imaging identify arterial cerebral infarction in term neonates? Arch Dis Child Fetal Neonatal Ed 2005;90(3):F252–6.

25. Paley MN, Hart AR, Lait M, et al. An MR-compatible neonatal incubator. Br J Radiol 2012;85(1015):952–8.

26. Barkovich MJ, Xu D, Desikan RS, et al. Pediatric neuro MRI: tricks to minimize sedation. Pediatr Radiol 2018;48(1):50–5.

27. Artunduaga M, Liu CA, Morin CE, et al. Safety challenges related to the use of sedation and general anesthesia in pediatric patients undergoing magnetic resonance imaging examinations. Pediatr Radiol 2021;51(5):724–35.

28. Kozak BM, Jaimes C, Kirsch J, et al. MRI techniques to decrease imaging times in children. Radiographics 2020;40(2):485–502.

29. Warach SM, Boska M, Welch KMA. Pitfalls and potential of clinical diffusion-weighted MR imaging in acute stroke. Stroke 1997;28(3):481–2.

30. Wagenaar N, van der Aa NE, Groenendaal F, et al. MR imaging for accurate prediction of outcome after perinatal arterial ischemic stroke: sooner not necessarily better. Eur J Paediatr Neurol 2017;21(4):666–70.

31. van der Aa NE, Benders MJ, Vincken KL, et al. The course of apparent diffusion coefficient values following perinatal arterial ischemic stroke. PLoS One 2013; 8(2):e56784.

32. Dudink J, Mercuri E, Al-Nakib L, et al. Evolution of unilateral perinatal arterial ischemic stroke on conventional and diffusion-weighted MR imaging. AJNR Am J Neuroradiol 2009;30(5):998–1004.

33. Husson B, Hertz-Pannier L, Adamsbaum C, et al. MR angiography findings in infants with neonatal arterial ischemic stroke in the middle cerebral artery territory: a prospective study using circle of Willis MR angiography. Eur J Radiol 2016; 85(7):1329–35.

34. Boudes E, Gilbert G, Leppert IR, et al. Measurement of brain perfusion in newborns: pulsed arterial spin labeling (PASL) versus pseudo-continuous arterial spin labeling (pCASL). Neuroimage Clin 2014;6:126–33.

35. Watson CG, Dehaes M, Gagoski BA, et al. Arterial spin labeling perfusion magnetic resonance imaging performed in acute perinatal stroke reveals hyperperfusion associated with ischemic injury. Stroke 2016;47(6):1514–9.

36. Lin DD, Kleinman JT, Wityk RJ, et al. Crossed cerebellar diaschisis in acute stroke detected by dynamic susceptibility contrast MR perfusion imaging. AJNR Am J Neuroradiol 2009;30(4):710–5.

37. Mah S, deVeber G, Wei XC, et al. Cerebellar atrophy in childhood arterial ischemic stroke: acute diffusion MRI biomarkers. Stroke 2013;44(9):2468–74.

38. Kamiya K, Sato N, Nakata Y, et al. Postoperative transient reduced diffusion in the ipsilateral striatum and thalamus. AJNR Am J Neuroradiol 2013;34(3):524–32.

39. Kirton A, Shroff M, Visvanathan T, et al. Quantified corticospinal tract diffusion restriction predicts neonatal stroke outcome. Stroke 2007;38(3):974–80.

40. Govaert P, Zingman A, Jung YH, et al. Network injury to pulvinar with neonatal arterial ischemic stroke. Neuroimage 2008;39(4):1850–7.

41. Ferriero DM, Fullerton HJ, Bernard TJ, et al. Management of stroke in neonates and children: a scientific statement from the American heart association/American stroke association. Stroke Mar 2019;50(3):e51–96.

42. Fluss J, Dinomais M, Chabrier S. Perinatal stroke syndromes: similarities and diversities in aetiology, outcome and management. Eur J Paediatr Neurol 2019; 23(3):368–83.

43. Kirton A, Shroff M, Pontigon A-M, et al. Risk factors and presentations of periventricular venous infarction vs arterial presumed perinatal ischemic stroke. Arch Neurol 2010;67(7):842–8.

44. Kirton A, Deveber G, Pontigon AM, et al. Presumed perinatal ischemic stroke: vascular classification predicts outcomes. Ann Neurol 2008;63(4):436–43.

45. Ilves P, Laugesaar R, Loorits D, et al. Presumed perinatal stroke: risk factors, clinical and radiological findings. J Child Neurol 2016;31(5):621–8.

46. Mirsky DM, Stence NV, Powers AM, et al. Imaging of fetal ventriculomegaly. Pediatr Radiol 2020;50(13):1948–58.

47. Nau S, McCourt EA, Maloney JA, et al. COL4A1 mutations in two infants with congenital cataracts and porencephaly: an ophthalmologic perspective. J AAPOS 2019;23(4):246–8.

48. Rattani A, Lim J, Mistry AM, et al. Incidence of epilepsy and associated risk factors in perinatal ischemic stroke survivors. Pediatr Neurol 2019;90:44–55.

49. Srivastava R, Shaw OEF, Armstrong E, et al. Patterns of brain injury in perinatal arterial ischemic stroke and the development of infantile spasms. J Child Neurol 2021;36(7):583–8.

50. Wiedemann A, Pastore-Wapp M, Slavova N, et al. Impact of stroke volume on motor outcome in neonatal arterial ischemic stroke. Eur J Paediatr Neurol 2020;25: 97–105.

51. Craig BT, Carlson HL, Kirton A. Thalamic diaschisis following perinatal stroke is associated with clinical disability. Neuroimage Clin 2019;21:101660.

52. Bosenbark DD, Krivitzky L, Ichord R, et al. Clinical predictors of attention and executive functioning outcomes in children after perinatal arterial ischemic stroke. Pediatr Neurol 2017;69:79–86.

53. Wagenaar N, Martinez-Biarge M, van der Aa NE, et al. Neurodevelopment after perinatal arterial ischemic stroke. Pediatrics 2018;142(3):e20174164.

54. Bernson-Leung ME, Boyd TK, Meserve EE, et al. Placental pathology in neonatal stroke: a retrospective case-control study. J Pediatr 2018;195:39–47 e5.

Imaging of Microcephaly

Chukwudi Okafor, MD, Sangam Kanekar, MD*

KEYWORDS

- Microcephaly • Microcephaly primary hereditary (MCPH)
- Microcephaly with simplified gyral pattern (MSGP) • Microlissensephaly
- Congenital cytomegalovirus • Zika virus infection

KEY POINTS

- Microcephaly is defined when the occipitofrontal circumference (OFC) of the head is less than two standard deviations below the average for age (or gestational age, if identified prenatally) and sex. Similarly, severe microcephaly is defined as an OFC that is less than three standard deviations below the average
- Microcephaly is primary, whereby it is present at birth or identified prenatally, and secondary, whereby a child is born with a normal OFC but subsequently demonstrates altered, abnormal growth
- Primary microcephaly largely results in a small brain and improperly developed secondary to genetic or chromosomal abnormalities while secondary microcephaly is when the brain is on a course of normal development, but a disease process disrupts this process.

INTRODUCTION

One of the most common definitions of microcephaly cited is that of an occipitofrontal circumference (OFC) of the head that is less than two standard deviations below the average for age (or gestational age, if identified prenatally) and sex.[1] Similarly, severe microcephaly is defined as an OFC that is less than three standard deviations below the average.[1,2] Microcephaly is not a diagnosis, but rather, a finding that is secondary to a multitude of etiologies that can be categorized as prenatal versus postnatal, genetic versus environmental, and congenital versus acquired.[3]

Depending on the exact definition used, and the population to which said definition is applied toward, the incidence of microcephaly varies. Worldwide, it is believed to occur at a rate of 0.5 to 20 per 10,000 live births.[1] However, in recent years, that number is believed to have increased with the start of the Zika virus outbreak, circa 2015. Indeed, the number of microcephaly live births in Brazil, one of the countries worst affected by the outbreak, reached a peak of approximately 50 per 10,000 live births.[4] The virus spread to surrounding countries in both North and South America; however,

Radiology Research, Division of Neuroradiology, Penn State Health, Penn State College of Medicine, Mail Code H066 500 University Drive, Hershey, PA 17033, USA
* Corresponding author.
E-mail address: skanekar@pennstatehealth.psu.edu

Clin Perinatol 49 (2022) 693–713
https://doi.org/10.1016/j.clp.2022.04.004
0095-5108/22/© 2022 Elsevier Inc. All rights reserved.
perinatology.theclinics.com

the full extent to which an increase in incidence can be attributed to the outbreak has yet to be identified. Nonetheless, the outbreak did spark further interest in studying the incidence of microcephaly, and in maintaining its surveillance in hopes of preparing for future outbreaks.[5]

To further clinical management, there have been attempts made to delineate whether microcephaly is *primary*, whereby it is present at birth or identified prenatally, and *secondary*, whereby a child is born with a normal OFC but subsequently demonstrates altered, abnormal growth.[2,6] Conceptually, this distinction helps to facilitate the understanding of different etiologies of microcephaly, but it does not account for the significant amounts of overlap between its presentations. For instance, a small OFC noted at birth implies an insult to the brain occurred prenatally, but it does not actually confirm if the brain was ever developing properly. As such, Fenichel in 2009 classifies[7] primary microcephaly as a finding relating to conditions that result in a brain that is small and improperly developed secondary to genetic or chromosomal abnormalities. Secondary microcephaly is when the brain is on a course of normal development, but a disease process disrupts this process.[7] These classifications more accurately identify potential causes of microcephaly and inspire the pursuit of further understanding.

CLINICAL EVALUATIONS AND CHALLENGES

Unfortunately, there is no universal diagnostic algorithm in place to characterize pediatric microcephaly. A wide variability exists among institutions regarding its evaluation, even among university centers with dedicated pediatric neurology departments.[6] Despite this, multiple sources state that a multidisciplinary team that includes at least a neurologist/pediatric neurologist, geneticist, and dysmorphologist is necessary.[1,3] Detailed and thorough medical histories should be taken, including that of pregnancy course and perinatal exposures, growth chart tracking, and family genealogy through at least 3 generations.[3] Social histories, such as that regarding maternal nutritional deprivation and travel to Zika virus-endemic areas, are also important to obtain.

The earliest point in time in which microcephaly may be detected is about halfway through the 2nd trimester in pregnancy via ultrasound, whereby the OFC can be calculated by obtaining both the biparietal (BPD) and occipitofrontal (OFD) diameters.[2] This is assuming that abnormalities in brain development are perceptible at that time, which is, accordingly, dependent on the particular etiology. In this context, antenatal and postnatal brain magnetic resonance imaging (MRI) is increasingly being used as a modality that is sensitive enough to find structural abnormalities that may suggest a particular diagnosis. Indeed, identification of certain patterns of brain injury on MRI can allow clinicians to direct diagnostic workup toward certain metabolic screenings or genetic testing. Alternatively, it may allow for the cessation of further unnecessary testing.[6] In fact, a retrospective study conducted by von der Hagen and colleagues[6] found that within their cohort of patients who had MRIs completed, diagnoses of autosomal recessive primary microcephaly, lissencephaly, mitochondriopathies were eventually made.

IMAGING CRITERIA

As previously mentioned, the earliest point in time at which microcephaly can be identified is around 18 to 22 weeks gestational age, and at present, ultrasound and MRI are the primary modalities capable of detecting microcephaly in the fetus and neonate.

Ultrasound is the first-line imaging modality used to assess fetal growth and anatomy during pregnancy. Sonographic equipment considered necessary to complete an examination include the following: ultrasound machine with real-time grayscale capabilities and capacity to print/store images, transabdominal transducers in the 3 to 5 MHz range (preferably curvilinear transducers, as they contour to a gravid abdomen and give a wide field of view[8]), electronic calipers, freeze-frame capabilities, and adjustable acoustic power output controls with output display standards.[9]

When examining the fetal head, four standard views are assessed, all of which are obtained in the axial plane: falx, transventricular, cavum, and posterior fossa/transcerebellar.[8] The falx view displays the falx cerebri as an echogenic, linear structure lying between the cerebral hemispheres. The transventricular view is obtained at the level of the cavum septum pellucidum, so as to demonstrate its positioning between the lateral ventricles and to demonstrate ventriculomegaly, if present.[8] The posterior fossa view is obtained at the level of the midbrain, with the transducer tilted toward the occiput, allowing for the visualization of the cisterna magna, cerebellar hemispheres and cerebellar vermis.[8] Finally, the cavum view is obtained at the level of the thalamus, displaying the cavum septum pellucidum as a box-like structure between the frontal horns of the lateral ventricles.

Of all of these views, the cavum view allows for an objective assessment of microcephaly, as it is the view that permits the measurement of both the BPD and head circumference (ie, OFC). These measurements are a typical part of the fetal biometric assessment during the 2nd trimester fetal ultrasound examination. BPD is measured by placing electronic calipers on either outer lateral edge of the skull at its widest part, using an angle perpendicular to the falx cerebri.[9] The OFC can subsequently be calculated by additionally obtaining the OFD by placing calipers in the center of the bone echo at both the frontal and occipital bones, then entering both the BPD and OFD values into the following equation: OFC (or head circumference) = 1.62 x (BPD + OFD).[9] The value obtained from this equation is then checked against reference tables listing normal OFC for gestational age and sex.

As mentioned previously, MRI is increasingly being included as part of the diagnostic evaluation for children with microcephaly. At present, there are no agreed-upon criteria or imaging parameters that explicitly identify microcephaly on MRI. That being said, there are findings that are commonly associated.

One example of commonly seen imaging finding is reduced complexity of brain gyration. In 2010, Vermeulen and colleagues created an MRI-based classification system to identify whether or not 12 infants with clinically identified microcephaly have a simplified brain gyration pattern. A 3-point subjective visual scale was established to grade the complexity of gyration: normal, simple, and severely simplified. A similar normal versus abnormal scale was created for basal ganglia and structures within the posterior fossa. Both scales were evaluated against a more objective morphologic analysis via the calculation of the gyral index, and this set of data was compared against data obtained from normocephalic controls. They found that their microcephalic cohort collectively demonstrated a gyral index that was much smaller than the normocephalic cohort.[10] Furthermore, they saw that their visual scale was accurate, as the assessment of simple and severely simple gyration correlated with the values obtained via the gyral index.[10]

It follows that multiple neuro-migrational abnormalities are, therefore, detectable on MRI. In infants found to have suffered from prenatal cytomegalovirus (CMV) infection with subsequent microcephaly, findings such as lissencephaly (smooth brain surface from the absence of brain sulcation), schizencephaly (congenital cleft extending from the cerebral ventricles to the cortical surface, lined with gray matter), and polymicrogyria (gray matter gyration composed of multiple small, abnormal gyri with irregular white–gray matter junction interface) are seen.[11] White matter abnormalities, such as extensive areas of delayed myelination or dysmyelination, can be seen in microcephalic infants with a history of Zika virus and CMV infection.[12]

Given the ability of MRI to find associated findings of microcephaly, attempts have been made to see if more objective findings can be made to explicitly establish microcephaly on MRI. One such attempt was carried out by Vannucci and colleagues in 2011.[13] The investigators retrospectively studied the MRIs of a cohort of 21 microcephalic patients with ages ranging from 2 weeks to 8.5 years old, obtaining craniometric measurements and ratios, and compared the data to that of an age/weight/sex-matched control cohort to seek out differences, if any were present. Data analysis revealed that there was a statistically significant difference between the groups regarding the ratio of the sagittal maximal cerebral height and axial maximal cerebral width (SCH/ACW), with the microcephalic cohort having a smaller ratio.[13] Similar significant findings were seen with the calculated sagittal frontal pole-cerebellar pole to sagittal maximal cerebral length ratio (FCP/SCL), ultimately indicating a longer frontal lobe to cerebellar pole length than frontal lobe to occipital pole length in the microcephalic cohort.[13]

Furthermore, these investigators were also able to establish that there was a statistically significant difference in brain volume in microcephalic patients when compared with their normocephalic counterparts, whereby the former was found to have reduced cerebral and cerebellar volumes among 1 to 2 years old and 2.5 to 8.5 years old age groups.[13] Collectively, these findings suggest MRI can augment and/or potentially confirm the detection of microcephaly as seen on ultrasound, and underscore the value of both modalities in the overall diagnostic evaluation.

Imaging Findings of Microcephaly Classifications

As previously stated, and as demonstrated in **Box 1** in the prior section, there is an innumerable amount of etiologies of pediatric microcephaly, too many to individually discuss in detail within this article. We, therefore, will attempt to describe the imaging findings of representative members of the different classes and display examples later in discussion.

Genetic and Chromosomal Anomalies

There are many causes of microcephaly that have a genetic basis, and therefore involve some level of Mendelian inheritance. Regardless of the particular gene(s) involved, the vast majority are due to processes that result in an imbalance between neuro-progenitor cell production and cell death.[3] They may be broadly classified into primary autosomal recessive microcephaly.

(MCPH) which is mostly due to disorders of progenitor cell proliferation; and Microcephaly with DNA repair deficiency.

Microcephaly Primary Hereditary (MCPH) or Autosomal recessive primary microcephaly or Microcephaly primary hereditary. One of the most studied entities within this group is microcephaly primary hereditary (MCPH), or primary autosomal recessive microcephaly, historically known as microcephalia vera. MCPH is a genetically and clinically heterogeneous disease. MCPH microcephaly is nonprogressive primary microcephaly. Brain size during birth is determined by both the proliferation rate and cell death rate during neurogenesis. This is a form of microcephaly now known to be associated with at least 12 different genetic loci.[3] Across the globe these 12 MCPH loci (MCPH1-MCPH12) have been mapped and contain the following genes: Microcephalin, WDR62, cyclin-dependent kinase 5 regulatory associated protein 2 (CDK5RAP2), CASC5, microcephaly associated protein (ASPM), CENPJ, SCL/TAL1-

---

Box 1
Causes of microcephaly

Genetic and Chromosomal Anomalies
  Genetic causes of microcephaly
  • Isolated
  • Autosomal recessive microcephaly
  • Autosomal dominant microcephaly
  • X-linked microcephaly
  Chromosomal disorders
  • Trisomy 21
  • Trisomy 13
  • Trisomy 18
  Contiguous gene deletion syndromes
  • 4p deletion (Wolf–Hirschhorn) syndrome
  • 7q11.23 deletion (Williams) syndrome
  • 17p13.3 deletion (Miller–Dieker lissencephaly syndrome
  • 5p15.2 deletion Cri-du-chat syndrome

Structural Brain Anomalies (Defect in Development)
• Neural tube defects (anencephaly, hydranencephaly, encephalocele)
• Defective cellular migration
• Defective neurulation
• Defective prosencephalization
• Agenesis of the corpus callosum
• Holoprosencephaly spectrum

Metabolic Causes (Genetic Etiology)
• Phenylketonuria
• Glycine encephalopathy
• Urea cycle disorders
• Organic aciduria
• Congenital disorders of glycosylation syndrome (CDG)
• Galactosemia
• Glucose transporter defect (GLUT1)
• Leukodystrophies, for example, Pelizaeus–Merzbacher diseases
• Mitochondriopathies
• Menkes diseases
• Neuronal ceroid lipofuscinosis (NCL)
• Peroxisomal and Lysosomal disorders
• Molybdenum cofactor deficiency and sulfite oxidase deficiency

Exogenic Factors/Environmental Causes of Microcephaly
• Intrauterine Infection (Toxoplasmosis, rubella, cytomegalovirus, herpes simplex, varicella zoster virus, syphilis, human immunodeficiency, virus)
• Teratogens (Alcohol, cocaine, antiepileptic drugs, lead/mercury intoxication, radiation)
• Vascular (Stroke, Intracranial hemorrhage)
• Perinatal brain injuries
• Hypoxic-ischemic encephalopathy
• Meningitis and encephalitis
• Postnatal chronic systemic diseases
• Malnutrition

---

interrupting locus (STIL), CEP135, CEP152, ZNF335, PHC1, and CDK6. It is hypothesized that the MCPH gene mutations lead to disturbed mitotic spindle orientation, premature chromosomal condensation, signaling response as a result of damaged DNA, microtubule dynamics, transcriptional control, or a few other hidden centrosomal mechanisms that can regulate the number of neurons produced by neuronal precursor cells.[14]

Affected patients show head circumference (HC) of at least 4 SD below the age- and sex-matched means; variable cognitive impairment, speech delay, hyperactivity, and attention deficit; no neurologic signs except mild seizures and pyramidal signs; absence of consistent associated anomalies, except facial dysmorphism secondary to narrow, sloping forehead. In primary microcephaly syndromes with the exception of MCPH1, height, weight, and growth velocity are typically within the normal range.[3,15] MRI brain shows reduced brain volumes for age affecting both cortex and white matter,[16] with a lack of specific findings (**Fig. 1**). Recently, it has been found that additional nonspecific abnormalities also arise, such as polymicrogyria, periventricular neuronal heterotopia, ventriculomegaly, agenesis of the corpus callosum, and brainstem hypoplasia.[16]

Microcephaly with Simplified Gyral Pattern (MSGP): Some primary microcephalies show an abnormally simplified gyral pattern without the thickening of the cerebral cortex; this group has been referred to as MSGP. The term "simplified gyral pattern" is most often used to describe a reduced number of gyri and shallow sulci with a normal cortical thickness.[17] MSGP is thought to be due to the result of reduced cell proliferation or increased apoptosis. It is postulated that decreased neuronal proliferation results in fewer cortical neurons and, thus, fewer axons exiting the cortex; this result might cause decreased tension arising from axons and, consequently, fewer and more shallow sulci. Clinically children with MSG may have more severe mental retardation, neurodevelopmental delay, and other associated central nervous system malformations than those with primary microcephaly. On MR, brain shows microcephaly with a reduced number of gyri and shallow sulci with a normal cortical thickness (**Fig. 2**). These findings are often associated with developmental brain anomalies, such as corpus callosal hypogenesis and hypoplasia, periventricular nodular heterotopia, and delayed myelination.[17]

Structural Brain Anomalies (Defects in Development)

Neuronal progenitor cell creation and migration are distinct processes that occur simultaneously during fetal development. It follows, therefore, that factors that control either process have a significant impact on the other. Indeed, factors involved with progenitor cell proliferation also regulate cortical neuron migration, and this may explain why defects in either process are associated with etiologies of microcephaly.[3] Congenital malformations commonly associated with microcephaly include neural tube defects, holoprosencephaly, atelencephaly, lissencephaly, schizencephaly, polymicrogyria, macrogyria, and fetal brain disruption sequence.

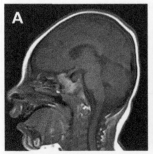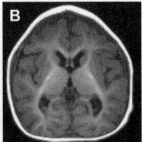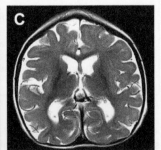

Fig. 1. Autosomal recessive Primary Microcephaly. Sag T1WI (A) shows head circumference of 3 SD below the age- and sex-matched means. Sagittal T1 demonstrate decreased craniofacial ratio and slanted forehead with otherwise normal brain and posterior fossa. Axial T1 (B) and T2 (C) images show a small but structural normal brain and normal myelination.

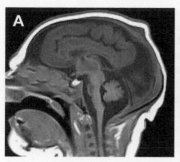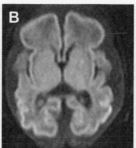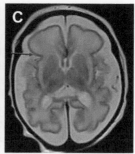

Fig. 2. Microcephaly with Simplified Gyral Pattern (MSGP). Sag T1 (A), axial FLAIR (B) and T2 (C) weighted images show head circumference of 4 SD below the age- and sex-matched means. MRI brain shows reduced brain volumes for age affecting both cortex and white matter with simplified brain gyration (*red arrows*).

Neural tube defects

Neural tube defects (NTD) are one of the most common malformations of the central nervous system. NTD can be classified depending on which stage of the neurulation is affected. Primary neurulation tube defects could be either because of tube closure or mesodermal defects, (anencephaly Craniorachischisis, Myelomeningocele), whereas secondary neurulation defects are mainly spinal and are seen in the lumbosacral region (Encephalocele, Meningocele).

Anencephaly occurs when the cephalic end of the embryonic neural tube fails to close, resulting in an absence of the calvarium and brain (Cater and colleagues, 2020). On prenatal ultrasound, these findings are usually apparent at some point halfway during the second trimester, and reveal a lack of neural tissue above the bilateral orbits.[8] Polyhydramnios, frog-like facies, and ill-defined soft tissue echoes superior to the orbits may also be present.[8]

Cephalocele

Cephaloceles are congenital defects in the cranium and dura with protrusion of the intracranial structures. Depending on the content of the sac, they are classified into 4 categories[1]: cranial meningocele, defined as the protrusion of leptomeninges and CSF[2]; cranial glioceles, defined as glial lined cysts[3]; meningoencephalocele, defined as the herniation of leptomeninges, CSF, and brain parenchyma.[8] On prenatal ultrasound, encephalocele feature a mixed cystic and solid tissue lesion protruding through a calvarial defect. It should be noted that, at times, differentiating between any one of these entities may be difficult to do on ultrasound alone; MRI would be necessary in those cases to delineate the neural contents. Postnatal neuroimaging is performed to evaluate the intracranial components of the malformation and identify any associated brain or vascular anomalies. Other cerebral malformations associated with encephalocele include complete or partial agenesis of the corpus callosum, myelomeningocele, hydrocephalus, corpus callosal abnormalities, and cerebral dysgenesis.

Corpus callosum agenesis

Another structural defect that can result in or contribute to the finding of microcephaly is agenesis of the corpus callosum (ACC). Clinically, affected patients often demonstrate learning disabilities, some with concurrent epilepsy due to focal heterotopia.[7] On imaging, ACC can be partial or complete and is often seen with an intact anterior commissure on MRI.[18] On prenatal ultrasound, an early clue to the presence of ACC is the nonvisualization of the cavum septum pellucidum on axial views.[8] Additionally, nonobstructive hydrocephalus, with colpocephaly (teardrop configuration to the occipital horns of the lateral ventricles), are often seen with ACC.[8] Notably, on both MRI and ultrasound, nondevelopment of the cingulate gyrus is also present, allowing for deep brain gyri to radially extend from the margins of the ventricular system to the cerebral surface.[18] Furthermore, on MRI coronal views, ill-defined bundles of white matter, known as Probst bundles, can be appreciated along the medial borders of the lateral ventricles[18]; these are congregates of the neurons that failed to migrate properly to form the corpus callosum.

Holoprosencephaly

Holoprosencephaly (HPE) results when there is a failure of the prosencephalon, or forebrain, to divide into the cerebral hemispheres early on during gestation, usually by the 4th or 5th week. There are multiple forms; however, there are 3 characteristically distinct forms, with increasing levels of severity: lobar, semilobar, and alobar.[8] HPE is associated with midline facial abnormalities, including cleft palate/lip, hypotelorism, and cyclopia.

In alobar HPE, there is a complete failure of prosencephalic cleavage, which results in a singular midline forebrain and monoventricle, appreciable on both ultrasound and MRI.[19] The contours of the forebrain can take on multiple shapes, including that of a ball, cup, or pancake; the ball form consists of the cerebral tissue completely encircling the monoventricle, and the latter 2 forms display decreasing amounts of circumferential enclosure of the monoventricle[19] (**Fig. 3**). Notably, multiple cerebral structures are absent, including the corpus callosum, anterior commissure, cavum septum pellucidum, and interhemispheric fissure, with a variable presence of the optic nerves.[7,19] The basal ganglia, hypothalamic and thalamic nuclei are fused in the midline, and the presence of fused midline structures and a monoventricle are key conspicuous features noted on ultrasound, and further characterized on MRI.[19]

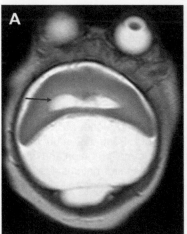 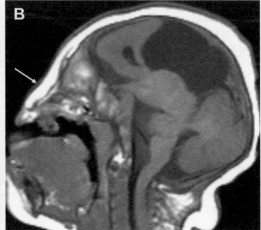

Fig. 3. Alobar holoprosencephaly and microcephaly: Axial T2 (A) and Sag T1 (B) weighted images show multiple features of holoprosencephaly including absent interhemispheric fissure, horseshoe-shaped monoventricle (*red arrow*), absent falx, absent septum pellucidum. Sagittal image shows agenesis of the corpus callosum and features of microcephaly including decreased craniofacial ratio and slanted frontal bone (*yellow arrow*).

In comparison to alobar HPE, the diagnosis of both semilobar and lobar HPE are considerably less straightforward. Semilobar HPE occurs when there is partial separation of the forebrain, occurring along a posterior-to-anterior basis. The cerebral falx and interhemispheric fissure are often present posteriorly, and the corpus callosum is also partially present.[19] The amount of separation can vary. Importantly, the deep nuclei (thalamic and hypothalamic) are also variably separated.[19] In lobar HPE, separation of the forebrain is nearly complete, and the interhemispheric fissure and cerebral falx can be appreciated along almost the entire midline,[19] and the deep nuclei are usually separated. The distinction between semilobar and lobar HPE is not definite, but findings are classified as lobar if, on either ultrasound or MRI, the 3rd ventricle is appreciated, and rudimentary frontal horns and posterior regions of the corpus callosum are present.[19]

Decreased Proliferation/Increased Apoptosis: Microcephaly and Microlissencephaly

Microcephaly due to defect in the proliferation may be classified into 3 different types: (a) microcephaly with normal to thin cortex, (b) microcephaly with thick cortex (microlissencephaly) (**Fig. 4**), and (c) microcephaly with polymicrogyria or other malformation of cortical development.[20] Microcephaly with normal to thin cortex is seen most frequently with autosomal-recessive inherited disorders and is further classified into 2 subtypes. The first subtype includes patients with normal to slightly short stature, higher function, and a mutation involving at least 1 of 6 specific loci on the MCPH gene. No clinical or imaging signs can effectively differentiate these particular loci. The second subtype includes patients with normal or slightly short stature and very poor function. Examples include Amish-type lethal microcephaly (SLC25A19 mutations on chromosome 17q25.3) and microcephaly with periventricular nodular heterotopia (ARFGEF2 mutations), microlissencephaly, as the name suggests, shows microcephaly with a smooth thickened cortex. In most cases, microlissencephaly has syndromic associations.[20,21] CT or MRI typically shows small overall brain size and fewer than normal gyri with abnormally shallow sulci. There is a overall reduction in the white matter with the preservation of normal myelination. In addition to these findings, microlissencephaly also shows complete/near-complete agyria with thickened cortex. Corpus callosal agenesis and/or cerebellar hypoplasia may also be present.

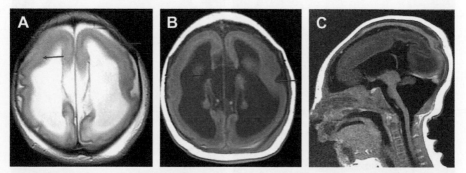

Fig. 4. . Microlissencephaly. Axial T2 (A), and axial T1 (B) WI denote presence of lissencephaly (red arrows) in the setting of microcephaly. T2 and T1 weighted MR demonstrate smooth cortex with ventriculomegaly. Sagittal T1 weighted (C) MR shows decreased craniofacial ratio with slanted frontal bone. Cerebellar hypoplasia is also present.

Malformations Attributable to Abnormal Neuronal Migration Lissencephaly

Lissencephaly (LIS; lissen = smooth and leucon = brain) is a severe form of abnormal neuroral migration characterized by an absence of gyri with a thickened cortex (agyria) or the presence of few broad fat gyri with a thickened cortex (pachygyria), both leading to a relatively smooth featureless brain. The basic pathology in lissencephaly is an arrest of normal neuronal migration leading to a 4-layer cortex (instead of the normal 6 layers) that consists of: (i) an outer marginal layer, (ii) a superficial cellular layer (disorganized pyramidal neurons), (iii) a variable cell sparse layer (layer III), and (iv) a deep cellular layer composed of medium-sized and small neurons(20). As per the revised molecular genetics classification, lissencephaly is classified into the following categories: (a) LIS1 mutations, (b) DCX mutations, (c) ARX mutations, (d) RELN mutations, and (e) other lissencephaly/pachygyria syndromes with or without cerebellar hypoplasia.[20,22] On imaging, classical lissencephaly shows a smooth brain with the vertical orientation of the sylvian fissures giving the cerebrum a "**Fig. 8**" appearance on axial images (**Fig. 5**). Also present is an overall decrease in white matter throughout the cerebrum. The degree of malformation and distribution of the gyral pattern depends primarily on the severity of the mutation.[20,22] Patients with the LIS1 defect typically present with a more pronounced pattern of lissencephaly (agyria) in the parietooccipital region and pachygyria in the frontal region, while those with the DCX mutation tend to exhibit asymmetrically prominent lissencephaly in the anterior regions.

Metabolic Causes and Leukodystrophies

There are many leukodystrophies and inborn errors of metabolism that are associated with pediatric microcephaly, yet the prevalence of distinct conditions in microcephalic children is not established.[2] Typically, a lack or malfunction of an enzyme, or enzymes, in a given metabolic pathway allows for the accumulation of organic metabolites that alter the function of neurons and eventual death leading to a reduction in the volume of

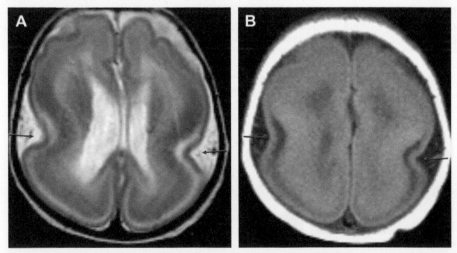

Fig. 5. Microcephaly with lissencephaly. Axial T2 (A) and DWI (B) WI show a thickened, agyric cortex, shallow vertically oriented sylvian fissures, giving figure of 8 appearance (red arrows). There is severely diminished cerebral white matter.

the brain parenchyma. This may occur in the pre or postnatal period and accounts for the varied presentations of entities in this category. Metabolic disorders associated with microcephaly include Untreated maternal phenylketonuria, aminoaciduria (phenylketonuria), adenylosuccinate lyase deficiency, cerebral glucose transporter (GLUT1) deficiency, methylmalonic aciduria, urea cycle disorders (eg, citrullinemia), and certain storage diseases (eg, neuronal ceroid lipofuscinosis). Inborn errors of metabolism more often lead to secondary microcephaly. Targeted metabolic studies are performed based on the patient's medical and family history, clinical examination, and neuroimaging.

Mitochondriopathies. The mitochondriopathies are a heterogeneous group of conditions that result from mitochondrial dysfunction. A characteristic example associated with microcephaly is Amish lethal microcephaly. Essentially isolated to the Lancaster Amish community of Lancaster, PA, it is a very rare condition that results in severe microcephaly and early onset developmental delay, and markedly elevated levels of urinary and serum 2-ketoglutarate in times of metabolic stress (eg, illness).[23] The key defect isolates to a mutation of the SLC25A19 gene, which encodes for a deoxynucleotide carrier in the inner mitochondrial membrane.[24] Classical imaging finding seen on MRI brain is a smooth, immature brain similar to that of a 20-week fetus except for a moderate degree of cerebellar vermal hypoplasia. Other imaging findings may include partial agenesis of the corpus callosum, lissencephaly, abnormally large cisterna magna communicating with the 4th ventricle, cerebellar hypoplasia, and global cerebral atrophy.[23,24]

Pyruvate dehydrogenase complex deficiency: The pyruvate dehydrogenase complex is composed of 3 enzymes that ultimately convert pyruvate into downstream metabolites that partake in the Krebs cycle. Phosphoglycerate dehydrogenase deficiency is an autosomal recessive disorder caused by a defect in the synthesis of L-serine. It is characterized by hypomyelination, congenital microcephaly, psychomotor retardation, and intractable seizures.[25] White matter volume loss is evident on brain MRI, and spastic quadriplegia ensues. A diagnosis is made by analyzing CSF amino acid levels, with the characteristic abnormalities best appreciated in the fasting state. The typical pattern reveals low levels of serine, glycine, and 5-methyltetrahydrofolate.

On MRI imaging during the prenatal period, characteristic findings include ventriculomegaly, parenchymal pseudocyst formation, significant white matter volume loss, partial or complete loss of the corpus callosum, hypoplasia of the brainstem, and lack of cortical gyration.[25] The putamen and caudate nucleus are the most frequently affected, but the globus pallidus, subthalamic nucleus, dentate nucleus, substantia nigra, tegmentum of pons, periaqueductal gray, red nucleus, medulla, and other brainstem structures are also frequently involved. These areas are edematous during the acute stage and show hyperintensity on T2 or FLAIR images.

Leukodystrophies. Leukodystrophies are a heterogeneous group of disorders that primarily affect white matter. They may arise from the disordered formation of myelin (dysmyelination) or from the breakdown of myelin (demyelination). Leukodystrophies with microcephaly are commonly seen with Aicardi–Goutieres Syndrome, Cockayne Syndrome; 3-methylglutaconic aciduria type 1, methylenetetrahydrofolate reductase deficiency; oculodentodigital dysplasia with cerebral white matter abnormalities; Pelizaeus–Merzbacher-like disease; RARS-related hypomyelination.

Pelizaeus–Merzbacher disease (PMD): Transferred through either autosomal or X-linked recessive inheritance, this extremely rare disorder clinically results in abnormal eye movements/nystagmus, spasticity, delayed psychomotor development, and extrapyramidal hyperkinesias.[26] MRI characteristically displays a virtually complete lack of normal myelination with resultant high T2 signal intensity throughout the deep white matter, extending into the subcortical U fibers[26]; in some cases, imaging reveals a more heterogeneous pattern of myelination such that the brain displays an overall "tigroid" appearance on MRI.[26] Interestingly, in 2016, Meng and colleagues[27] recently found a more direct link between PMD-like diseases and microcephaly. They were able to identify in 5 different patients that the presence of a loss-of-function mutation in the PYCR2 gene, one that codes for an enzyme that catalyzes proline biosynthesis, results in a dysmyelinating form of leukodystrophy that causes progressive postnatal microcephaly and severe developmental delay.[26] Indeed, across multiple patients over time, the presence of progressive global cerebral atrophy and white matter loss, and agenesis of the corpus callosum were apparent.[26]

Neuronal Ceroid Lipofuscinoses. Neuronal ceroid-lipofuscinosis (NCL) is one of the most common neurodegenerative disorders of childhood. The first symptom of the affected child is the failure of vision. The child might also develop muscular hypotonia, microcephaly, ataxia, choreoathetosis, stereotyped hand movements, myoclonic jerks, epilepsy, irritability, and visual failure.[28] The impairment of palmitoyl protein thioesterase 1 (PPT1) leads to the accumulation of ceroid lipopigment in lysosomes of neurons, inducing deleterious effects on the functioning of neurons that leads to neuronal death. The pathologic hallmark of NCL is neuronal lipofuscin storage and neuronal loss leading to severe atrophy of the brain, with moderate to severe loss of myelin and significant astrogliosis.

CT scan of the brain shows severe atrophy; cerebral is more severe than the cerebellum. There is severe thinning of the cortex with diffuse hypodensity of the white matter. On MRI, the white matter shows high signal intensity on T2-weighted image in all stages of the disease (**Fig. 6**). These changes are thought to be due to a combination of delayed and disturbed myelination, increasingly severe gliosis, and some myelin loss.[28]

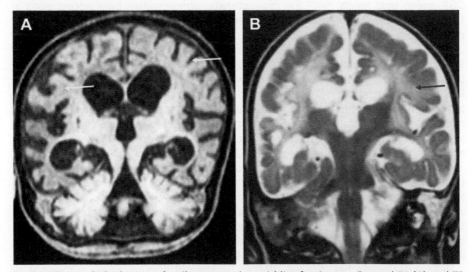

Fig. 6. Microcephaly due to Infantile neuronal ceroid lipofuscinoses. Coronal T1 (A) and T2 (B) images show advanced brain atrophy (yellow arrows) for age with large ventricles and sulci. Supratentorial white matter is diffusely hyperintense (red arrow) on T2 weighted image.

Miscellaneous and Environmental Causes of Microcephaly

Intrauterine Infections. Maternal exposure to a number of viral, bacterial, and parasitic infectious agents is a well-documented cause of pediatric microcephaly. That said, overall, congenital infection is far from the most common underlying causative diagnosis.[29] Before the emergence of Zika virus, "TORCH" agents (*Toxoplasma gondii*, rubella virus, and cytomegalovirus) were the most common causes of the infection-induced microcephaly. All these pathogens are neurotropic to the fetal CNS cells leading to brain destruction with calcifications, microcephaly, sensorineural hearing loss, and ophthalmologic abnormalities in addition to microcephaly.[29] Blood workup and imaging are commonly used in the diagnosis of a suspected case of intrauterine infection. The most commonly used test is enzyme-linked immunosorbent assay (ELISA). It is important to note that positive serology testing for virus-specific immunoglobulinM (IgM) and immunoglobulinG (IgG) antibodies does not necessarily mean that the fetus will be affected by the pathogen. Imaging with antenatal ultrasound and/or fetal MRI is very useful in documenting structural abnormalities.

Congenital cytomegalovirus (CMV) infection is one of the most common congenital viral infections worldwide and is the most common in the US.[11] Infants born to mothers with primary CMV infection during pregnancy have, on average, the risk of congenital infection in the order of 30% to 40%, while those born following non-primary maternal infection have a risk in the order of 1% to 2% (USG practice guidelines). The vast majority of those infected display no symptoms, and there is often no maternal–fetal transfer. Maternal patients who are immunocompromised face an increased risk of fetal transfer.[30] In those patients, transfer to and infection of the fetus can occur at any time, but a greater risk of severe neurologic damage is present when it occurs in the first or second trimesters.[30] Clinical features can vary depending on when the fetus is exposed, but it is understood that the earlier exposure occurs during gestation, the more severe they can become. Symptoms include sensorineural hearing loss, chorioretinitis leading to vision impairment, seizures, and cognitive impairment.[11]

Microcephaly is appreciated in more than 25% of patients with congenital CMV infection, and it represents one of the many forms of cerebral atrophy seen with this condition; when identified, either explicitly on physical examination or implicitly on imaging via global volume loss, it portends a poor neurologic outcome if the patient is symptomatic (Fink and colleagues, 2010). Additional imaging findings include dystrophic periventricular and punctate basal ganglia calcifications, migrational abnormalities (eg, lissencephaly, polymicrogyria), ventriculomegaly with or without septations, and T2 hyperintense white matter lesions related to delayed myelination[11,29] **(Fig. 7)**. Regarding white matter abnormalities, it has been found that the largest of the lesions are found in the deep white matter of the parietal lobes, particularly when there are no significant gyral abnormalities identified.[31] Other associated imaging findings include ophthalmologic abnormalities (chorioretinitis, retinal atrophy, and microphthalmia, often unilateral), thrombocytopenia, petechiae, purpura hepatosplenomegaly, jaundice, and hyperbilirubinemia.

Toxoplasmosis is another similarly infectious agent capable of maternal–fetal transfer. Similar to CMV infection, most in the general population who come into contact with it display no symptoms. If symptomatic, maternal patients typically display nonspecific lymphadenopathy and fever. Affected newborns can display symptoms that demonstrate a range of severity related to when parasitic contact with the fetus occurred; it has been found that the earlier (ie, first or second trimester) fetal infection

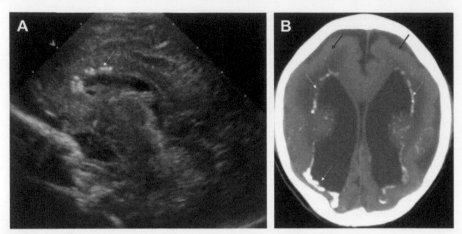

Fig. 7. Intrauterine cytomegalovirus infection with microcephaly. Sag view of the cranial ultrasound (A) shows speckled periventricular calcification. Axial CT scan (B) of the brain shows dense periventricular calcification (yellow arrows). Also seen is migrational abnormalities (lissencephaly)(red arrows) in the bilateral cerebral parenchyma.

occurs, the more severe symptoms tend to be.[30] Clinical findings include microcephaly, developmental delay, seizures, chorioretinitis, and infantile anemia and jaundice.[30] Microcephaly is noted in 5% to 15% of severely symptomatic congenitally infected infants, and microphthalmia in 1% to 2%.

In utero, characteristic imaging findings on ultrasound include scattered echogenic cerebral nodules in no particular location. These correspond to calcifications appreciated on CT/MRI; unlike in CMV, these nodular calcifications arise secondary to necrosis.[29] Other imaging findings include hydrocephalus, ventriculomegaly, and chorioretinitis; and hepatosplenomegaly (**Fig. 8**). The interpretation of toxoplasma

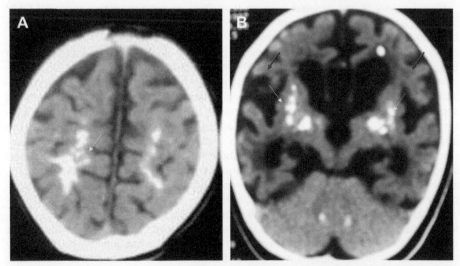

Fig. 8. Microcephaly due to intrauterine toxoplasmosis infection. Axial (A) and coronal (B) images of the CT show coarse calcification (yellow arrows) scattered throughout the cerebral white matter. Also note atrophic changes (red arrows) in the bilateral cerebral hemispheres.

test results may be challenging. Diagnosis of maternal toxoplasmosis infections can be made by testing maternal serum, including toxoplasma IgM and IgG.

Zika Virus Infection. The Zika virus is an arbovirus transmitted by mosquitos. This virus has been commonly associated with congenital infections of the central nervous system and has greatly increased the rates of microcephaly. Infected patients present with fever, small joint pain, myalgia, maculopapular rash, retro-orbital headache, and conjunctivitis. The diagnosis of Zika virus infection is based on the demonstration of the virus in the blood (acute phase) and urine (after the first week of symptoms) by using real-time reverse transcription-polymerase chain reaction (RT-PCR).[32]

Most common imaging findings seen in prenatal ultrasonography is microcephaly. Other findings which may be encountered are cortical and/or periventricular calcifications, cerebral atrophy, ventriculomegaly, corpus callosum abnormalities, brainstem hypoplasia, enlarged cisterna magna, craniofacial disproportion, and redundant scalp skin in the occipital region. In suspected cases, fetal MRI may be performed for a better demonstration of the cortical gyral abnormalities, polymicrogyria, agyria (lissencephaly), and pachygyria (**Fig. 9**).

Postnatal evaluation with USG may be challenging due to premature closures of fontanelles. However, US still remains the first modality of the choice in the evaluation of the brain parenchyma and associated anomalies such as thinning of the parenchyma, punctiform calcifications, and dysgenesis of the corpus callosum.[33,34] MRI is more sensitive in defining the brain malformation in infant with Zika virus infection. Cross-sectional imaging shows microcephaly with craniosynostosis, and junctional calcifications between the cortex and the subcortical white matter. MRI may also show decreased brain volume, and diffuse cortical atrophy characterized by diffuse cortical thinning, enlarged supratentorial subarachnoid space, widely open sylvian fissures, and ventriculomegaly.[33,34] Delayed myelination and dysmyelination, agyria, extremely diminished volume of white matter, delayed myelination, small cerebellum, and enlarged lateral ventricles, have been described in these syndromes.

Teratogens. Ethanol is a well-known teratogen and is among the most commonly encountered teratogens in the US.[15] It has far-reaching clinical symptomatology, and can result in effects that last throughout infancy into childhood.[15] Demonstrating this, in 2012, Feldman and colleagues published a report on a prospective study on approximately 1000 neonates born between 1978 and 2005 who were prenatally exposed to ethanol in attempts to quantitatively define ethanol's effects on newborns, with regards to incidence of microcephaly and other dysmorphic features. They found that there was a 12% increase in the incidence of microcephaly in newborns with mothers who had at least 1 drink per day (on average) when compared with those

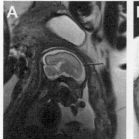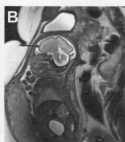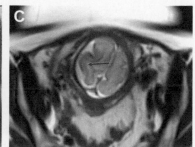

Fig. 9. Zica virus microcephaly: Sagittal (A,B) and axial (C) view of the head on fetal MRI shows microcephaly with BPD <1 percentile. There is simplified sulcation pattern given estimated gestational age of 30 weeks. Poorly delineated corpus collosum, possibly hypoplastic.

who averaged less per day. Additionally, these effects are the most significant in those who sustained those averages when consuming alcohol in the first trimester. Even higher incidences were noted with facial dysmorphism and decreases birth weight.[35]

In 2004, Riley and associates[36] conducted a review of the literature spanning over 10 years' worth of ongoing research on the imaging findings of patients who were diagnosed with either fetal alcohol syndrome (FAS) or fetal alcohol spectrum disorder (FASD). This was an attempt to thoroughly document the wide range of effects that ethanol exposure can have on the developing brain and to conglomerate the results of multiple studies into a succinct review. They found that one of the most consistent findings across multiple studies was the presence of microcephaly in either group of patients; indeed, it was commonly seen that there is a reduction in the size of the cranial vault in neonates following prenatal ethanol exposure.[36] Additionally, reduction in cerebellar volume was very commonly seen. Compared with nonaffected controls in various studies, patients with FAS were found to have a greater than 15% loss of cerebellar volume, and this was often focused on the anterior vermis.[36] Additional findings that were found include partial and complete agenesis of the corpus callosum, atrophy of the basal ganglia and caudate nucleus[36] (**Fig. 10**). Individual members of Riley's team of researchers also conducted studies assessing whether MRI volumetric analysis could detect differences between patients with FAS and normally developing children. In concert with colleagues from associated institutions, they found that there was a marked reduction in the size of both the temporal and parietal lobes, specifically involving the peri-Sylvian cortices.[36] Additional data from these studies revealed that the posterior regions of the corpus callosum connecting the bilateral peri-Sylvian cortices of the temporal and parietal lobes were the most atrophied in patients with FAS.[36]

In 2018, Petrelli and colleagues[37] attempted to further study the genetic and enzymatic pathways that fetal ethanol exposure effects to result in FAS. They demonstrated that ethanol exposure decreases the retinoic acid enzymatic activity which plays a role in the development of craniofacial abnormalities seen in FAS, which include microcephaly.[37]

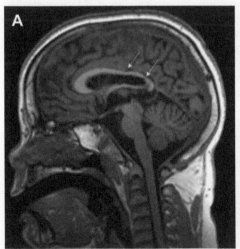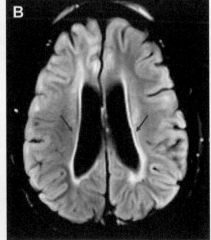

Fig. 10. Microcephaly due to Fetal alcohol syndrome. Sag T1 (A) and Axial FLAIR (B) images demonstrate abnormally elongated philtrum and thinned corpus callosum (yellow arrows) with microcephaly. There is ventriculomegaly of the lateral ventricles with patchy hyperintensity (red arrows) of the cerebral white matter.

Another class of teratogens associated with microcephaly and other neurologic malformations is antiepileptic drugs (AEDs). AEDs have been in use for seizure control for many decades by many people, including expectant women. Research into their teratogenic effects and postnatal complications dates back to the 1960s with the discovery of thalidomide embryonic toxicity.[38] More recent studies have attempted to quantitatively document their impact. In 2013, Veiby and colleagues[39] conducted a retrospective analysis on 2600 infants born to mothers who had been taking a mix of old- and new-generation AEDs for epilepsy and other related conditions during pregnancy. This cohort was compared with another group of more than 770,000 infants with no AED prenatal exposure. They found that overall, the risk of microcephaly was more than five times that of the general population (11.4% vs 2.4%), and that number was even higher for those taking older generation drugs, such as topiramate (14.9% vs 2.4%).[39]

The exposure of AEDs to the fetus in utero is associated with various neural tube defects.[8] These include findings such as anencephaly and the cephaloceles, the latter of which can be seen in the different presentations of spina bifida.[8] It is believed that the exposure to AEDs can negatively affect the migration of neuronal progenitor cells that lead to neural tube defects. However, AEDs may affect processes that control progenitor cell creation as well. Indeed, prenatal AED exposure has been linked with the occurrence of global cerebellar hypoplasia. In this imaging finding, the cerebellum displays a normal or near-normal shape, but there is a marked reduction in its volume, and the surrounding subarachnoid spaces are abnormally prominent. On imaging major congenital malformations found in pregnancies exposed to carbamazepine, valproate, and phenytoin include neural tube defects, facial clefts, cardiac defects, hypospadias, and skeletal abnormalities. Treatment with valproic acid has a greater risk of spina bifida, atrial septal defects, cleft palate, and craniosynostosis, while carbamazepine shows a greater risk of spina bifida.

Intracranial Hemorrhage (ICH). ICH can occur in either the prenatal or postnatal periods. One of the most common etiologies for prenatal ICH is germinal matrix hemorrhages. The germinal matrix is a densely cellular and vascularized focus of periventricular cerebral tissue that is the site of neuronal and glial differentiation in the fetal brain. Its walls are relatively weak compared with surrounding tissue and, thus, prone to injury. Severity can vary from a self-limiting finding on prenatal ultrasound (most commonly a hyperechoic collection in the caudothalamic groove) to intraventricular hemorrhage with obstructive hydrocephalus and parenchymal extension.[40] In cases of the latter, neuronal death can occur, and result in cystic encephalomalacia that communicates with the ventricular system.[8]

In cases of postnatal hemorrhage, nonaccidental causes of ICH are, unfortunately, commonly encountered in the pediatric population. An estimated 24.6 cases per 100,000 children under the age of 1 year occur each year.[41] Both morbidity and mortality are high, and it can lead to long-term neurologic consequences, including epilepsy, vision loss and impairment, and neurodevelopmental delay.[41] Lo et al also demonstrated that microcephaly and significant cerebral atrophy were common in the previously treated for nonaccidental trauma. On imaging, these patients show microcephaly, diffuse thickening of the calvarium, cerebral atrophy or chronic changes in contusions, diffuse axonal injury, and hypoxic-ischemic injury.

Hypoxic-Ischemic Injury/Hypoxic-Ischemic Encephalopathy (HIE). Not much is known about the pathophysiology of HIE, but it is agreed on that both the lack of blood flow and decreased oxygen content of blood leads to abnormal cerebral autoregulation and injury.[42,43] As stated in the prior section, hypoxic-ischemic injury and resultant HIE can result from nonaccidental trauma, but it can also arise from other insults, such

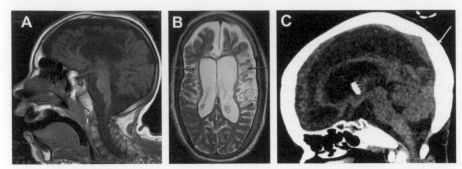

Fig. 11. Microcephaly secondary to diffuse Hypoxic Ischemic Injury. Sag T1 (A) and axial T2 (B) images show diffuse bilateral encephalomalacia with severe loss of white matter (red arrows) and dilatation of lateral ventricles. There is severe atrophy of corpus callosum and microcephaly. Sagittal reconstructed image of CT scan (C) shows severe encephalomalacia, microcephaly and diffuse thickening of the calvarium (yellow arrow).

as maternal infection, maternal pulmonary embolism, pneumonia, severe anemia, fetal bradycardia, and much more.[42]

In premature infants, if HIE is suspected, findings of leukomalacia are typically seen in the periventricular white matter in cases of mild to moderate hypoperfusion, whereas in severe cases, leukomalacia is appreciated in areas of high metabolic activity, which include the thalami, brainstem, and cerebellum.[42] Oftentimes, making this diagnosis is challenging based on the stage of myelination present, as normal adult-type myelination patterns are not seen until around 2 years of age. Areas of concern initially appear as hyperechoic foci on ultrasound, with corresponding hyperintensity on T1 and T2 MRI sequences; these same areas later develop cystic change over time, appearing as anechoic on ultrasound and solely T2 hyperintense on MRI. In many cases, there is eventual loss of cerebral/cerebellar parenchyma, with resultant ex-vacuo ventriculomegaly, and loss of white matter in the periventricular regions and corpus callosum[42] (**Fig. 11**). In infants who are born at full term, HIE from mild to moderate hypoperfusion results in injury to the vascular watershed zones between the anterior-middle and middle-posterior cerebral arteries, and in the thalami, hippocampi, brainstem, and corticospinal tracts in cases of severe injury.[42] This is discussed in detail under the imaging of premature infants in this issue.

SUMMARY

Microcephaly is a frequent clinical sign associated with numerous disorders of diverse etiology. Defining the exact cause of microcephaly is very challenging clinically. However, it is important to pinpoint the exact cause and diagnosis, for counseling the patient and the affected family, to understand the clinical course, and recurrence risk. It takes a multidisciplinary approach to classify and understand the exact cause of the microcephaly. Besides the thorough physical examination, laboratory tests, and genetic counseling, imaging plays a vital role in classifying the types, severity, and understand the risk of recurrence.

CASE IN POINT

- Microcephaly is not a diagnosis, but rather, a finding that is secondary to a multitude of etiologies that can be categorized as prenatal versus postnatal, genetic versus environmental, and congenital versus acquired.

- Microcephaly is primary, whereby it is present at birth or identified prenatally, and secondary, whereby a child is born with a normal OFC but subsequently demonstrates altered, abnormal growth
- Multidisciplinary team that includes a neurologist/pediatric neurologist, geneticist, and dysmorphologist is necessary for identifying the underlying cause of the microcephaly.

DISCLOSURE

The authors have nothing to disclose.

REFERENCES

1. Elgamal EA, Salih MA. Disorders of head shape and size. Clin Child Neurol 2020;957–99. https://doi.org/10.1007/978-3-319-43153-6_33.
2. Becerra-Solano LE, Mateos-Sánchez L, López-Muñoz E. Microcephaly, an etiopathogenic vision. Pediatr Neonatal 2021;62(4):354–60.
3. Passemard S, Kaindl A, Verloes A. Microcephaly. Handbook Clin Neurol 2013;3: 129–41. https://doi.org/10.1016/b978-0-444-53497-2.09992-7.
4. de Oliveira WK, de França GV, Carmo EH, et al. Infection-related microcephaly after the 2015 and 2016 zika virus outbreaks in Brazil: a Surveillance-based analysis. Lancet 2017;390(10097):861–70.
5. Morris SK, Farrar DS, Miller SP, et al. Population-based surveillance of severe microcephaly and congenital zika syndrome in Canada. Arch Dis Child 2021; 106(9):855–61.
6. von der Hagen M, Pivarcsi M, Liebe J, et al. Diagnostic approach to microcephaly in childhood: a two-center study and review of the literature. Developmental Med Child Neurol 2014;56(8):732–41.
7. Fenichel, G. M. (2009). Disorders of cranial volume and shape. In Clinical pediatric neurology a signs and symptoms approach (6th ed., pp. 369–386). essay, Elsevier-Saunders.
8. Cater SW, Boyd BK, Ghate SV. Abnormalities of the fetal central nervous system: prenatal US diagnosis with postnatal correlation. RadioGraphics 2020;40(5): 1458–72.
9. Salomon LJ, Alfirevic Z, Berghella V, et al. Practice guidelines for performance of the routine mid-trimester fetal ultrasound scan. Ultrasound Obstet Gynecol 2010; 37(1):116–26.
10. Vermeulen RJ, Wilke M, Horber V, et al. Microcephaly with simplified gyral pattern: MRI classification. Neurology 2010;74(5):386–91.
11. Fink KR, Thapa MM, Ishak GE, et al. Neuroimaging of pediatric central nervous system cytomegalovirus infection. RadioGraphics 2010;30(7):1779–96.
12. Ribeiro BG, Werner H, Lopes FP, et al. Central Nervous System Effects of intrauterine zika virus infection: a pictorial review. RadioGraphics 2017;37(6): 1840–50.
13. Vannucci RC, Barron TF, Vannucci SJ. Craniometric measures of microcephaly using MRI. Early Hum Dev 2012;88(3):135–40.
14. Mochida GH. Genetics and biology of microcephaly and Lissencephaly. Semin Pediatr Neurol 2009;16(3):120–6.
15. Abuelo D. Microcephaly syndromes. Semin Pediatr Neurol 2007;14(3):118–27.
16. Zaqout S, Morris-Rosendahl D, Kaindl A. Autosomal recessive primary microcephaly (MCPH): an Update. Neuropediatrics 2017;48(03):135–42.

17. Adachi Y, Poduri A, Kawaguch A, et al. Congenital microcephaly with a simplified gyral pattern: associated findings and their significance. AJNR Am J Neuroradiol 2011;32(6):1123–9.

18. Choudhri AF, Cohen HL, Siddiqui A, et al. Twenty-five diagnoses on midline images of the brain: from fetus to child to adult. RadioGraphics 2018;38(1):218–35.

19. Winter TC, Kennedy AM, Woodward PJ. Holoprosencephaly: a survey of the entity, with embryology and fetal imaging. RadioGraphics 2015;35(1):275–90.

20. Barkovich AJ, Kuzniecky RI, Jackson GD, et al. A developmental and genetic classification for malformations of cortical development. Neurology 2005;65: 1873–87.

21. Barkovich AJ, Ferriero DM, Barr RM, et al. Microlissencephaly: a heterogeneous malformation of cortical development. Neuropediatrics 1998;29:113–9.

22. Kanekar Sangam, Gent Michael. Malformations of cortical development. Semin Ultrasound CT MR 2011;32(3):211–27.

23. Kelley RI, Robinson D, Puffenberger EG, et al. Amish lethal microcephaly: a new metabolic disorder with severe congenital microcephaly and 2-ketoglutaric aciduria. Am J Med Genet 2002;112(4):318–26.

24. Siu VM, Ratko S, Prasad AN, et al. Amish microcephaly: long-term survival and biochemical characterization. Am J Med Genet A 2010;152A(7):1747–51.

25. Gonçalves FG, Alves CA, Heuer B, et al. Primary mitochondrial disorders of the pediatric central nervous system: neuroimaging findings. RadioGraphics 2020; 40(7):2042–67.

26. Cheon J-E, Kim I-O, Hwang YS, et al. Leukodystrophy in children: a pictorial review of mr imaging features. RadioGraphics 2002;22(3):461–76.

27. Meng L, Donti T, Xia F, et al. Homozygous variants in pyrroline-5-carboxylate reductase 2 (PYCR2) in patients with progressive microcephaly and hypomyelinating leukodystrophy. Am J Med Genet Part A 2016;173(2):460–70.

28. Seitz D, Grodd W, Schwab A, et al. MR imaging and Localized Proton MR Spectroscopy in late infantile neuronal ceroid lipofuscinosis. Am J Neuroradiology 1998;19(7):1373–7.

29. Levine D, Jani JC, Castro-Aragon I, et al. How does imaging of congenital zika compare with imaging of other torch infections? Radiology 2017;285(3):744–61.

30. Frenkel LD, Gomez F, Sabahi F. The pathogenesis of microcephaly resulting from congenital infections: why is my baby's Head so small? Eur J Clin Microbiol Infect Dis 2017;37(2):209–26.

31. van der Knaap MS, Vermeulen G, Barkhof F, et al. Pattern of white matter abnormalities at MR imaging: use of polymerase chain reaction testing of Guthrie cards to link pattern with congenital cytomegalovirus infection. Radiology 2004;230(2): 529–36.

32. Bianca Guedes Ribeiro, Werner Heron, et al. Central nervous system effects of intrauterine zika virus infection. A Pictorial Rev Radiographics 2017;37(6): 1840–50. https://doi.org/10.1148/rg.2017170023.

33. Werner H, Fazecas T, Guedes B, et al. Intrauterine Zika virus infection and microcephaly: correlation of perinatal imaging and three-dimensional virtual physical models. Ultrasound Obstet Gynecol 2016;47(5):657–60.

34. Soares de Oliveira-Szejnfeld P, Levine D, Melo AS, et al. Congenital brain abnormalities and Zika virus: what the radiologist can expect to see prenatally and postnatally. Radiology 2016;281(1):203–18.

35. Norman Andria L, Crocker Nicole, Mattson Sarah N, et al. Neuroimaging and fetal alcohol spectrum disorders. Dev Disabil Res Rev 2009;15(3):209–17.

36. Riley EP, McGee CL, Sowell ER. Teratogenic effects of alcohol: a decade of brain imaging. Am J Med Genet 2004;127C(1):35–41.
37. Petrelli B, Bendelac L, Hicks GG, et al. Insights into retinoic acid deficiency and the induction of Craniofacial Malformations and microcephaly in fetal alcohol spectrum disorder. Genesis 2019;57(1). https://doi.org/10.1002/dvg.23278.
38. Tomson T, Battino D. Teratogenic effects of antiepileptic drugs. Lancet Neurol 2012;11(9):803–13.
39. Veiby G, Daltveit AK, Engelsen BA, et al. Fetal growth restriction and birth defects with newer and older antiepileptic drugs during pregnancy. J Neurol 2014;261(3):579–88.
40. Castillo M. Neuroradiology companion: Methods, guidelines, and imaging Fundamentals. Lippincott Williams & Wilkins; 2006.
41. Lo TY, Mcphillips M, Minns RA, et al. Cerebral atrophy following shaken impact syndrome and other non-accidental head injury (Nahi). Pediatr Rehabil 2003;6(1):47–55.
42. Chao CP, Zaleski CG, Patton AC. Neonatal hypoxic-ischemic encephalopathy: Multimodality imaging findings. RadioGraphics 2006;26(suppl_1). https://doi.org/10.1148/rg.26si065504.
43. Gunda D, Cornwell BO, Dahmoush HM, et al. Pediatric central nervous system imaging of nonaccidental trauma: beyond subdural hematomas. RadioGraphics 2018;39(1):213–28.

Imaging of Macrocephaly

Ilana Neuberger, MD*, Nicholas V. Stence, MD, John A. Maloney, MD,
Christina J. White, DO, David M. Mirsky, MD

KEYWORDS

- Macrocephaly • Hydrocephalus • Megalencephaly • Abusive head trauma

KEY POINTS

- Imaging modality and role in the evaluation of macrocephaly.
- Differential diagnoses for macrocephaly by anatomic compartment.
- Typical neuroimaging features for a wide range of associated conditions.

INTRODUCTION

Macrocephaly is a frequently encountered physical examination finding in the pediatric population. The differential diagnosis of underlying etiologies is broad and encompasses a wide spectrum of neurologic outcomes, from normal to devastating. Imaging plays an important role in both diagnosis and management. This article provides a review of neuroimaging findings in infant with macrocephaly.

DISCUSSION
Definition and Evaluation

Head circumference is obtained by encircling the head with measuring tape to include an area 1 to 2 cm above the glabella anteriorly (ie, just above the eyebrows) and the most prominent portion of the occiput posteriorly. It is routinely measured throughout the first 3 years of a normal child's life and at any pediatric age in a child who presents with neurologic or developmental concerns. It is an important data point in pediatric evaluation, particularly in infancy. It is during this time that normal cranial vault development is occurring, and the fontanelles and sutures are open, allowing the head size to easily expand with increased intracranial pressure. With time, the fontanelles and sutures narrow, ultimately closing, resulting in a more rigid structure and thereby limiting the head's ability to change size due to intracranial pathology.[1–4]

Macrocephaly is defined as a head circumference greater than 2 standard deviations above the mean for age and gender. It can also be diagnosed when sequential

Department of Radiology, Children's Hospital Colorado, University of Colorado, 13123 East
16th Avenue, Box 125 Aurora, CO 80045, USA
* Corresponding author.
E-mail address: ilana.neuberger@childrenscolorado.org

Clin Perinatol 49 (2022) 715–734
https://doi.org/10.1016/j.clp.2022.05.006
0095-5108/22/© 2022 Elsevier Inc. All rights reserved.

measurements increase in percentiles or when the head circumference increases by more than 2 cm per month in an infant less than 6 months old.[1] Macrocephaly is a commonly encountered diagnosis, with an estimated incidence of up to 5% of the pediatric population. Because there are currently no official recommendations from the American Academy of Pediatrics or the American College of Radiology (ACR) to guide imaging evaluation for the macrocephalic infant, clinicians are often faced with the question of when and how to image. Clinically, this group of patients has a wide range of presentations, from the neurologically normal to the obviously syndromic, with a variable likelihood that an abnormal imaging finding is present.

Most of the patients with asymptomatic, incidentally diagnosed macrocephaly do not harbor underlying pathology; most commonly the macrocephaly is familial or idiopathic in etiology. Parental head measurements and/or screening with neonatal head ultrasound is, therefore, a practical approach in this population.[1] Head ultrasound has the benefit of reasonable diagnostic accuracy without necessitating ionizing radiation or sedation; noting the limited utility in older infants, > approximately 6 months, due to the smaller acoustic windows from closing fontanelles.[5] If benign macrocephaly is confirmed by ultrasound, no further imaging (CT or MRI) is indicated.[1,4,6] Alternatively, rapid brain MRI may be used in this clinical setting. It offers superior diagnostic accuracy compared with ultrasound and also does not expose the child to radiation or necessitate sedation.[7,8] It is, however, limited by institutional availability and technique/quality.

Macrocephalic patients with developmental delay, neurologic symptoms, or syndromic appearance, warrant more advanced cross-sectional imaging with CT or MRI despite the accompanying risks, specifically, the increased oncologic risk from ionizing radiation with CT,[9] and the more recently reported complications from procedural sedation/anesthesia.[10–12] CT is of particular use in the urgent clinical setting, as it is fast, readily accessible, and of lower cost. When there is high clinical concern for intracranial pathology, particularly when there is a concern for an underlying genetic abnormality or syndrome, a complete brain MRI is the most appropriate imaging procedure for further evaluation.

Causes of Macrocephaly

Although most cases of macrocephaly in infants are familial or idiopathic in etiology, the differential diagnosis for infant macrocephaly remains broad. We will approach the imaging differential through anatomic compartments: extra-axial spaces, ventricles, calvarium, and parenchyma (Table 1). Expansion or enlargement of any of these compartments may lead to a large head circumference, noting that there can be an overlap with some diagnoses that involve more than one compartment. For example, parenchymal overgrowth is often associated with enlarged ventricles.

Enlarged Extraaxial Spaces

Benign enlargement of the subarachnoid spaces of infancy (BESS) is a self-limited condition that spontaneously resolves without treatment or sequelae. It is estimated to account for 57% to 75% of macrocephalic infants.[2,13–15] Clinically, infants present between 2 and 7 months of age with a rapid increase in head circumference that crosses percentiles and a neurologically normal or minimally delayed cognitive development.[16] The head size stabilizes by approximately 18 months and returns to normal by 2 to 3 years of age. It is thought to be due to the reduced ability of the immature arachnoid granulations to absorb cerebrospinal fluid (CSF).

On imaging, there will be symmetric enlargement of the subarachnoid spaces, particularly along the frontal convexities, as well as widening of the interhemispheric

Table 1
Causes of macrocephaly with classic associated neuroimaging features

Category	Disorder	Neuroimaging
Extra-axial Spaces		
	BESS	Enlarged subarachnoid space
	Subdural hematoma	Findings associated with nonaccidental trauma
	Glutaric aciduria type 1	Open sylvian fissures, abnormal basal ganglia, may have subdural hematomas
Ventricles (Hydrocephalus)		
Congenital	Aqueductal stenosis	Supratentorial ventriculomegaly with normal-sized fourth ventricle
	Chiari II	Small posterior fossa with hindbrain herniation; myelomeningocele
	Dandy–Walker malformation	Large posterior fossa with 4th ventricle cystic enlargement and cerebellar vermian hypoplasia
	Obstructive cyst	Cyst following CSF on all sequences
Acquired	Posthemorrhagic/infectious	Complex multicompartmental hydrocephalus with septations/adhesions
	Tumor	Often posterior fossa or midline mass
	Vein of Galen malformation	Large midline venous varix with arteriovenous shunting
Bone		
	Achondroplasia	Frontal bossing and depressed nasion; small skull base/foramen magnum
	Thalassemia/Sickle Cell	Thick calvarium with "hair on end"
	Bone overgrowth	Thick calvarium, can have ground glass density in fibrous dysplasia
Parenchyma (Megalencephaly)		
Metabolic		

(continued on next page)

Table 1
(continued)

Category	Disorder	Neuroimaging
Leukodystrophy	Alexander	Frontal predominant white matter and basal ganglia signal abnormality with periventricular rind of enhancement (Garland)
	Canavan	Elevated NAA on Spectroscopy, Diffuse
	MLC	Diffusely abnormal white matter with frontotemporal subcortical cysts
Organic Acid	GTA1	As above
	L2-D2	Subcortical frontal lobe signal abnormality becoming confluent and diffuse; basal ganglia and dentate nuclei involvement
Lysosomal	MPS	Enlarged perivascular spaces with periventricular white matter signal abnormality
Developmental		
PI3K-AKT-MTOR		HME, focal megalencephaly, diffuse megalencephaly, cerebellar overgrowth leading to Chiari 1 deformity, polymicrogyria, thickened corpus callosum
PHTS (PTEN)	Macrocephaly/autism	Multifocal white matter signal abnormality, periventricular trigone, with prominent perivascular spaces, subtle polymicrogyria
	Cowden, BRRS	± Lhermitte-Duclos
PROS (PI3KCA)	CLOVES	± HME, focal megalencephaly
	KTS	± HME, focal megalencephaly
	MCAP	Megalencephaly, thick corpus callosum, cerebral asymmetry and/or perisylvian polymicrogyria; ± enlarged cerebellum → Chiari 1

(continued on next page)

Table 1 (continued)		
Category	Disorder	Neuroimaging
AKT3, CCND2, PIK3R2	MPPH	Same as MCAP
AKT1	Proteus	± HME, focal megalencephaly
TSC1/TSC2	TSC	Tubers, Subependymal nodules, SEGA
Ras/MAPK	NF1	Myelin vacuolization in deep gray matter, mesial temporal lobes, brainstem, and cerebellum; Optic pathway gliomas
Transcriptional	Soto	Ventriculomegaly, Callosal abnormalities

sulcus. Mild supratentorial ventriculomegaly can also be seen. The enlarged extra-axial spaces should also follow CSF appearance on all modalities. Notably, the mass effect on the underlying parenchyma should not be present. The enlarged extra-axial spaces can be confirmed as subarachnoid, rather than subdural, by identifying bridging vessels traversing the spaces, either by ultrasound or MRI (**Fig. 1**). On CT, it may be difficult to differentiate subarachnoid from subdural space enlargement.[17] If feasible, a rapid brain MRI is useful to distinguish these compartments, especially if rapid FLAIR and FFE sequences are performed. The presence of a subdural collection is clinically relevant as it may be the result of abusive head trauma. That said, there is an increased prevalence of small incidental subdural collections in the setting of BESS. The prevalence of these incidental subdural collections correlates with the degree of subarachnoid space enlargement. Regardless, a clinical work-up for possible nonaccidental trauma is advised in all cases of BESS and subdural collection.[13,18]

Abusive Head Trauma (AHT) may present as macrocephaly due to underlying subdural collections.[13,17] A subset of these infants may be asymptomatic, underscoring the importance of detecting these subdural collections to prevent a more devastating injury.[19] Complete evaluation by a child protective team, including clinical and social history, radiographic skeletal survey, and ophthalmologic examination is crucial.

Subdural hematomas are seen in approximately 80% of AHT cases. Bridging vein injury, from rotational and/or acceleration/deceleration forces, is thought to be responsible for these subdural hematomas. Often there is concomitant disruption of the arachnoid membrane. This allows for CSF to mix with the subdural hemorrhage, leading to a wide variety of appearances on imaging, including mixed density. Dating subdural collections is thus challenging and not advised.

On imaging, subdural hematomas are crescentic collections, often along the cerebral convexities, falx, and tentorium (**Fig. 2**). They can be identified by ultrasound, CT, and MRI. The presence of a bridging vein injury can result in a characteristic appearance on susceptibility-weighted imaging (SWI), particularly at the vertex, termed the "lollipop" sign.[20] In AHT, often there are other radiologic findings such as traumatic and/or hypoxic-ischemic brain injury, cervical spine injury, and classic skeletal fractures. Susceptibility-weighted imaging, which is sensitive for the identification of blood

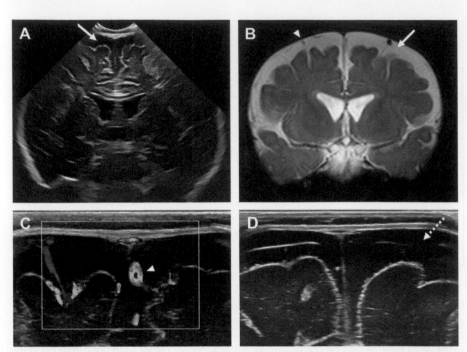

Fig. 1. 5 months old with benign enlargement of the subarachnoid spaces of infancy (A–C). (A) Grayscale ultrasound image demonstrates enlarged extra-axial spaces (*white arrow*) overlying the parasagittal convexities with expected (B) bridging vessels (white *arrowhead*) on color Doppler confirming that this is the subarachnoid space. (C) Coronal T2-weighted image from rapid brain MRI shows similar subarachnoid space enlargement, as well as mildly prominent ventricles. (D) 4 months old with subdural collections. Grayscale ultrasound image depicts subdural collections (*dashed arrow*) to contrast with the enlarged subarachnoid space.

products, can also be helpful for visualizing retinal hemorrhages, though ophthalmologic examination remains the gold standard.

Glutaric Aciduria Type 1 is a rare autosomal recessive mitochondrial disease caused by a deficiency in glutaryl-coenzyme A dehydrogenase resulting in the accumulation

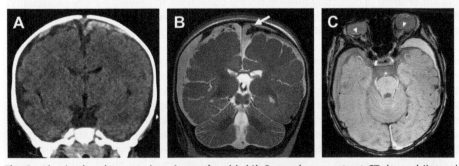

Fig. 2. Abusive head trauma in a 4 months old. (A) Coronal noncontrast CT shows bilateral mixed density subdural hematomas over the cerebral convexities. (B) Coronal T2-weighted image demonstrates linear signal abnormality from the subdural blood indicative of bridging vein injury (*arrow*). (C) Retinal hemorrhages (*arrowheads*) can be identified on axial susceptibility-weighted images.

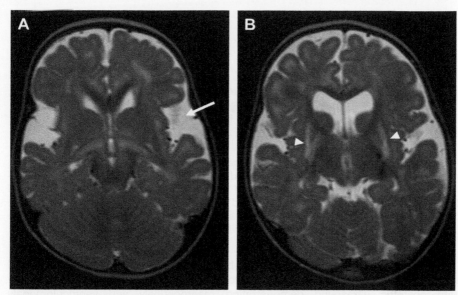

Fig. 3. 13 months old with glutaric aciduria type 1. Axial T2-weighted images demonstrate (A) enlarged open sylvian fissures (*arrow*) and (B) atrophy with signal abnormality in the basal ganglia (*arrowheads*).

of glutaric acids in the brain. Patients may present initially with either acute encephalopathy or gradual neurologic deterioration. Ultimately, they go on to have a combination of both.[21]

Neuroimaging features include the enlargement of the subarachnoid spaces overlying the frontal and temporal lobes, with an open or under-opercularized appearance of the sylvian fissures (**Fig. 3**). This expansion of the arachnoid space reflects frontotemporal opercular hypoplasia rather than cyst formation. There is also progressive signal abnormality and atrophy within the basal ganglia, particularly the putamen and caudate, as well as the white matter.[22] Subdural hygromas and hematomas can be identified in up to 20% to 30% of these patients, making this entity crucial to differentiate from nonaccidental trauma.[21]

Ventriculomegaly (hydrocephalus)

While ventricular enlargement is not invariably synonymous with hydrocephalus, when it is encountered in the context of macrocephaly, it is usually interchangeable. Clinically, infants with hydrocephalus present with lethargy, irritability, emesis, sundowning (restricted upgaze), frontal bossing, and/or bulging fontanelles. On imaging, there will be outward bowing and dilation of the third ventricular margins, particularly the floor and anterior and posterior recesses. The lateral ventricular temporal horns are also ballooned with medial compression of the hippocampi. Subarachnoid spaces are often small and effaced. Acute and subacute hydrocephalus typically will have periventricular T2 prolongation indicating a failure of normal parenchymal CSF drainage and accumulation of fluid in the interstitial spaces (**Fig. 4**). The normal unmyelinated periventricular white matter in infants may make interstitial edema more difficult to discern than in older children and adults. In patients with long-standing hydrocephalus, frontal bossing and calvarial thinning with prominent convolutional markings ("copper beaten skull") may be identified on radiographs or CT.

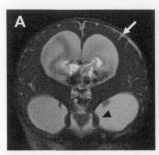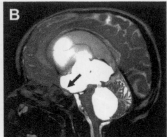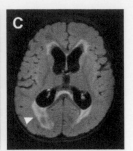

Fig. 4. Typical imaging features of hydrocephalus. (*A*) Coronal T2-weighted image demonstrates dilated temporal horns with medial displacement and compression of the hippocampi (*black arrowhead*), and effacement of the cerebral sulci (*white arrow*). (*B*) Sagittal T2-weighted image shows an enlarged third ventricle with inferior displacement of the third ventricular floor and ballooning of the anterior (*black arrow*) and posterior recesses. (*C*) Axial FLAIR with periventricular edema (*white arrowhead*).

Causes of hydrocephalus can broadly be divided into congenital/developmental and acquired etiologies.[23] Congenital hydrocephalus is often identified prenatally with obstetric ultrasound demonstrating macrocephaly and ventriculomegaly (**Fig. 5**). Further characterization with fetal MRI is helpful to better visualize structural brain malformations and associated abnormalities, allowing for improved prognostic accuracy and family counseling.[24–28]

Aqueductal stenosis (AS), a common cause of congenital hydrocephalus, results in significant macrocephaly. On imaging, there is an enlargement of the lateral and third ventricles, with a normal-sized fourth ventricle (see **Fig. 5**A). The cerebral aqueduct may be funneled in appearance, with superior dilation and inferior narrowing. The aqueductal occlusion, often a thin web or adhesion, is best visualized on postnatal imaging, using high-resolution, heavily T2-weighted sequences.[29]

AS may be present in isolation or associated with other brain malformations. It can also have genetic origins. X-linked AS is the most common heritable form of hydrocephalus and is caused by mutations in the L1CAM gene. Imaging may reveal associated syndromic abnormalities such as corpus callosal dysgenesis and limb anomalies (eg, adducted thumbs).[30] Rhomboencephalosynapsis, a brain malformation with incomplete cleavage of the cerebellar hemispheres, is present in up to 2/3 of cases of aqueductal stenosis. The degree of cerebellar vermian hypoplasia/aplasia correlates with clinical severity. Dystroglycanopathies, also associated with AS, are a heterogenous group of congenital muscular dystrophies. The most severe of which, Walker–Warburg syndrome, demonstrates a dysmorphic Z-shaped brainstem, cerebellar polymicrogyria with cysts, and diffuse cobblestone lissencephaly.

Chiari II malformation is a frequently encountered cause of macrocephaly, especially in the prenatal time period. Patients will present with ventriculomegaly because of obstruction to CSF flow at the level of the foramen magnum. The characteristic small posterior fossa with hindbrain herniation, a towering cerebellum, and tectal beaking is a result of CSF leakage through an open neural tube defect of the spine, most commonly myelomeningocele (see **Fig. 5**B). There is frequently associated callosal dysgenesis and gray matter heterotopia. This is an important diagnosis to make prenatally as in-utero repair of the open spinal dysraphism decreases the need for postnatal CSF diversion and can improve neurologic outcomes.[31,32]

Dandy–Walker malformation, another developmental cause of macrocephaly, is characterized by an enlarged posterior fossa with marked cystic enlargement of the

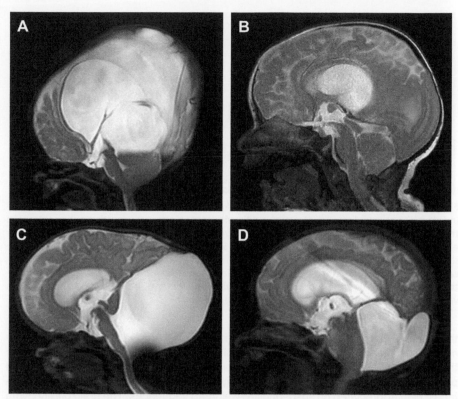

Fig. 5. Congenital hydrocephalus. Sagittal T2-weighted images demonstrate (*A*) aqueductal stenosis with severe supratentorial ventriculomegaly, normal-sized fourth ventricle, and aqueductal occlusion; (*B*) Chiari II malformation (shunted) with small posterior fossa, hindbrain herniation, and tectal beaking; (*C*) Dandy–Walker malformation with cystic enlargement of the fourth ventricle and posterior fossa, and a rotated cerebellar vermian remnant; and (*D*) Retrocerebellar arachnoid cyst compresses the cerebellum and fourth ventricle causing supratentorial ventricular enlargement.

fourth ventricle, and cerebellar vermian agenesis/hypogenesis (see **Fig. 5**C). The tentorium is displaced superiorly, with the torcular Herophili positioned above the lambdoid suture (torcular-lambdoid inversion). Other posterior fossa cystic anomalies, namely vermian hypoplasia, Blake's pouch remnant/cyst, and mega cisterna magna, have sometimes been referred to as the Dandy–Walker continuum or variant, but this verbiage is confusing given the different etiologies and clinical outcomes and should, therefore, be avoided.

Developmental cysts, typically arachnoid cysts, can also cause hydrocephalus due to the direct mass effect leading to macrocephaly (see **Fig. 5**D). It is important to differentiate these from other more severe cystic-associated entities, such as a true Dandy–Walker malformation.

Posthemorrhagic and postinfectious hydrocephalus are frequently encountered acquired causes of macrocephaly. Perinatal hemorrhage is especially common in premature neonates from germinal matrix hemorrhage and periventricular venous infarcts. In the acute period, hemorrhage is present at the caudothalamic notches and may fill/expand the ventricular system. Periventricular venous infarction, part of

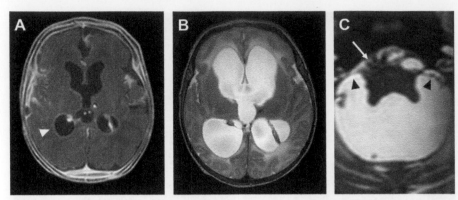

Fig. 6. One week old with *E. Coli* meningitis. (*A*) Postcontrast T1-weighted axial image early in infectious course demonstrates meningitis with leptomeningeal contrast enhancement in the sylvian fissures, greater on the right, and ventriculitis with posterior lateral ventricular ependymal enhancement (*white arrowhead*). Six weeks later, (*B*) axial T2-weighted image shows the development of lateral and third ventricular enlargement compatible with hydrocephalus. (*C*) High-resolution T2-weighted axial image through the fourth ventricle illustrates basal cistern adhesion formation (*white arrow*) and obstruction of the fourth ventricular outlet foramina (*black arrowheads*).

the germinal matrix hemorrhage spectrum, manifests as hemorrhage in the deep white matter, particularly along the lateral ventricular bodies, and is thought to develop from the compression/obstruction of the subependymal veins. With time, the acute blood products resolve to leave hemosiderin lining the leptomeningeal and ependymal surfaces, best appreciated on susceptibility-weighted sequences. The brain parenchyma will lose volume, often with the development of cystic encephalomalacia and ex-vacuo enlargement of the ventricular system. The evolving blood products may lead to the obstruction of CSF circulation and absorption from ependymal and arachnoid scarring, resulting in a complex pattern of multicompartmental hydrocephalus. Up to 15% of these children eventually need ventriculoperitoneal shunting.[33]

Postinfectious hydrocephalus develops similarly, with the inflammation of the arachnoid and ependyma causing scarring. Imaging during the acute infection often demonstrates leptomeningeal enhancement, indicating meningitis. Additional findings can be seen depending on the infectious agent and compartment involved. Ventricular ependymal enhancement and layering intraventricular diffusion-restricting debris indicate ventriculitis (**Fig. 6**A). Both parenchymal and extra-axial abscesses can develop, as well as areas of cerebritis and ischemia. Over time, parenchymal volume loss with or without cystic encephalomalacia may develop, as well as hydrocephalus (see **Fig. 6**B). High-resolution heavily T2-weighted imaging may demonstrate adhesions, particularly in the basal cisterns (see **Fig. 6**C).

Given the risk of developing hydrocephalus after both infection and hemorrhage, these neonates are closely followed by head circumference measurements and serial brain ultrasounds. Ventricular size may be misleading in this context due to the confounding presence of atrophy-related ventriculomegaly, therefore, particular attention to the ventricular morphology and head size is necessary to evaluate for coexisting hydrocephalus.

Intracranial masses cause hydrocephalus, and thus macrocephaly, through mass effect/obstruction, venous hypertension, meningeal infiltration, CSF overproduction, and/or altered CSF composition (**Fig. 7**).[23] Early childhood tumors are often centered

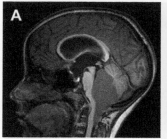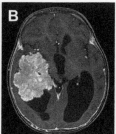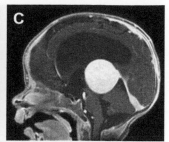

Fig. 7. Obstructive hydrocephalus. (*A*) Sagittal T1-weighted image shows a posterior fossa ependymoma causing obstructive hydrocephalus at the level of the fourth ventricle. (*B*) Axial T1-weighted postcontrast image illustrates a choroid plexus papilloma causing hydrocephalus due to CSF overproduction. (*C*) Sagittal T1-weighted postcontrast depicts an enlarged midline venous varix with mass effect resulting in hydrocephalus compatible with a vein of Galen malformation.

in the posterior fossa and therefore present with hydrocephalus from fourth ventricle outlet obstruction. The most common tumor pathologies are astrocytoma, medulloblastoma, and ependymoma. Atypical teratoid rhabdoid tumor is difficult to differentiate from medulloblastoma by imaging and is an important consideration in the infant time period. Tectal gliomas and pineal region masses (eg, germinoma, pineoblastoma, and teratoma) can also cause obstructive hydrocephalus due to the mass effect on the cerebral aqueduct. Choroid plexus papillomas and carcinomas cause hydrocephalus through a combination of CSF overproduction and obstruction. Vascular masses, such as the *vein of Galen malformation,* may cause hydrocephalus from a combination of venous hypertension due to abnormal arteriovenous shunting as well as mass effect from the enlarged vessels.

Bone

Achondroplasia is an autosomal dominant condition caused by an abnormality of fibroblast growth factor receptor 3 (FGFR3). A defect in enchondral bone formation results in a hypoplastic skull base and enlargement of the membranous cranial vault (**Fig. 8**A). These patients have marked macrocephaly at birth with frontal bossing and nasion depression. They have characteristic spinal and extraspinal anomalies and a predisposition for developing atlantoaxial instability. Head size may be further enlarged by hydrocephalus from a stenotic foramen magnum limiting CSF circulation and hypoplastic jugular foramen causing venous hypertension.[34]

Calvarial thickening and enlargement are a potential cause of macrocephaly. Extramedullary hematopoiesis, such as from *sickle cell anemia* and *thalassemia,* has a characteristic "hair-on-end" appearance (see **Fig. 8**B). *Osteopetrosis* and *fibrous dysplasia* may also cause macrocephaly through bony overgrowth.

Parenchyma (megalencephaly)

Megalonocphaly is defined as the overgrowth of the brain parenchyma that exceeds the age-related mean by 2 or more standard deviations. It is useful to categorize the many causative disorders into metabolic and developmental (anatomic) megalencephaly. While metabolic megalencephaly is often caused by an accumulation of abnormal metabolites, developmental megalencephaly is due to increased size and/or number of cells related to mutations in signal mediators that regulate cell growth, migration, and replication during development. Both metabolic and developmental

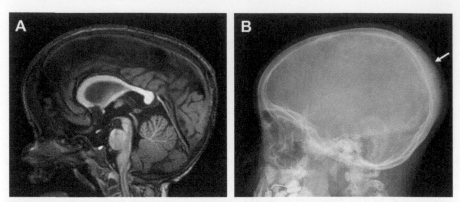

Fig. 8. Osseous causes of macrocephaly. (*A*) Sagittal T1-weighted image demonstrates typical findings of achondroplasia with a disproportionately enlarged membranous cranial vault relative to a hypoplastic skull base. (*B*) Lateral radiograph of a sickle cell patient depicts calvarial thickening with vertical striations representing the "hair on end" appearance (*white arrow*) from marrow hyperplasia.

megalencephaly are genetic in etiology. Metabolic disorders are often due to germline mutations, resulting in diffuse and homogeneous abnormalities. Whereas focal malformations, such as hemimegalencephaly and focal megalencephaly, are more common with developmental conditions, and may be the result of somatic mosaicism.

Metabolic megalencephaly

Metabolic megalencephaly is a heterogeneous group of disorders that can be broadly divided into leukoencephalopathy, organic acid disorders, and lysosomal storage diseases (**Fig. 9**). Of these categories, imaging plays a more central role in the diagnosis of leukoencephalopathy, particularly *Alexander disease.* It is caused by an autosomal dominant mutation resulting in the accumulation of glial fibrillary acidic protein (GFAP) within astrocytes. The infantile or classical type is the most common and presents with macrocephaly, seizures, and rapid neurologic deterioration.[35] Presence of 4 of the 5 MRI criteria establishes the diagnosis: extensive cerebral white matter abnormalities most prominent in the frontal lobes; a frontal periventricular rind of T1 and T2 shortening (garland); abnormal signal intensity in the basal ganglia and thalami; abnormal signal intensity in the medulla and midbrain; and contrast enhancement of one or more of the ventricular ependyma, periventricular rim, frontal white matter, optic chiasm, fornix, basal ganglia, thalamus, dentate nucleus, or brainstem.[36]

Canavan disease is an autosomal recessive disorder due to deficiency of aspartoacylase, which results in the accumulation of N-acetylaspartate (NAA). Children with Canavan disease are often normal for the first few months of life, start having developmental delay from 3 to 6 months with ongoing skill regression, hypotonia, and eventual spasticity.[37] Similar to the clinical disease progression, early imaging may be normal with diffuse signal abnormality developing throughout the cerebral and cerebellar white matter, noting relative sparing of the corpus callosum. The deep gray matter, particularly the globus pallidus, and brainstem may also be involved. The hallmark of this disorder is an abnormal MR spectroscopy which demonstrates an elevated NAA peak. Familiarity with a normal infant MR spectroscopy is crucial for this interpretation since an elevated NAA peak in an infant may resemble that of a normal adult. This elevated NAA peak on MR spectroscopy may be the only abnormal finding by imaging early in life.[38,39]

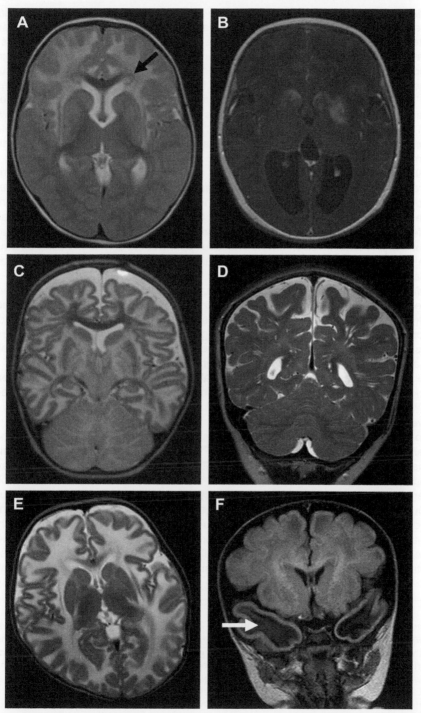

Fig. 9. Metabolic megalencephaly. (*A, B*) Alexander Disease in a 16 months old. (*A*) Axial T2-weighted image shows frontal predominant white matter signal abnormality, basal ganglia T2 hyperintensity, and a frontal periventricular rind of T2 hypointensity (*black arrow*). (*B*)

Megalencephalic leukoencephalopathy with subcortical cysts (MLC) is usually caused by a mutation in the MLC1 gene and inherited in an autosomal recessive pattern. It presents with macrocephaly in the first year of life and mild gross motor skill delay. This relatively mild initial clinical presentation contrasts with the extensive signal abnormality on MRI, which is characterized by homogeneous swelling and diffuse hyperintense signal on T2-weighted images involving much of the cerebral white matter. There are distinctive subcortical cysts in the anterior temporal and frontoparietal lobes. The disease most often progresses to develop ataxia and dysarthria, with MRI demonstrating evolving volume loss.[37,40] A second phenotype with clinical improvement rather than deterioration has been identified, with corresponding normalization on MRI.[41]

Glutaric aciduria type 1 is an organic acid disorder discussed above in the enlarged extra-axial spaces section. *L-2-Hydroxyglutaric Aciduria and D2-Hydroxyglutaric Aciduria* is a slowly progressive neurodegenerative disorder caused by an autosomal recessive mitochondrial enzyme deficiency. On imaging, multifocal signal abnormality preferentially involving the subcortical frontal lobes progresses to more confluent and diffuse white matter involvement with relative sparing of the central white matter structures. The basal ganglia and dentate nuclei are affected, while the brainstem and cerebellar white matter are spared.[42]

Mucopolysaccharidoses, such as Hurler and Hunter syndromes, may develop macrocephaly, at least in part from ventriculomegaly and a propensity to slowly develop hydrocephalus. On MRI, the perivascular spaces are enlarged with nonspecific patchy or confluent periventricular white matter signal abnormality. Other lysosomal disorders, such as *GM2 gangliosidosis (Tay-Sachs and Sandhoff)* and *Krabbe,* are also associated with macrocephaly, and demonstrate thalamic hyperdensity on CT as well as variable additional areas of signal abnormality. The presence of optic nerve thickening and cranial/cauda equina nerve enhancement indicates Krabbe disease.

Developmental megalencephaly

Two cellular pathways account for the largest number of megalencephaly syndromes: Ras/mitogen-activated protein kinase (MAPK) and PI3K-AKT-mTOR. They are functionally related and are associated with multiple essential cellular functions. The syndromes resulting from the dysregulation of either pathway demonstrate overlapping phenotypic features involving many organ systems, including but not limited to cutaneous stigmata, vascular malformations, overgrowth (focal and/or diffuse), and tumor predisposition (benign and malignant). Our understanding of these disorders and their genetic/molecular foundation has undergone recent substantial advancement with much of the phenotypic diversity and focality explained by the presence of mosaic mutations. These postzygotic mutations result in localized cell expression, explaining

---

Postcontrast T1-weighted axial demonstrates heterogeneous enhancement in the basal ganglia, greater on the left. (*C*) Canavan Disease in a 1 year old. Diffuse T2 hyperintensity in the cerebral and cerebellar white matter, globus pallidi, and brainstem with relative sparing of the corpus callosum is seen on an axial T2-weighted image. There is a hallmark elevation of NAA on MR spectroscopy (not pictured). (*D*) Hunter syndrome in a 2 years old. Coronal T2-weighted image demonstrates enlarged perivascular spaces with patchy white matter signal abnormality. (*E, F*) Megalencephalic leukoencephalopathy with subcortical cysts in a 6 months old with mild developmental delay. Extensive white matter T2 hyperintensity is present the on axial image (*E*) and characteristic anterior temporal cortical cysts are visualized as a suppressed signal on coronal FLAIR image (F, *white arrow*).

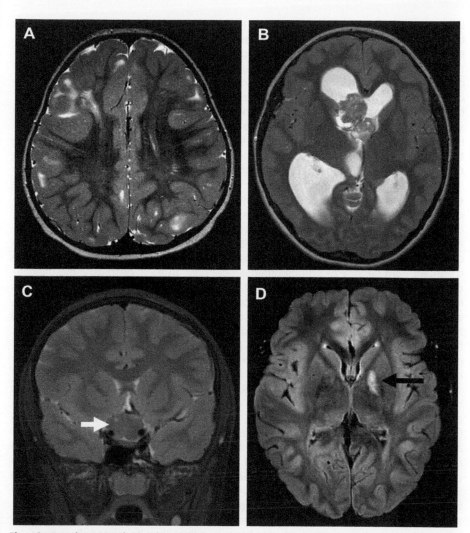

Fig. 10. Developmental megalencephaly. Two years old with tuberous sclerosis complex. (*A*) Axial T2-weighted images demonstrate typical tubers with expansile T2 hyperintensity centered in the subcortical white matter. (*B*) A mass at the foramen of Monro compatible with subependymal giant cell astrocytoma is seen with findings of hydrocephalus. Three years old with neurofibromatosis type 1. (*C*) Coronal T2-weighted sequence shows an optic pathway glioma (*white arrow*), while a typical myelin vacuolization focus is identified in the left basal ganglia on (*D*) axial FLAIR (*black arrow*).

the variability and focality of these related histopathologic brain abnormalities: generalized megalencephaly, hemimegalencephaly (HME), focal megalencephaly, tubers in tuberous sclerosis, and focal cortical dysplasia.

A complete evaluation of these disorders and their genetic underpinnings is beyond the scope of this review, so we will focus on some of the more common disorders and pathways. Two of the most familiar disorders demonstrate classic cutaneous stigmata and pathognomonic neuroimaging, *neurofibromatosis type 1* (NF1) and *tuberous sclerosis complex* (TSC) (**Fig. 10**). Both dysregulate the mTOR pathway, through unopposed Ras activity as a result of the NF1 gene mutation in NF1, and through loss of function mutations in TSC1 or TSC2 genes in TSC. Brain imaging in NF1 demonstrates foci of myelin vacuolization with nonenhancing T2 prolongation in typical locations, including the deep gray matter, mesial temporal lobes, brainstem, and cerebellum. There is an increased frequency of developing brain gliomas, particularly optic pathway gliomas. TSC is characterized by multifocal cortical and subcortical tubers, often demonstrating classic radial lines extending to the ventricular margins, and subependymal nodules. Enhancing masses representing WHO grade 1 subependymal giant cell tumors can develop at the foramen of Monro. If the lesion causes ventricular obstruction, hydrocephalus may develop, and further contribute to macrocephaly, with a pattern of asymmetric lateral ventriculomegaly.

PIK3CA-related overgrowth spectrum (PROS) is a group of syndromes demonstrating phenotypic overlap and continuum, including but not limited to *CLOVES* syndrome (congenital lipomatous asymmetric overgrowth of the trunk, lymphatic, capillary, venous, and combined-type vascular malformations, epidermal nevi, skeletal and spinal anomalies), *KTS* (Klippel–Trenaunay syndrome) and *MCAP* (megalencephaly-capillary malformation).[43] There is variable brain involvement in these disorders from generalized diffuse megalencephaly, to focal dysplastic megalencephaly, to asymmetric or classic HME. HME is not unique to PROS as it also occurs in isolation and in conjunction with many other disorders, including Proteus syndrome, which is the result of an AKT1 mutation. It is characterized by overgrowth of a cerebral hemisphere with ipsilateral severe cortical dysplasia, white matter signal abnormality, and hypertrophy, and dysmorphic lateral ventriculomegaly (**Fig. 11**A). The cerebellum may also be involved. Clinically, HME predisposes patients to intractable early-onset epilepsy.

Among the disorders grouped in PROS, MCAP has a more uniform appearance on neuroimaging, characterized by marked diffuse megalencephaly, often with corpus callosal thickening, cerebral asymmetry, and/or bilateral perisylvian polymicrogyria (see **Fig. 11**B). An enlarged cerebellum causing posterior fossa crowding may be present, which in turn can result in a Chiari 1 deformity (see **Fig. 11**C). Development of hydrocephalus has also been described. Imaging surveillance has, therefore, been proposed at 6-month intervals until 2 years of age with subsequent 3-yearly scans to monitor for the necessity of surgical decompression and/or CSF diversion.[44] Cutaneous vascular malformations (typically capillary malformations) are present in MCAP, often on the face. Other features characteristic of PROS, namely polydactyly/syndactyly and focal somatic overgrowth, are typically milder than its related disorders.

Megalencephaly-polymicrogyria-polydactyly-hydrocephalus (MPPH) and MCAP have considerable overlap, demonstrating similar neuroimaging features. MPPH is also caused by mutations in the PI3K-AKT-mTOR pathway, often involving PIK3R2 and AKT3. Hydrocephalus and postaxial polydactyly are variable manifestations of MPPH, present in about half of individuals.

The *PTEN hamartoma tumor syndrome (PHTS)* is another umbrella term that encompasses disorders resulting from mutations in PTEN (a tumor-suppressor gene), which causes the downregulation of the same PI3K/AKT/mTOR pathway. There is a wide phenotypic range, which includes the well-known tumor predisposition syndromes, *Bannayan–Riley–Ruvalcaba syndrome* (BRRS), and *Cowden syndrome*. Both syndromes result in an increased frequency of breast, thyroid, and endometrial cancers, as well as benign multisystem lesions. BRRS is more common in children, while Cowden syndrome is often diagnosed later in life. From a brain imaging perspective, *Lhermitte-Duclos* disease (cerebellar dysplastic gangliocytoma) is the most distinct entity, both in association with Cowden syndrome and as an isolated manifestation of PHTS.

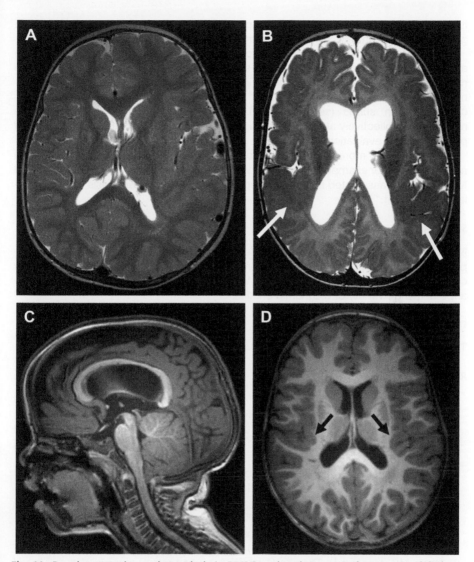

Fig. 11. Developmental megalencephaly in PIK3CA-related overgrowth spectrum. (*A*) Three years old with CLOVES syndrome (congenital lipomatous asymmetric overgrowth of the trunk, lymphatic, capillary, venous, and combined-type vascular malformations, epidermal nevi, skeletal and spinal anomalies). Axial T2-weighted image demonstrates features of hemimegalencephaly with asymmetric overgrowth of the left cerebral hemisphere and cortical dysplasia; (*B*) 4 months old with megalencephaly-capillary malformation. Axial T2-weighted image depicts bilateral polymicrogyria (*white arrows*) and enlarged ventricles; (*C*) 11 months old with Klippel–Trenaunay syndrome. Sagittal T1 weighted image shows ventricular enlargement and an enlarged cerebellum resulting in posterior fossa crowding and Chiari I deformity. PTEN mutation (*D*) in a 3 years old with autism and macrocephaly. Axial T1-weighted image shows subtle bilateral peri-sylvian polymicrogyria (*black arrows*).

It is characterized by focal mass-like expansion of the cerebellar folia maintaining a gyriform striated pattern. Occasionally, mild enhancement is present.

In addition, PTEN mutations account for the largest single gene defect identified in autistic children with macrocephaly. MRI shows megalencephaly with multifocal white matter signal abnormality, preferentially in the periventricular trigone, and accompanying prominent perivascular spaces.[45–47] Up to 50% of these patients have polymicrogyria, often subtle (see **Fig. 11**D).[48] While individually these findings are nonspecific, collectively and in the setting of autism with macrocephaly, they should prompt genetic evaluation.

There are other more common syndromes that have nonspecific or even normal neuroimaging. For example, *cerebral gigantism* (Sotos syndrome) has distinctive facial features, while associated imaging findings include callosal dysgenesis and ventricular enlargement.[49]

SUMMARY

Neuroimaging can guide the imaging differential and treatment of pediatric macrocephaly. An anatomic compartmental approach is helpful, as the enlargement of any component can result in macrocephaly. We have illustrated the characteristic appearance of a wide variety of diagnostic entities.

DISCLOSURE

The authors have nothing to disclose.

REFERENCES

1. Yilmazbas P, Gokcay G, Eren T, et al. Macrocephaly diagnosed during well child visits. Pediatr Int 2018;60(5):474–7.
2. Medina LS, Frawley K, Zurakowski D, et al. Children with macrocrania: clinical and imaging predictors of disorders requiring surgery. AJNR Am J Neuroradiol 2001;22(3):564–70.
3. Sampson MA, Berg AD, Huber JN, et al. Necessity of intracranial imaging in infants and children with macrocephaly. Pediatr Neurol 2019;93:21–6.
4. Thomas CN, Kolbe AB, Binkovitz LA, et al. Asymptomatic macrocephaly: to scan or not to scan. Pediatr Radiol 2021;51(5):811–21.
5. Smith R, Leonidas JC, Maytal J. The value of head ultrasound in infants with macrocephaly. Pediatr Radiol 1998;28(3):143–6.
6. Haws ME, Linscott L, Thomas C, et al. A retrospective analysis of the utility of head computed tomography and/or magnetic resonance imaging in the management of benign macrocrania. J Pediatr 2017;182:283–289 e1.
7. Lindberg DM, Stence NV, Grubenhoff JA, et al. Feasibility and accuracy of fast MRI versus CT for traumatic brain injury in young children. Pediatrics 2019; 144(4). https://doi.org/10.1542/peds.2019-0419.
8. Tekes A, Senglaub SS, Ahn ES, et al. Ultrafast brain MRI can be used for indications beyond shunted hydrocephalus in pediatric patients. AJNR Am J Neuroradiol 2018;39(8):1515–8.
9. Pearce HT. A tried and true advocate: SCMA President Andrew J. Pate, MD 2012-2013. J S C Med Assoc 2013;109(1):1.
10. Bosnjak ZJ, Logan S, Liu Y, et al. Recent insights into molecular mechanisms of propofol-induced developmental neurotoxicity: implications for the protective strategies. Anesth Analg 2016;123(5):1286–96.

11. Loepke AW. Developmental neurotoxicity of sedatives and anesthetics: a concern for neonatal and pediatric critical care medicine? Pediatr Crit Care Med 2010; 11(2):217–26.
12. Havidich JE, Beach M, Dierdorf SF, et al. Preterm versus term children: analysis of sedation/anesthesia adverse events and longitudinal risk. Pediatrics 2016;137(3): e20150463.
13. Tucker J, Choudhary AK, Piatt J. Macrocephaly in infancy: benign enlargement of the subarachnoid spaces and subdural collections. J Neurosurg Pediatr 2016; 18(1):16–20.
14. Alper G, Ekinci G, Yilmaz Y, et al. Magnetic resonance imaging characteristics of benign macrocephaly in children. J Child Neurol 1999;14(10):678–82.
15. Greiner MV, Richards TJ, Care MM, et al. Prevalence of subdural collections in children with macrocrania. AJNR Am J Neuroradiol 2013;34(12):2373–8.
16. Zahl SM, Egge A, Helseth E, et al. Quality of life and physician-reported developmental, cognitive, and social problems in children with benign external hydrocephalus-long-term follow-up. Childs Nerv Syst 2019;35(2):245–50.
17. Care MM. Macrocephaly and subdural collections. Pediatr Radiol 2021;51(6): 891–7.
18. Hansen JB, Frazier T, Moffatt M, et al. Evaluations for abuse in young children with subdural hemorrhages: findings based on symptom severity and benign enlargement of the subarachnoid spaces. J Neurosurg Pediatr 2018;21(1):31–7.
19. Feldman KW, Sugar NF, Browd SR. Initial clinical presentation of children with acute and chronic versus acute subdural hemorrhage resulting from abusive head trauma. J Neurosurg Pediatr 2015;16(2):177–85.
20. Choudhary AK, Bradford R, Dias MS, et al. Venous injury in abusive head trauma. Pediatr Radiol Nov 2015;45(12):1803–13.
21. Hoffmann GF, Athanassopoulos S, Burlina AB, et al. Clinical course, early diagnosis, treatment, and prevention of disease in glutaryl-CoA dehydrogenase deficiency. Neuropediatrics 1996;27(3):115–23.
22. Hedlund GL, Longo N, Pasquali M. Glutaric acidemia type 1. Am J Med Genet C Semin Med Genet 2006;142C(2):86–94.
23. Kahle KT, Kulkarni AV, Limbrick DD Jr, et al. Hydrocephalus in children. Lancet 2016;387(10020):788–99.
24. Neuberger I, Garcia J, Meyers ML, et al. Imaging of congenital central nervous system infections. Pediatr Radiol 2018;48(4):513–23.
25. Benacerraf BR, Shipp TD, Bromley B, et al. What does magnetic resonance imaging add to the prenatal sonographic diagnosis of ventriculomegaly? J Ultrasound Med 2007;26(11):1513–22.
26. Griffiths PD, Reeves MJ, Morris JE, et al. A prospective study of fetuses with isolated ventriculomegaly investigated by antenatal sonography and in utero MR imaging. AJNR Am J Neuroradiol 2010;31(1):106–11.
27. Manganaro L, Savelli S, Francioso A, et al. Role of fetal MRI in the diagnosis of cerebral ventriculomegaly assessed by ultrasonography. Radiol Med 2009; 114(7):1013–23.
28. Morris JE, Rickard S, Paley MNJ, et al. The value of in-utero magnetic resonance imaging in ultrasound diagnosed foetal isolated cerebral ventriculomegaly. Clin Radiol 2007;62(2):140–4.
29. Mirsky DM, Stence NV, Powers AM, et al. Imaging of fetal ventriculomegaly. Pediatr Radiol 2020;50(13):1948–58.
30. Kenwrick S, Jouet M, Donnai D. X linked hydrocephalus and MASA syndrome. J Med Genet 1996;33(1):59–65.

31. Adzick NS, Thom EA, Spong CY, et al. A randomized trial of prenatal versus post-natal repair of myelomeningocele. N Engl J Med 2011;364(11):993–1004.
32. Tulipan N, Wellons JC 3rd, Thom EA, et al. Prenatal surgery for myelomeningo-cele and the need for cerebrospinal fluid shunt placement. J Neurosurg Pediatr 2015;16(6):613–20.
33. Kazan S, Gura A, Ucar T, et al. Hydrocephalus after intraventricular hemorrhage in preterm and low-birth weight infants: analysis of associated risk factors for ven-triculoperitoneal shunting. Surg Neurol 2005;64(Suppl 2):S77–81, discus-sion S81.
34. Gordon N. The neurological complications of achondroplasia. Brain Dev 2000; 22(1):3–7.
35. Sarkar S, Sinha R, Chakraborty A, et al. Infantile alexander disease: case report and review of literature. J Clin Diagn Res 2017;11(6):ZD14–5.
36. van der Knaap MS, Ramesh V, Schiffmann R, et al. Alexander disease: ventricular garlands and abnormalities of the medulla and spinal cord. Neurology 2006; 66(4):494–8.
37. Renaud DL. Leukoencephalopathies associated with macrocephaly. Semin Neu-rol 2012;32(1):34–41.
38. Orru E, Calloni SF, Tekes A, et al. The child with macrocephaly: differential diag-nosis and neuroimaging findings. AJR Am J Roentgenol 2018;210(4):848–59.
39. De Bernardo G, Giordano M, Sordino D, et al. Early diagnosis of Canavan syn-drome: how can we get there? BMJ Case Rep 2015;2015. https://doi.org/10. 1136/bcr-2014-208755.
40. van der Knaap MS, Boor I, Estevez R. Megalencephalic leukoencephalopathy with subcortical cysts: chronic white matter oedema due to a defect in brain ion and water homoeostasis. Lancet Neurol 2012;11(11):973–85.
41. van der Knaap MS, Lai V, Kohler W, et al. Megalencephalic leukoencephalopathy with cysts without MLC1 defect. Ann Neurol 2010;67(6):834–7.
42. Seijo-Martinez M, Navarro C, Castro del Rio M, et al. L-2-hydroxyglutaric aciduria: clinical, neuroimaging, and neuropathological findings. Arch Neurol 2005;62(4): 666–70.
43. Keppler-Noreuil KM, Rios JJ, Parker VE, et al. PIK3CA-related overgrowth spec-trum (PROS): diagnostic and testing eligibility criteria, differential diagnosis, and evaluation. Am J Med Genet A 2015;167A(2):287–95.
44. Conway RL, Pressman BD, Dobyns WB, et al. Neuroimaging findings in macrocephaly-capillary malformation: a longitudinal study of 17 patients. Am J Med Genet A 2007;143A(24):2981–3008.
45. Butler MG, Dasouki MJ, Zhou XP, et al. Subset of individuals with autism spec-trum disorders and extreme macrocephaly associated with germline PTEN tumour suppressor gene mutations. J Med Genet 2005;42(4):318–21.
46. Buxbaum JD, Cai G, Chaste P, et al. Mutation screening of the PTEN gene in pa-tients with autism spectrum disorders and macrocephaly. Am J Med Genet B Neuropsychiatr Genet 2007;144B(4):484–91.
47. Vanderver A, Tonduti D, Kahn I, et al. Characteristic brain magnetic resonance imaging pattern in patients with macrocephaly and PTEN mutations. Am J Med Genet A 2014;164A(3):627–33.
48. Shao DD, Achkar CM, Lai A, et al. Polymicrogyria is associated with pathogenic variants in PTEN. Ann Neurol 2020;88(6):1153–64.
49. Olney AH. Macrocephaly syndromes. Semin Pediatr Neurol 2007;14(3):128–35.

Imaging of Hypoxic-Ischemic Injury (in the Era of Cooling)

Judith A. Gadde, DO, MBA[a,b,c],*, Andrea C. Pardo, MD[d], Corey S. Bregman, MD[a,b,c], Maura E. Ryan, MD[a,b,c]

KEYWORDS

- Hypoxic-ischemic injury • Therapeutic hypothermia • MRI • Prognosis

KEY POINTS

- Hypoxic-ischemic injury (HII) is a major worldwide contributor of term neonatal mortality and long-term morbidity in high, middle, and low-income countries.
- At present, therapeutic hypothermia is the only therapy with efficacy in reducing severe disability or death in infants with moderate to severe encephalopathy.
- Magnetic resonance imaging (MRI) is important in the workup for patients affected by HII due to its ability to assist with prognostication for infants' families.
- US is often the first-line imaging evaluation for many neonates with suspected intracranial abnormalities.

INTRODUCTION

Hypoxic-ischemic injury (HII) is a major worldwide contributor to term neonatal mortality and long-term morbidity in high, middle, and low-income countries. HII occurs in 2 per 1000 live births in high income countries and may be ten times higher in middle and low-income countries[1,2] and is one of the most common neurologic complaints in the neonatal intensive care unit (NICU).[3,4] HII is a significant worldwide contributor to the pathogenesis of cerebral palsy[5] and other neurodevelopmental disabilities.[6] Several cellular processes are responsible for neuronal damage during HII, including abnormalities of intracellular homeostasis, excitotoxicity, free radical formation, mitochondrial impairment, inflammation and apoptosis.[7,8] HII is clinically diagnosed by the presence of neonatal encephalopathy associated to metabolic acidosis, multiorgan system dysfunction usually associated with a sentinel event and low Apgar scores.[9] At present, therapeutic hypothermia (33.5° Celsius for 72 hours) is the only therapy

[a] Ann & Robert H. Lurie Children's Hospital of Chicago, 225 East Chicago Avenue, Box 9, Chicago, IL 60611, USA; [b] Medical Imaging Department; [c] Northwestern University Feinberg School of Medicine; [d] Ruth D. and Ken M. Davee Pediatric Neurocritical Care Program, Ann & Robert H. Lurie Children's Hospital of Chicago, Northwestern University Feinberg School of Medicine, 225 East Chicago Avenue, Box 51, Chicago, IL 60611, USA
* Corresponding author.
E-mail address: jgadde@luriechildrens.org

Clin Perinatol 49 (2022) 735–749
https://doi.org/10.1016/j.clp.2022.05.007
0095-5108/22/© 2022 Elsevier Inc. All rights reserved.
perinatology.theclinics.com

that has demonstrated efficacy reducing severe disability or death in infants with moderate to severe encephalopathy in several randomized controlled clinical trials.[10–13] Therapeutic hypothermia may provide its protective effect by impacting intracellular signaling, inflammation and cell death.[14] There is a substantial body of literature on biomarkers for the prognostication of neurodevelopmental outcome and death in infants with HII, among these, magnetic resonance imaging (MRI) and magnetic resonance spectroscopy (MRS) play an important role in the management of infants and counseling of families with infants affected by HII. Typically, infants are evaluated with neuroimaging anywhere from day of life (DOL) 2 to DOL 14. With the implementation of therapeutic hypothermia, there is an increasing number of data evaluating the role of different neuroimaging modalities and their applicability in infants with HII, there is a broad variation in the timing of neuroimaging and its prognostic utility as well as limitations for prognostic evaluation.

CLINICAL ASSOCIATIONS OF NEUROIMAGING AND OUTCOME

Before the standard use of therapeutic hypothermia for the treatment of neonatal HII, several authors have described the natural history of infants with perinatal asphyxia and correlated the imaging patterns with specific neurodevelopmental outcomes[15–18] and as a result of clinical trials have further allowed a direct comparison of infants receiving therapeutic hypothermia vs those that did not, providing an extensive description of the neuroimaging evolution in HII. Grading systems were developed to evaluate the role of specific patterns of injury and outcomes. For instance, basal ganglia abnormalities in T1 and T2 sequences correlated with increasing rates of motor impairment in neonates with HII at 3 months, as well as feeding and communication impairments[19] and abnormal scores in T1 and T2 sequences in watershed areas showed abnormal cognitive outcomes at age 12 months.[20] Findings of abnormal T1 and T2 signal in the posterior limb of the internal capsule (PLIC) correlate with abnormal neuromotor outcomes at 12 months and inability to ambulate by 2 years of age.[17,21] Involvement of the brainstem is independently associated to death at 9 months.[21] Furthermore, findings of restricted diffusion in gray matter including basal ganglia and cortex are associated with abnormal neurodevelopmental outcome at both, 2 years of age and school-age.[22] Diffusion restriction has shown to be more sensitive than T1 and T2 changes for the evaluation of injury in infants with HII, demonstrating utility earlier in the clinical course, it becomes apparent as early as day of life 1 and maximal between days 2 and 3 of life and then "pseudo-normalizes" on days 6 to 8.[23] Findings of spectroscopy have demonstrated to be highly predictive of outcomes, specifically, lactate to N-acetyl-aspartate ratio (NAA) have good positive predictive and negative predictive values for the prognostication of adverse neurodevelopmental outcomes.[24]

POSTTHERAPEUTIC HYPOTHERMIA ERA

Controlled randomized studies for the use of therapeutic hypothermia allowed the evaluation of the impact of hypothermia on outcomes demonstrating efficacy for decreased mortality and severe disability as well as its impact on neuroimaging patterns. From these studies, it has become apparent that there is an impact on the diffusivity values of neonates receiving hypothermia versus those that did not, showing that the findings of diffusion restriction were delayed in infants that received therapeutic hypothermia "pseudo-normalizing" after 11 to 12 days of age.[25] Additional studies comparing apparent diffusion coefficients (ADC) also noted that there was a reduction of ADC values in those infants that received therapeutic hypothermia,[26] regardless, these studies demonstrate that abnormalities noted on MRI remain valid as a prognostic indicator for adverse neurodevelopmental outcome with a high degree of sensitivity and specificity.[27] Additionally, findings of diffusion restriction and ADC in the brainstem after hypothermia were not only associated with increased mortality, but also longer hospital stay in surviving neonates.[28] Notably, the findings of MRS have not seemed to be affected by therapeutic hypothermia and are significantly sensitive and specific to predict abnormal neurodevelopmental outcome.[29–32] Outside of clinical trials, and in clinical practice, magnetic resonance (MR) has consistently performed well as a biomarker for adverse neurodevelopmental outcomes with a high negative predictive value.[33] The standard clinical use of therapeutic hypothermia has generated questions and new evidence regarding the timing for neuroimaging to be used for prognostication. The clinical trials that evaluated the use of therapeutic hypothermia used MRI performed around 2 weeks of age (late MRI) demonstrating good sensitivity and specificity for outcome prediction, there have been several studies documenting evidence that DWI and ADC values are abnormal earlier in infants with HII and they had high sensitivity to predict the adverse neurodevelopmental outcome.[34,35] In addition, a normal MRI after hypothermia was predictive of a favorable developmental outcome.[36] Several studies have since compared the use of MRI performed in the first 2 to 3 days (early MRI) of life and how this impacted prognostication, demonstrating that early MRI was able to detect later brain injury accurately,[37–39] with similar findings noted for the use of early MRS.[40,41]

ULTRASOUND

Due to accessibility and convenience, head ultrasound (US) is often the first-line imaging evaluation for many neonates with suspected intracranial abnormalities. Unlike cross-sectional imaging, US can be conducted portably in the ICU, eliminating the concerns and challenges of transporting critically ill neonates to imaging suites. Additionally, US is widely available and does not require sedation or exposure to ionizing radiation.

Ischemic injury classically results in increased echogenicity of the parenchyma in US (**Fig. 1**), although it should be noted that increased echogenicity is not specific for ischemia and can be seen with areas of hemorrhage as well. US findings of HII also may include evidence of cerebral swelling with sulcal effacement, burring of the interhemispheric fissure, and narrowed ventricles (**Fig. 2**). Doppler imaging of the intracranial vessels may demonstrate increased resistive indices, although this is not specific for HII.

US provides excellent assessment of the ventricles and is highly sensitive for germinal maxtrix hemorrhages, as well as later cystic changes and periventricular leukomalacia that develop as sequelae of HII.[42] However, the sensitivity and specificity of US for acute parenchymal injury are less, particularly when compared with MR.[43] US may underestimate the degree of parenchymal injury and changes may be difficult to appreciate in less severe cases[44] (**Fig. 3**). Additionally, as both hemorrhage and ischemia can have a similar echogenic appearance, the specificity of US is also inferior to MR

Although there is little debate that MR is the gold standard for the evaluation of HII,[45–47] the true accuracy of US in the evaluation of HII remains controversial. This may in part be due to the greater operator and interpreter variability of US in comparison to CT or MRI and US is likely more accurate in experienced centers.[48] Additionally, older assessments of the sensitivity of US may be limited as modern technical improvements such as cine imaging and the use of high-resolution linear transducers can increase the performance of US.

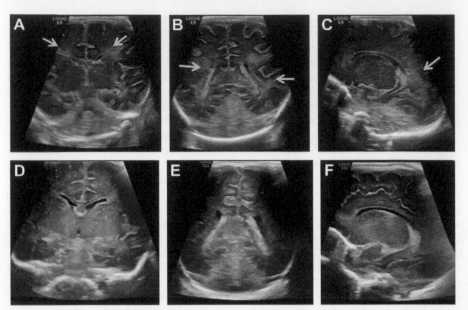

Fig. 1. top row: coronal (*A, B*) and sagittal (*C*) US of severe HII in a 2-day old 37-week boy with abruption. There is increased echogenicity in the parenchyma (*arrows*), most prominently in the posterior parietal periventricular white matter. The extraaxial spaces are preserved. Bottom row: coronal (*D, E*) and sagittal (*F*) US of a comparison normal head US in a term neonate.

COMPUTED TOMOGRAPHY

Computed tomography (CT) is often readily available and can provide faster imaging, easier monitoring, and fewer equipment safety concerns in comparison to MR. Exposure to ionizing radiation is also a theoretic risk, although the negative effects of a single CT performed with appropriate pediatric parameters are likely minimal.[49,50]

However, although CT imaging has a high sensitivity for acute hemorrhage, it provides the only limited evaluation of the neonatal parenchyma, particularly when compared with the diagnostic value of MR.[51] This is in part due to the normal low density of unmyelinated white matter in the neonatal brain, which can both mimic and obscure hypodensity related to ischemic injury and edema (**Figs. 4** and **5**).

Due to the relative insensitivity to ischemic injury, CT typically has a very limited role in the evaluation of HII[42] (**Fig. 6**).

MAGNETIC RESONANCE IMAGING

Magnetic resonance imaging is important in the workup for patients affected by HII due to its ability to assist with prognostication for infant's families. A standard brain MRI without contrast should be performed including MR spectroscopy (see the section later in discussion). ASL (arterial spin labeled) perfusion imaging can also be performed for further assessment, which is ideal given the lack of need for intravenous contrast.

Timing of Imaging

The American College of Obstetrics and Gynecology (ACOG) guidelines recommend 2 MRIs of the brain to evaluate the timing of neonatal cerebral injury.[9,39] These

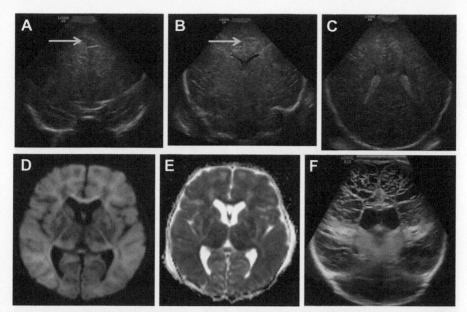

Fig. 2. Severe HII in a term infant with a history of nuchal cord, status postcooling. Coronal US images on the day of life 3 (*A, B, C*) demonstrate diffuse cerebral swelling with efface-ment of the sulci and an indistinct interhemispheric fissure (*arrow*). The Ventricles are com-pressed and there is a poor distinction between the cortices and white matter. MRI DWI (*D*) and ADC (*E*) imaging at day of life 6 show corresponding injury with diffusion restriction throughout the bilateral cortices, white matter, basal ganglia, and thalami. Follow-up US at 4 months (*F*) demonstrates sequelae of injury with developing cystic encephalomalacia and ventricular enlargement due to volume loss.

guidelines assume that an early MRI assists in timing the injury, while a later MRI dem-onstrates the extent of the injury.[39] O'Kane and colleagues[39] performed a prospective longitudinal cohort study to evaluate the agreement between the early and late MRI, as well as to assess the ability of the early MRI to predict outcomes, of the brain in newborn infants with HII after undergoing therapeutic hypothermia. The results sug-gested that a single MRI performed during the first week of life is adequate to assess brain injury and offer prognosis.[39]

If diffusion imaging is performed in the first 24 hours of life, it may yield false-negative results and underestimate the amount of injury.[52] As previously stated, administration of therapeutic hypothermia can alter the timing of pseudonormalization of diffusion imaging.[39] Pseudonormalization typically occurs around 5 to 7 days of life without therapeutic hypothermia, compared with 8 to 12 days of life with therapeutic hypothermia.[53]

Patterns of Injury

Patterns of injury will depend on the gestational age of the neonate, that is, term, pre-term, or an older child, as well as the degree of hypotension.[52] **(Table 1)**. Mild to mod-erate hypotension in premature infants will often cause injury to the periventricular and deep white matter while sparing the cerebral cortex and subcortical white matter often evolving to periventricular leukomalacia after 2 to 6 weeks[54] **(Fig. 7)**. Areas of T1 hyperintensity may be depicted in areas of larger T2 hyperintensity. These foci may subsequently demonstrate cavitation/necrosis with central areas of T1 hypointensity.

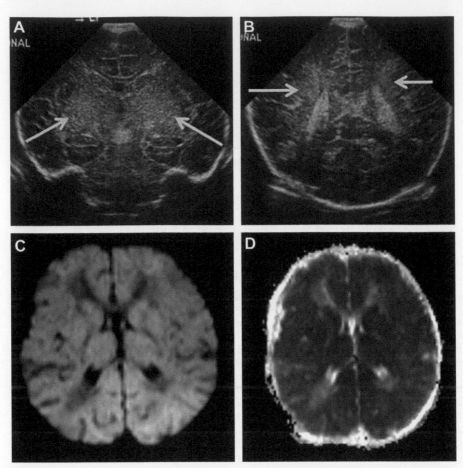

Fig. 3. Severe HII in a term baby girl after emergent cesarean section due to abruption. Coronal US (*A*, *B*) on day of life 3 demonstrates subtle increased echogenicity of the deep gray matter and periventricular white matter (*arrows*) as well as mild compression of the sulci and ventricles. DWI (*C*) and ADC (*D*) MR images on day of life 4 show extensive diffusion restriction throughout the hemispheric cortices, white matter, basal ganglia, and thalami.

A similar degree of hypotension in term infants will typically cause injury to the watershed regions with areas of T2 hyperintensity and restricted diffusion (**Fig. 8**).

On the other hand, profound/severe hypotension will typically cause injury to the areas of highest metabolic demand, which includes the thalami, basal ganglia, and brainstem in preterm neonates.[52] Term neonates who undergo profound hypotension will often have injury to their dorsal brainstem, anterior cerebellar vermis, thalami, basal ganglia, corticospinal tracts, and perirolandic cortex.[52] Areas of gray matter injury will often demonstrate T1 hyperintensity, variable T2 signal, and restricted diffusion. White matter injury will typically demonstrate T1 hypointensity, T2 hyperintensity, and restricted diffusion (**Fig. 9**).

MAGNETIC RESONANCE SPECTROSCOPY

MR spectroscopy spectroscopy offers an additional tool to the clinicians and diagnosticians caring for neonates suspected to have sustained HII. Soon after descriptions of

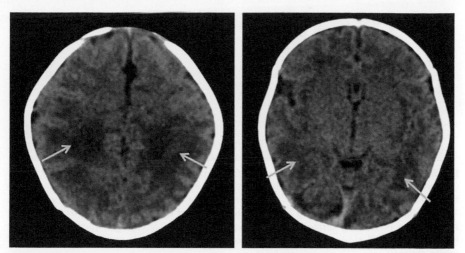

Fig. 4. Normal CT in a 6-day-old term infant. Patchy low density in the bihemispheric white matter (*arrows*) reflects normal unmyelinated white matter. Normal parenchyma was confirmed on MRI the following day.

MR patterns in infants with asphyxia began being defined, investigations into the utility of MR spectroscopy in these patients began as well. Early researchers argued that elevated lactate to creatine ratio by proton MR spectroscopy in asphyxiated infants results from the disruption of energy metabolism and suggested it can be used to identify infants who could benefit from neuronal rescue therapies.[55]

MR spectroscopy also has the advantage of identifying potential injury in the first 24 hours, before conventional anatomic imaging may show the characteristic findings of hypoxic injury. The spectroscopic abnormality is often evident on the first day of injury but may continue to become further evident over the next 4 to 5 days, before beginning to normalize.[23] One thing to still keep in mind if imaging at a time that falls between 24 and 48 hours is a brief pseudonormalization period which may occur between the initial episode of lactate development secondary to hypoxemia from the

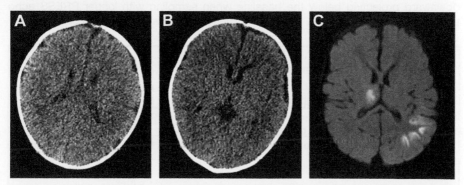

Fig. 5. Ischemia in a term neonate with seizures. CT (*A, B*) demonstrates diffuse, symmetric hemispheric low density typical of unmyelinated white matter and an unremarkable CT appearance of the deep gray matter. DWI imaging on same day MRI (*C*) revealed acute ischemic changes in the left parietal parenchyma and right thalamus, occult on the CT.

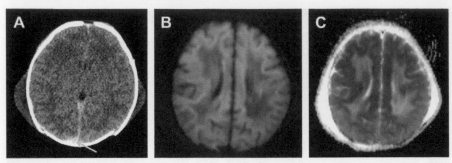

Fig. 6. HII in a term neonate with seizures. CT (*A*) demonstrates diffuse low density of the white matter, although this is difficult to distinguish from normal unmyelinated white matter. There is cerebral swelling with effacement of the sulci and relatively small ventricles. There is biparietal scalp swelling and a small amount of high-density parturition subdural hemorrhage posteriorly (*arrow*). DWI (*B*) and ADC (*C*) MR imaging demonstrates severe ischemia with diffusion restriction throughout the bihemispheric cortices and subcortical white matter.

primary injury versus a later lactate generation phase known as secondary energy failure.[56]

Higher lactate to choline ratio in the basal ganglia has shown to be predictive of worse clinical outcomes. Elevation of choline to creatine ratio and decreased NAA has also been identified as associated markers for HII in full-term infants.[23,57] Briefly it is mentioned that additional metabolite ratios have also been considered for the evaluation such as choline to creatinine and glutamine to glutamate.[56] However, the detection of lactate has largely been the mainstay of clinical MR spectroscopy in these patients.

Spectroscopy is performed with single-voxel point resolved spectroscopy (PRESS) technique. The voxel placement when performing Spectroscopy in neonatal HII is typically one sample acquisition overlying the deep gray matter nuclei to include the thalamus and lentiform nucleus, with a second sample acquisition overlying the watershed zone in the deep white matter. Positioning of the lactate doublet on spectroscopic sampling is characteristically centered at 1.31 ppm. The peak is upright projecting above the baseline in sampling with short PRESS echo times, however, is downward projecting below the baseline when sampling with longer PRESS echo times above 135 ms[24] (**Figs. 10** and **11**). These parameters hold in the case of 1.5 T

Table 1 Patterns of hypoxic-ischemic encephalopathy		
Age of Child	**Mild to Moderate Hypotension**	**Profound/Severe Hypotension**
Preterm neonate (up to 32 wk gestation)	Periventricular/deep white matter injury	Thalamic, basal ganglia, brainstem injury
Term neonate (34–36 wk gestation)	Cortex and white matter injury	Dorsal brainstem, thalamus, basal ganglia, corticospinal tracts, and perirolandic cortex
Older child (greater than 4–6 mo postnatal)	Parasagittal watershed injury	Basal ganglia and diffuse cortical injury (sparing perirolandic and thalamus)

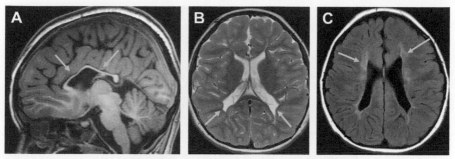

Fig. 7. Periventricular leukomalacia in a 7-year-old female with infantile spasm born via c-section at 35 weeks gestation for fetal decelerations followed by therapeutic hypothermia. Sagittal T1-weighted image (A) shows diffuse thinning of the corpus callosum (arrows). Axial T2-weighted image (B) shows irregular borders of the bodies and trigones of the lateral ventricles (arrows). Axial T2 FLAIR image (C) demonstrates abnormal T2 FLAIR hyperintensity in the periventricular white matter (arrows).

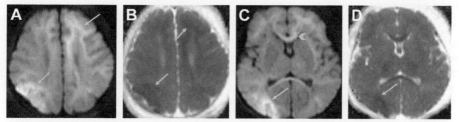

Fig. 8. 4-day-old female born at 40 weeks gestation complicated by maternal fever and fetal tachycardia status posthead cooling. DWI (A, C) and ADC (B, D) demonstrate restricted diffusion in the watershed regions of the bilateral cerebral hemispheres (arrows), as well as in the corpus callosum (arrowheads).

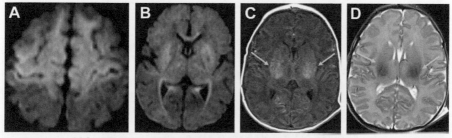

Fig. 9. 4-day-old female born at 38 weeks gestation via crash c-section for fetal bradycardia and placental abruption status posttherapeutic hypothermia. DWI (A, B) demonstrates restricted diffusion in the bilateral perirolandic regions, frontal lobes, basal ganglia, corpus callosum, and periventricular white matter. Axial T1-weighted image (C) shows abnormal T1 hyperintensity in the bilateral posterior putamen and ventrolateral thalami (arrows). Axial T2-weighted image (D) demonstrates abnormal T2 hypointensity in the bilateral posterior putamen and ventrolateral thalami (arrows).

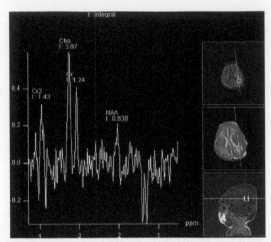

Fig. 10. Term infant with HII status posttherapeutic hypothermia imaged at 5 days on 1.5 T with PRES 135 ms, transferred from outside hospital with hypoglycemia, acidosis, respiratory distress, encephalopathy. Note inverted lactate doublet at 1.3 ppm in both voxels over the basal ganglia and deep white matter.

MRI imaging. However, in the case of 3T MRI imaging there is a known pitfall that lactate peaks can be diminished in their magnitude above baseline, though doubling of the PRESS echo times restores this lactate signal.[58] In such cases when spectroscopy is performed at 3T field strength with a doubled echo time, the inversion of lactate which is observed at 1.5 T field strength will not occur (**Figs. 12** and **13**).

Of note, minimal lactate has been noted in the watershed zones of neonates, particularly in infants born premature, without any history of hypoxic injury or other neurologic disease process.[57,59] Gestational age at delivery must be considered in a patient as lactate presence alone is not specific to HII in such cases.

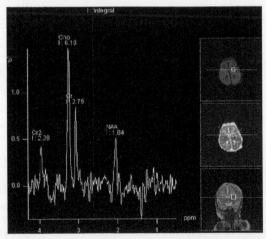

Fig. 11. Term infant with HII status posttherapeutic hypothermia imaged at 5 days on 1.5 T with PRES 135 ms, transferred from outside hospital with hypoglycemia, acidosis, respiratory distress, encephalopathy. Note inverted lactate doublet at 1.3 ppm in both voxels over the basal ganglia and deep white matter.

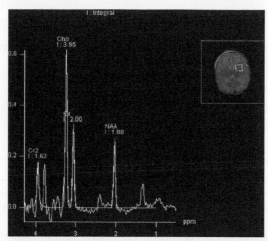

Fig. 12. Term infant with HII status posttherapeutic hypothermia imaged on day 8, transferred from OSH for meconium aspiration. Performed on 3T with PRES of 270 ms. Note the above baseline lactate doublet at 1.3 ppm in both voxels over the basal ganglia and deep white matter when performed at long press on 3T.

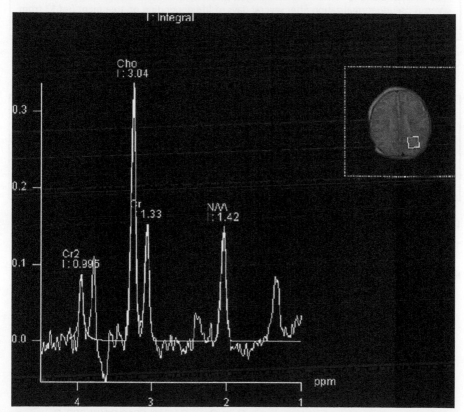

Fig. 13. Term infant with HII status posttherapeutic hypothermia imaged on day 8, transferred from OSH for meconium aspiration. Performed on 3T with PRES of 270 ms. Note the above baseline lactate doublet at 1.3 ppm in both voxels over the basal ganglia and deep white matter when performed at long press on 3T.

SUMMARY

HII is a major worldwide contributor to term neonatal mortality and long-term morbidity. At present, therapeutic hypothermia is the only therapy that has demonstrated efficacy in reducing severe disability or death in infants with moderate to severe encephalopathy. US may be first-line imaging due to its availability. However, MRI and MRS are more sensitive to acute parenchymal injury and offer prognostic information.

BEST PRACTICES

- Therapeutic hypothermia is the only therapy that has demonstrated efficacy reducing severe disability or death in infants with moderate to severe encephalopathy (ref 10-13 from bibliography).
- Lactate to N-acetyl-aspartate ratio (NAA) have good positive predictive and negative predictive values for the prognostication of adverse neurodevelopmental outcomes (ref 24 from bibliography).
- Appropriate timing of MRI will depend upon if therapeutic hypothermia has been administered due to concerns of false-negative results within the first 24 hours of life versus pseudonormalization after several days of life depending on treatment (ref 53 from bibliography).

CLINICS CARE POINTS

- Hypoxic-ischemic injury is clinically diagnosed by the presence of neonatal encephalopathy associated to metabolic acidosis, multiorgan system dysfunction associated with a sentinel event and low Apgar scores.
- Diffusion restriction has shown to be more sensitive than T1 and T2 changs for the evaluation of injury in infants with HII.
- US may underestimate the degree of parenchymal injury.

DISCLOSURES

The authors have no disclosures.

REFERENCES

1. Moshiro R, Mdoe P, Perlman JM. A global view of neonatal asphyxia and resuscitation. Front Pediatr 2019;7:489.
2. Hug L, Alexander M, You D, et al. National, regional, and global levels and trends in neonatal mortality between 1990 and 2017, with scenario-based projections to 2030: a systematic analysis. Lancet Glob Health 2019;7(6):e710-20.
3. Glass HC, Bonifacio SL, Peloquin S, et al. Neurocritical care for neonates. Neurocrit Care 2010;12(3):421-9.
4. Glass HC, Ferriero DM, Rowitch DH, et al. The neurointensive nursery: concept, development, and insights gained. Curr Opin Pediatr 2019;31(2):202-9.
5. Oskoui M, Coutinho F, Dykeman J, et al. An update on the prevalence of cerebral palsy: a systematic review and meta-analysis. Develop Med Child Neurol 2013; 55(6):509-19.

6. Lee-Kelland R, Jary S, Tonks J, et al. School-age outcomes of children without cerebral palsy cooled for neonatal hypoxic-ischaemic encephalopathy in 2008-2010. Arch Dis Child Fetal Neonatal Ed 2020;105:8–13.
7. Vexler ZS, Ferriero DM. Molecular and biochemical mechanisms of perinatal brain injury. Semin Neonatal 2001;6(2):99–108.
8. Hagberg H, David Edwards A, Groenendaal F. Perinatal brain damage: the term infant. Neurobiol Dis 2016;92(Pt A):102–12.
9. ACOG. Neonatal encephalopathy and neurologic outcome, second edition. Obstet Gynecol 2014;123(4):896–901.
10. Committee on F, Newborn, Papile LA, et al. Hypothermia and neonatal encephalopathy. Pediatrics 2014;133(6):1146–50.
11. Azzopardi DV, Strohm B, Edwards AD, et al. Moderate hypothermia to treat perinatal asphyxial encephalopathy. N Engl J Med 2009;361(14):1349–58.
12. Shankaran S, Laptook AR, Ehrenkranz RA, et al. Whole-body hypothermia for neonates with hypoxic-ischemic encephalopathy. N Engl J Med 2005;353(15):1574–84.
13. Jacobs SE, Berg M, Hunt R, et al. Cooling for newborns with hypoxic ischaemic encephalopathy. Cochrane Database Syst Rev 2013;1(1):CD003311.
14. Davidson JO, Gonzalez F, Gressens P, et al. Update on mechanisms of the pathophysiology of neonatal encephalopathy. Semin Fetal Neonatal Med 2021;26(5):101267.
15. Christophe C, Clercx A, Blum D, et al. Early MR detection of cortical and subcortical hypoxic-ischemic encephalopathy in full-term-infants. Pediatr Radiol 1994;24(8):581–4.
16. Rutherford MA, Pennock JM, Dubowitz LM. Cranial ultrasound and magnetic resonance imaging in hypoxic-ischaemic encephalopathy: a comparison with outcome. Develop Med Child Neurol 1994;36(9):813–25.
17. Rutherford MA, Pennock JM, Counsell SJ, et al. Abnormal magnetic resonance signal in the internal capsule predicts poor neurodevelopmental outcome in infants with hypoxic-ischemic encephalopathy. Pediatrics 1998;102(2 Pt 1):323–8.
18. Kaufman SA, Miller SP, Ferriero DM, et al. Encephalopathy as a predictor of magnetic resonance imaging abnormalities in asphyxiated newborns. Pediatr Neurol 2003;28(5):342–6.
19. Martinez-Biarge M, Diez-Sebastian J, Wusthoff CJ, et al. Feeding and communication impairments in infants with central grey matter lesions following perinatal hypoxic-ischaemic injury. Europ J Paediatr Neurol 2012;16(6):688–96.
20. Barkovich AJ, Hajnal BL, Vigneron D, et al. Prediction of neuromotor outcome in perinatal asphyxia: evaluation of MR scoring systems. AJNR Am J Neuroradiol 1998;19(1):143–9.
21. Martinez-Biarge M, Diez-Sebastian J, Kapellou O, et al. Predicting motor outcome and death in term hypoxic-ischemic encephalopathy. Neurology 2011;76(24):2055–61.
22. Weeke LC, Groenendaal F, Mudigonda K, et al. A novel magnetic resonance imaging score predicts neurodevelopmental outcome after perinatal asphyxia and therapeutic hypothermia. J Pediatr 2018;102:33 40.e2.
23. Barkovich AJ, Miller SP, Bartha A, et al. MR imaging, MR spectroscopy, and diffusion tensor imaging of sequential studies in neonates with encephalopathy. AJNR Am J Neuroradiol 2006;27(3):533–47.
24. Barkovich AJ, Baranski K, Vigneron D, et al. Proton MR spectroscopy for the evaluation of brain injury in asphyxiated, term neonates. AJNR Am J Neuroradiol 1999;20(8):1399–405.

25. Bednarek N, Mathur A, Inder T, et al. Impact of therapeutic hypothermia on MRI diffusion changes in neonatal encephalopathy. Neurology 2012;78(18):1420–7.

26. Imai K, de Vries LS, Alderliesten T, et al. MRI changes in the thalamus and basal ganglia of full-term neonates with perinatal asphyxia. Neonatology 2018;114(3): 253–60.

27. Rutherford M, Ramenghi LA, Edwards AD, et al. Assessment of brain tissue injury after moderate hypothermia in neonates with hypoxic–ischaemic encephalopathy: a nested substudy of a randomised controlled trial. Lancet Neurol 2010; 9(1):39–45.

28. Sarkar SS, Gupta S, Bapuraj JR, et al. Brainstem hypoxic-ischemic lesions on MRI in infants treated with therapeutic cooling: effects on the length of stay and mortality. J Perinatol 2021;41(3):512–8.

29. Lucke AM, Shetty AN, Hagan JL, et al. Early proton magnetic resonance spectroscopy during and after therapeutic hypothermia in perinatal hypoxic-ischemic encephalopathy. Pediatr Radiol 2019;49(7):941–50.

30. Lally PJ, Montaldo P, Oliveira V, et al. Magnetic resonance spectroscopy assessment of brain injury after moderate hypothermia in neonatal encephalopathy: a prospective multicentre cohort study. Lancet Neurol 2019;18(1):35–45.

31. Alderliesten T, de Vries LS, Staats L, et al. MRI and spectroscopy in (near) term neonates with perinatal asphyxia and therapeutic hypothermia. Arch Dis Child Fetal Neonatal Ed 2017;102(2):F147–52.

32. Ancora G, Testa C, Grandi S, et al. Prognostic value of brain proton MR spectroscopy and diffusion tensor imaging in newborns with hypoxic-ischemic encephalopathy treated by brain cooling. Neuroradiology 2013;55(8):1017–25.

33. Tharmapoopathy P, Chisholm P, Barlas A, et al. In clinical practice, cerebral MRI in newborns is highly predictive of neurodevelopmental outcome after therapeutic hypothermia. Europ J Paediatr Neurol 2020;25:127–33.

34. Shankaran S, McDonald SA, Laptook AR, et al. Neonatal magnetic resonance imaging pattern of brain injury as a biomarker of childhood outcomes following a trial of hypothermia for neonatal hypoxic-ischemic encephalopathy. J Pediatr 2015;167(5):987–93.e3.

35. Shankaran S, Barnes PD, Hintz SR, et al. Brain injury following trial of hypothermia for neonatal hypoxic-ischaemic encephalopathy. Arch Dis Child Fetal Neonatal Ed 2012;97(6):F398–404.

36. Bach AM, Fang AY, Bonifacio S, et al. Early magnetic resonance imaging predicts 30-month outcomes after therapeutic hypothermia for neonatal encephalopathy. J Pediatr 2021;238:94–101.e1.

37. Wintermark P, Hansen A, Soul J, et al. Early versus late MRI in asphyxiated newborns treated with hypothermia. Arch Dis Child Fetal Neonatal Ed 2011;96(1): F36–44.

38. Charon V, Proisy M, Ferré JC, et al. Comparison of early and late MRI in neonatal hypoxic-ischemic encephalopathy using three assessment methods. Pediatr Radiol 2015;45(13):1988–2000.

39. O'Kane A, Vezina G, Chang T, et al. Early versus Late brain magnetic resonance imaging after neonatal hypoxic ischemic encephalopathy treated with therapeutic hypothermia. J Pediatr 2021;232:73–9.e2.

40. Barta H, Jermendy A, Kolossvary M, et al. Prognostic value of early, conventional proton magnetic resonance spectroscopy in cooled asphyxiated infants. BMC Pediatr 2018;18(1):302.

41. Shibasaki J, Niwa T, Piedvache A, et al. Comparison of predictive values of magnetic resonance biomarkers based on scan timing in neonatal encephalopathy following therapeutic hypothermia. J Pediatr 2021;239:101–9.e4.

42. Barkovich AJ. The encephalopathic neonate: choosing the proper imaging technique. AJNR Am J Neuroradiol 1997;18(10):1816–20.

43. Daneman A, Epelman M, Blaser S, et al. Imaging of the brain in full-term neonates: does sonography still play a role? Pediatr Radiol 2006;36(7):636–46.

44. Epelman M, Daneman A, Chauvin N, et al. Head Ultrasound and MR imaging in the evaluation of neonatal encephalopathy: competitive or complementary imaging studies? Magn Reson Imaging Clin N Am 2012;20(1):93–115.

45. Debillon T, N'Guyen S, Muet A, et al. Limitations of ultrasonography for diagnosing white matter damage in preterm infants. Arch Dis Child Fetal Neonatal Ed 2003;88(4):F275–9.

46. Blankenberg FG, Norbash AM, Lane B, et al. Neonatal intracranial ischemia and hemorrhage: diagnosis with US, CT, and MR imaging. Radiology 1996;199(1):253–9.

47. Maalouf EF, Duggan PJ, Counsell SJ, et al. Comparison of findings on cranial ultrasound and magnetic resonance imaging in preterm infants. Pediatrics 2001;107(4):719–27.

48. Sewell EK, Andescavage NN. Neuroimaging for neurodevelopmental prognostication in high-risk neonates. Clin Perinatol 2018;45(3):421–37.

49. Epelman M, Daneman A, Kellenberger CJ, et al. Neonatal encephalopathy: a prospective comparison of head US and MRI. Pediatr Radiol 2010;40(10):1640–50.

50. Hendee WR, O'Connor MK. Radiation risks of medical imaging: separating fact from fantasy. Radiology 2012;264(2):312–21.

51. Frush DP. Whats and whys with neonatal CT. Pediatrics 2014;133(6):e1738–9.

52. Barnette AR, Horbar JD, Soll RF, et al. Neuroimaging in the evaluation of neonatal encephalopathy. Pediatrics 2014;133(6):e1508–17.

53. James BA, Charles R. Brain and spine injuries in infancy and childhood. In: Zinner S, editor. Pediatric neuroimaging. 6th edition. Philadelphia: Wolters Kluwer; 2019. p. 263–404.

54. Chao CP, Zaleski CG, Patton AC. Neonatal hypoxic-ischemic encephalopathy: multimodality imaging findings. Radiographics 2006;26(Suppl 1):S159–72.

55. Hanrahan JD, Sargentoni J, Azzopardi D, et al. Cerebral metabolism within 18 Hours of birth asphyxia: a proton magnetic resonance spectroscopy study. Pediatr Res 1996;39(4):584–90.

56. Heinz ER, Provenzale JM. Imaging findings in neonatal hypoxia: a practical review. AJR Am J Roentgenol 2009;192(1):41–7.

57. Zarifi MK, Astrakas LG, Poussaint TY, et al. Prediction of adverse outcome with cerebral lactate level and apparent diffusion coefficient in infants with perinatal asphyxia. Radiology 2002;225(3):859–70.

58. Lange T, Dydak U, Roberts TPL, et al. Pitfalls in lactate measurements at 3T. Am J Neuroradiol 2006;27(4):895–901.

59. Leth H, Toft PB, Pryds O, et al. Brain lactate in preterm and growth-retarded neonates. Acta Paediatr 1995;84(5):495–0.

Intrauterine and Perinatal Infections

Jennifer A. Vaughn, MD[a,b,c,d,*], Luis F. Goncalves, MD[a,b,c,e], Patricia Cornejo, MD[a,b,c,d,e]

KEYWORDS

- Neonatal meningitis
- Meningoencephalitis
- MRI
- Ultrasound
- Fetal
- Congenital infection

KEY POINTS

- Clinical symptoms and signs in congenital and perinatal CNS infections are often absent or nonspecific; therefore, imaging plays a crucial role in identifying specific pathogens to target early treatment.
- Many of the congenitally acquired CNS infections have broader manifestations in other organ systems with certain findings suggestive of specific syndromes.
- Advances in fetal and neonatal ultrasound and MRI allow for earlier and more specific diagnoses if the radiologist is familiar with suggestive imaging patterns and works in close collaboration with the clinical teams.

INTRODUCTION

Despite continued advances in maternal–fetal medicine and the implementation of vaccination programs leading to more wide-spread immunization, congenital and perinatal central nervous system (CNS) infections remain a significant cause of long-term morbidity and mortality for affected fetuses and neonates. Infections during these time periods differ from those acquired later in childhood and adulthood due to a variety of factors including exposure to unique pathogens, immaturity of the CNS and diminished ability to mount immunologic response. These factors can lead to particular and recognizable patterns in imaging, with which radiologists and clinicians should be familiar. In this patient population, clinical symptoms and signs are often absent or nonspecific; therefore, imaging plays a crucial role in identifying specific

[a] Department of Radiology, Phoenix Children's Hospital, 1919 East Thomas Road, Phoenix, AZ 85016, USA; [b] University of Arizona College of Medicine, Phoenix, AZ, USA; [c] Creighton University School of Medicine, Phoenix, AZ, USA; [d] Barrows Neurological Institute, Phoenix, AZ, USA; [e] Mayo Clinic, Scottsdale, AZ, USA
* Corresponding author. Department of Radiology, Phoenix Children's Hospital, 1919 East Thomas Road, Phoenix, AZ 85016.
E-mail address: Jvaughn2@phoenixchildrens.com

Clin Perinatol 49 (2022) 751–770
https://doi.org/10.1016/j.clp.2022.05.008
0095-5108/22/© 2022 Elsevier Inc. All rights reserved.
perinatology.theclinics.com

pathogens to target early medical treatment, discerning secondary complications of generalized inflammation which may warrant additional medical or surgical treatment, differentiating infection from other conditions which clinically may present similarly and providing prognostic information for families.

Congenital and perinatal CNS infections are typically acquired by several distinct modes of transmission. Prenatally, pathogens may cross the placenta or ascend from the vaginal canal with increased risk in the setting of ruptured membranes. Some of the more commonly recognized entities transmitted trans-placentally include Toxoplasmosis, CMV, Rubella, Listeria, Syphilis, and Zika virus. Intrapartum infections are acquired via contact during delivery with the maternal rectovaginal flora including such organisms as group B streptococci and enteric gram-negative organisms, primarily *Escherichia coli*, or via contact with infected maternal secretions in the vaginal canal in the case of Herpes simplex virus (HSV). In the immediate postpartum period, infections are acquired via transmission from mother to infant such as TB, HIV, Parechovirus, and Enterovirus or from exposure to the hospital setting with increased host susceptibility in the setting of prematurity or underlying medical conditions such as fungal organisms such as Candida.

In most cases, the initial prenatal diagnosis relies on ultrasound and polymerase chain reaction. Infection may be suspected by common but nonspecific sonographic abnormalities including growth restriction (IUGR), ascites, hydrops, ventriculomegaly, microcephaly, intracranial calcifications hepatosplenomegaly, cardiac anomalies, hyperechoic bowel, placentomegaly and abnormal amniotic fluid with certain combinations of manifestations suggestive of specific syndromes. Patients should be referred for dedicated anatomic ultrasound including 3D imaging if anomalies are suspected with a targeted evaluation of all organ systems as many of the congenital CNS infections have broader manifestations. Fetal MRI, which is increasingly available, plays a complimentary role in permitting a more detailed evaluation and should include at minimum targeted imaging of both the brain and body using T2-weighted imaging in 3 planes, T1 imaging, gradient-echo imaging with echo-planar to detect blood and calcification and diffusion-weighted imaging (DWI).

Postnatally, neonates are most readily evaluated with ultrasound given the sonographic window afforded by the anterior fontanelle. Ultrasound can well depict the extra-axial spaces, evaluate for hemorrhage, and assess the size of the ventricles. It is also the most portable of all potential imaging modalities available, can be performed repeatedly due to the absence of ionization radiation and nonnecessity of sedation. When abnormalities are detected on ultrasound, MRI with consideration to the administration of intravenous contrast should be obtained for a more detailed evaluation of intracranial structures that ultrasound cannot depict well, including the brainstem and posterior fossa, and to fully characterize potential abnormalities detected. The use of DWI can characterize fluid collections with suspected purulence in the case of empyema and evaluate for stroke in the setting of meningoencephalitis. In the perinatal period, MRI can often be obtained without the need for sedation, especially at specialized tertiary centers with child life teams adept at feed and wrap/swaddle technique. Computed tomography (CT) plays a limited role in these neonates suspected of CNS infection in the acute setting though can be useful in the nonemergent characterization of intracranial calcifications characteristic of certain congenital infections.

This review aims to provide an overview of the characteristic imaging findings, when present, of the more common bacterial, viral, parasitic, and fungal infections acquired congenitally or in the immediate perinatal period as well as serve as an aid for clinicians seeking to optimize imaging timing and modality selection.

DISCUSSION
Intrauterine

Viruses

Cytomegalovirus. Cytomegalovirus (CMV) infection is the most common congenital infection in the United States affecting 0.5% to 2% of all live births.[1] CMV is the leading nonhereditary cause of sensorineural hearing loss and an important cause of neurodevelopmental disability. Vertical transmission can occur at any time during gestation with higher risk during primary maternal infections and higher risk of infecting the fetus during the third trimester. To date, there are no public health policies or management guidelines despite the frequency and impact of infection on the fetus and newborn. In suspected cases, the diagnosis is based on maternal serology, detection of CMV-DNA in amniotic fluid, and fetal blood and imaging. Early diagnosis of congenital CMV at birth or within 3 weeks of life is paramount in moderate to severe symptomatic infants as oral treatment with valganciclovir improves hearing and neurodevelopmental outcomes. Approximately 90% of infants with congenital CMV are asymptomatic at birth. Of these, 10% to 15% will develop neurologic sequelae. In the other 10% of cases, there are visible manifestations.[1]

On fetal ultrasound, the findings that suggest congenital CMV infection are ventriculomegaly, hyperechogenic bowel (**Fig. 1**), microcephaly, periventricular calcifications (**Fig. 2**), increased echogenicity of the intermediate zone of lamination (**Fig. 3**), pseudocysts, intraventricular adhesions, intrauterine growth retardation, thickened placenta with calcifications (**Fig. 4**) and oligohydramnios. The manifestations vary depending on the time of infection with more severe abnormalities identified in fetuses infected before the first half of the second trimester. Ventriculomegaly, defined as greater than 10 mm diameter of the atrium of the lateral ventricles, is a common and nonspecific prenatal finding with multiple etiologies. Cerebral calcifications are also nonspecific; however, it is the most common finding of congenital CMV, present in up to 70% of cases.[1] The calcifications can be thick or fine and are usually located at the periventricular zones. Early CMV infections interfere with normal proliferation and migration of the neurons resulting in microcephaly and malformations of cortical development. Microcephaly is commonly associated with periventricular calcifications and ventriculomegaly and is linked to poor prognosis due to psychomotor retardation. Late infections are associated with white matter abnormalities from myelin destruction

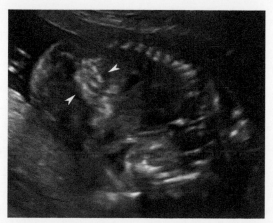

Fig. 1. CMV hyperechogenic bowel 20w5d. Coronal oblique images of the torso of a fetus at 20 weeks and 5 days show hyperechogenic fetal bowel (*arrowheads*).

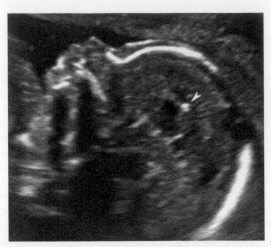

Fig. 2. CMV at 20 weeks and 5 days. Sagittal view of the fetal brain shows an echogenic periventricular calcification (arrow head).

and/or delayed myelination. The white matter involvement is typically posterior and spares the subcortical and periventricular zones with focal, regional, or confluent signal abnormalities. Periventricular cysts are commonly identified in the anterior temporal lobes in association with white matter abnormalities due to necrosis or hemorrhage of the germinal matrix.

Fetal MRI complements and enhances ultrasound diagnosis with a more detailed delineation of parenchymal abnormalities that are quite specific for congenital CMV infection when combined with other intracranial and extracranial manifestations. Anterior temporal lobe abnormalities, white matter lesions (**Fig. 5**A), disorders of cortical migration (**Fig. 5**B), and cerebellar dysplasia are better visualized with MRI. Also, detection of transitional abnormalities including anterior temporal lobe cysts and occipital horn adhesions may only be identified with fetal MRI as they can later resolve postnatally. Follow-up postnatally with MRI reveals similar findings (**Fig. 6**A–C).

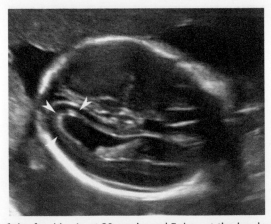

Fig. 3. Axial view of the fetal brain at 20 weeks and 5 days at the level of the lateral ventricles show hyperechogenic ventricular wall and intermediate zone (*arrowheads*).

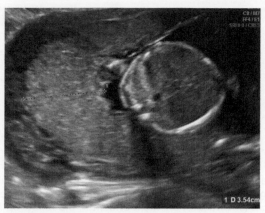

Fig. 4. CMV. Thickened placenta with calcs 20w5d. Transverse image of the uterus shows thickened placenta with calcifications at 20 weeks and 5 days.

Zika virus. Zika virus (ZIKV) is a mosquito borne neurotropic flavivirus. The infection can be transmitted during pregnancy or at the time of birth. The term congenital Zika syndrome (CZS) groups 5 distinctive features of the infection in utero including brain anomalies (microcephaly and calcifications), ocular anomalies (chorioretinal scars and pigmentary changes in the macula), congenital contractures and hypertonia.[2] ZIKV can cross multiple placental and fetal tissue barriers using complex mechanisms to evade and modulate the host immune system. The strong neurotropism of the virus and preferential involvement of neural progenitor cells causes massive cellular death and neurogenesis disruption. This mechanism of pathogenesis leads to a more severe spectrum of CNS anomalies compared with other congenital infections.

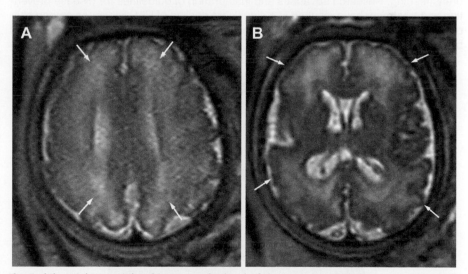

Fig. 5. (*A*). Axial T2-weighted image at the level of the corona radiata shows abnormal sulcation and greater than expected T2 hyper intense signal in the anterior frontal and posterior parietal white matter (*arrows*). Same patient. (*B*) Axial super resolution image at the level of the basal ganglia shows diffuse bihemispheric dysgyria with shallow and serrated morphology of the sulci (*arrows*).

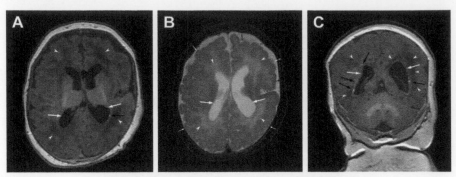

Fig. 6. Postnatal brain MRI at 2 months of age: Axial T1-weighted (*A*), axial T2-weighted (*B*) and coronal T1-weighted images (*C*). The bilateral sulcation abnormalities (*thin arrows*) and white matter changes (*arrowheads*) are more evident in the follow-up images. The lateral ventricles are mildly dilated and dysmorphic (*thick arrows*). There are also scattered punctuate calcifications in the periventricular white matter (*black arrows*).

Fetal ultrasound and MRI show a wide range of abnormalities including reduced brain volumes (**Fig. 7**), disorders of cortical development, callosal dysgenesis, gray-white matter junction calcifications (**Fig. 8**), dysmyelination, ventriculomegaly (see **Fig. 8**) and prominent extra-axial spaces. Decreased brainstem-cerebellar volumes, venous thrombosis, and lenticulostriate vasculopathy can also be seen.

Human immunodeficiency viruses. The human immunodeficiency viruses (HIV-1 and HIV-2) are 2 species of lentiviruses that attack the immune system by infecting and destroying the CD4-T cells, reducing the host's capacity to respond to other infections and diseases. Perinatal transmission can occur during pregnancy, childbirth, or breastfeeding. Research advances and instauration of guidelines for disease prevention and treatment have resulted in a significant decline of HIV diagnoses among children born in the US from 2014 to 2018 resulting in less than 1% of infections in 2018 being due to perinatal transmission.[2]

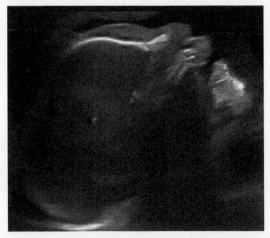

Fig. 7. Sagittal sonographic profile view of a 30-weeks fetus with Zika virus shows sloping forehead secondary to microcephaly. (*Courtesy of* F Peralta, MD, Sao Paulo, Brazil.)

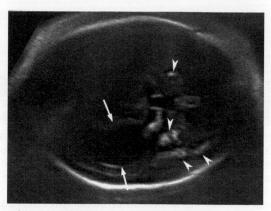

Fig. 8. Axial sonographic view of the head of a 30-weeks fetus with Zika virus shows ventriculomegaly (*arrows*) and intraparenchymal hyperechogenic foci consistent with calcification (*arrowheads*). (*Courtesy of* F Peralta, MD, Sao Paulo, Brazil.)

On imaging, there are no specific fetal anomalies associated with HIV infection. Brain atrophy and calcifications predominantly at the frontal subcortical white matter can be identified. Additional findings include lymphadenopathy and parotid lymphoepithelial cysts. If untreated, the infection progresses to autoimmune immunodeficiency syndrome (AIDS) associated with vasculopathy and increased risk of hemorrhagic infarcts in approximately 1% of children. Secondary infections and increased risk of neoplasms are less frequent in children; however, CMV encephalitis, fungal, varicella-zoster virus infections and CNS lymphoma can occur. Serial ultrasound follow-up is recommended to detect IUGR is known HIV-positive pregnancies.

Human herpes virus-3 (varicella-zoster virus) Varicella-Zoster (VZV) is a highly contagious Herpesvirus. The maternal infection is transmitted to fetus through the placenta and is more common with advanced maternal age. The type and severity of infection depend on the time of transmission. When infections occur during the first 20 weeks of gestation more serious complications can be expected which have been grouped as congenital varicella syndrome (CVS). Maternal infections close to the time of delivery cause neonatal varicella. Most cases of VZV infection can be diagnosed clinically or with the detection of viral DNA in amniocentesis at least 1 month after maternal infection to avoid false-negative results.

The imaging findings of congenital varicella syndrome are variable and nonspecific. To date, there are no reliable markers of fetal infection which makes it challenging to diagnose these cases with noninvasive methods. Serial ultrasound is recommended to document the development of fetal anomalies during pregnancy, however, the sensitivity and specificity of ultrasound to diagnose CVS are suboptimal and more invasive methods should be considered to confirm congenital infection. IUGR, oligohydramnios, polyhydramnios, hydrops, limb hypoplasia or contractures, CNS involvement, ocular involvement (**Fig. 9A**) and calcifications in different abdominal and pelvic organs (**Fig. 9B**) can be present. Parenchymal destruction, hydrocephalus (**Fig. 9C**), basal ganglia necrosis, cerebellar hypoplasia/aplasia, and polymicrogyria are the most common findings in the CNS. Echogenic debris in the amniotic fluid and specular reflections from the fetal skin are suggestive of vesicular rashes in the fetal skin. Cataracts and microphthalmia are noted with ocular involvement. Fetal MRI complements and refines the evaluation of most of these anomalies due to multiplanar imaging

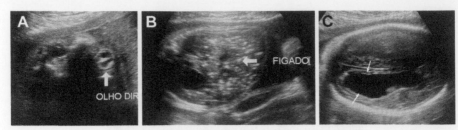

Fig. 9. Fetal varicella at 26 weeks. Courtesy of E M Tomaz da Cunha, MD, São Paulo, Brazil (*A*) Axial sonographic image at 26 weeks in a fetus with varicella demonstrates abnormal right eye with mixed echogenicity material in the posterior aspect of the globe consistent with vitreous hemorrhage and retinal detachment. (*B*). Axial sonographic image at 26 weeks in a fetus with varicella demonstrates a heavily calcified liver. (*C*). Axial sonographic image at 26 weeks in a fetus with varicella demonstrates lateral ventriculomegaly (*arrows*).

capabilities and superior soft-tissue resolution. The prognosis of congenital varicella syndrome is poor if VZ immunoglobulin or antiviral therapy are not administered to susceptible seronegative women with exposure to varicella. The neonatal mortality rates are as high as 31%. With the administration of therapy, the rates drop to 7%.[2] Recurrent aspiration pneumonia and respiratory failure are the principal causes of neonatal demise.

Parvovirus. Erythema infectiosum or 5th disease is a common infection caused by Parvovirus B19 (B19 V). Women at higher risk include mothers of school-age children, teachers, and daycare workers. During viral outbreaks, B19 V can infect up to 1% to 5% of pregnant women, with most of these infections resolving spontaneously without major complications.[3] The estimated risk of vertical transmission is 25%, with the likelihood of fetal infection being higher if seroconversion occurs during the first half of pregnancy.[3] B19 V is a potent inhibitor of erythropoiesis that targets erythroid progenitor cells leading to arrest the maturation of red blood cell precursors and apoptosis. The affected fetuses develop severe anemia, high-output cardiac failure, and nonimmune hydrops.Prior literature has reported up to 27% of cases of nonimmune hydrops in anatomically normal fetuses to be caused by B19 V infection.[4] The virus may also spread to cardiac myocytes and hepatocytes causing local inflammation which further deteriorates the cardiac function. The results of a systematic review of 35 observational studies involving 611 fetuses affected by B19 V (++), demonstrated that hydrops is the main determinant of mortality and adverse outcomes in congenital parvo B19 infections with a higher risk of miscarriage and perinatal death in fetuses affected with hydrops.[3] Hypoxic injuries from severe anemia, direct viral damage to microglial cells, intrauterine growth retardation and prematurity have been described.

Although, there is no randomized trial on the type or frequency of prenatal follow-up of fetuses at high risk, weekly ultrasound to evaluate hydrops and measurements of middle cerebral artery peak systolic velocity (MCA-PSV) are highly recommended. Abnormal MCA-PSV is a reliable indicator of fetal anemia. When values are 1.5 x higher than the median for gestational age, confirmation with percutaneous umbilical blood sampling should be considered. Other signs include cardiomegaly, hyperechoic bowel, ascites, polyhydramnios, meconium peritonitis, and enlarged placenta. For confirmed cases of severe fetal anemia, intrauterine blood transfusion with packed red blood cells has been shown to reduce perinatal morbidity and mortality.

Rubella. Congenital rubella syndrome (CRS) results from vertical transmission of the single-stranded RNA Togavirus rubella virus during the first 12 weeks of pregnancy.

The infection was common in children and nonimmunized adults before the vaccine development in 1969 and now extremely rare.[2] The consequences of CRS are devastating with increased risk of miscarriage, intrauterine demise, and severe birth defects. The clinical manifestations are diverse among survivors. The most frequent malformations reported in the fetus are microcephaly, congenital cataracts, microphthalmia, cardiac septal defects, pulmonary artery stenosis, and hepatosplenomegaly.[5] Amniotic fluid sampling for fetuses with suspected CRS should be performed 6 to 8 weeks after maternal infection.

Lymphocytic choriomeningitis virus Lymphocytic choriomeningitis virus (LCMV) is an underrecognized fetal pathogen distributed worldwide and transmitted to humans after exposure to urine, saliva, or nesting materials from infected rodents.[2] Additional forms of transmission include transplacental and organ transplantation. The incidence rates and estimates of geographic prevalence of LCMV infections are unknown.[2] The virus is strongly neurotropic and replicates in the meninges, choroid plexus, and ependyma. Postnatal infections usually manifest as aseptic meningitis or less frequently, encephalitis, meningoencephalitis, hydrocephalus, or myelitis. The symptoms can last several weeks with full recovery. Prenatal infections are more severe during the first trimester with higher rates of fetal demise. Second and third trimester infections can cause severe injury to the developing brain and retina. Hydrocephalus, periventricular calcifications, and chorioretinitis are the most common findings of congenital infection.[6] Additional findings include microcephaly, porencephalic cysts, encephalomalacia, cerebellar hypoplasia, and cortical migration abnormalities.

Chikungunya Chikungunya (CHIKV) is an RNA virus member of the genus Alphavirus and family Togaviridae. The cases of CHKV infection have dropped significantly after the most recent outbreak in the Caribbean and US in 2013 with no reported cases since 2016.[2] The CHIKV is transmitted to humans by the bite of infected mosquitos. Less common forms of transmission occur with infected blood or mother to child at the time of birth. In one study of pregnant patients with confirmed CHKV infection, pregnancy complications were seen in 20% of cases including premature delivery, premature rupture of membranes, decreased fetal movements, intrauterine deaths, and oligohydramnios.[7]

Parasitic

Toxoplasmosis
Toxoplasma Gondii is an obligate intracellular protozoan parasite with high rates of infection worldwide. Approximately 11% of the population 6 years and older have been infected with Toxoplasma in the United States.[2] Congenital infection ranges from 1 in 10,000 births in the United States to 1 in 1000 cases in endemic areas with hot, humid climates.[6] The parasite has a complex life cycle that includes 3 stages: the tachyzoite phase responsible for the acute infection with parasitic invasion and replication within host cells. The bradyzoite phase during the latent stage with cystic lesions found in different tissues and lastly, the sporozoite phase with resistant cysts released to the environment. Congenital infections occur during the tachyzoite phase. The most common routes of human transmission are the ingestion of contaminated food, goat's milk, water, or by accidental contact with cat's feces. Transplacental transmission causes congenital infection. The prevalence of maternal infection is 0.4% and out of these, 40% will develop congenital toxoplasmosis.[1] The risk of congenital infection is higher during the second half of pregnancy, while the severity of infection is greater during the first trimester and first half of second trimester.

Once maternal infection is confirmed, amniocentesis with PCR testing has high sensitivity and specificity to detect *T. gondii*. The classic triad of chorioretinitis, hydrocephalus, and intracranial calcifications only occur in less than 10% of infected fetuses. Abnormalities in ultrasound are more commonly detected during the third trimester. Imaging findings include ventriculomegaly, intracranial echogenic nodules/calcifications randomly distributed in the parenchyma (**Fig. 10**), periventricular and caudothalamic zones, different from CMV calcifications which have predilection for the periventricular white matter. Furthermore, periventricular cysts, microcephaly, and cortical migration abnormalities are more common with CMV while hydrocephalus and chorioretinitis are more common with toxoplasmosis. Non-CNS findings include intrauterine growth retardation, thickened placenta, hepatosplenomegaly, and echogenic foci in the liver. Treatment with spiramycin during the first trimester and a combination of pyrimethamine and sulfadiazine during the second and third trimesters is recommended. Prevention of infection before conception is critical, particularly in endemic areas. The prognosis depends on the time of congenital infection with higher risk of serious long-term sequelae during the first half of pregnancy including seizures, learning disabilities, hydrocephalus, motor and hearing deficits, and retinal scarring with impaired vision.

Bacterial

Syphilis

Syphilis is a sexually transmitted infection caused by the bacterium *Treponema pallidum*. The cases of congenital syphilis (CS) in the United States have increased significantly since 2012.[2] The American College of Obstetricians and Gynecologists and the American Academy of Pediatrics recommend screening of CS during the first prenatal visit and a second screening during 32 to 36 weeks in high-risk women. Fetal infections can occur at any disease stage and in any trimester. The most common imaging findings on ultrasound are hepatomegaly, placentomegaly, hydrops, and elevated peak systolic velocities in the middle cerebral artery, a marker of fetal anemia. Hepatic calcifications, and echogenic bowel are occasionally seen.[1] Once maternal infection is confirmed by serologic testing, treatment should be initiated according to the stage per CDC algorithms, ideally more than 30 days before delivery.[2] CS has a variety of clinical manifestations depending on the timing of childhood infection. Early congenital

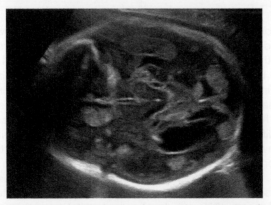

Fig. 10. Axial sonographic view of the brain of 29 weeks and 6 days fetus with confirmed toxoplasmosis shows multiple hyperechogenic lesions distributed randomly through the brain parenchyma. (*Courtesy of* J Abdalla, MD, Sao Paulo, Brazil.)

syphilis occurs in the first 2 years of life. Children present with hepatosplenomegaly, anemia, leukopenia, thrombocytopenia, mucosal and cartilage ulcerations (saddle nose deformity), periostitis, maculo-papular skin rash, renal failure, and CNS-ocular abnormalities. Late congenital syphilis can present with notched central incisors (Hutchinson teeth), multi-cuspid first molars (mulberry teeth), interstitial keratitis, hydrocephalus, seizures, 8th cranial nerve palsy, developmental delay, periostitis, and arthritis.

Perinatal

Bacterial
Escherichia coli, group B Streptococcus, Proteus, and Citrobacter. Neonatal bacterial sepsis is far more common than viral sepsis with a prevalence of approximately 1 to 10 in 1000 live births worldwide.[8] According to the timing of infection, neonatal sepsis is divided into early and late onset, with different modes of transmission and organisms responsible in each group. Early-onset sepsis is secondary to maternal intrapartum transmission and is defined when neonates return positive cultures for external pathogens during the first 7 days of life.[9] There has been a decreasing incidence of early-onset sepsis with GBS due to increased testing of the mother and administration of antenatal antibiotics however the incidence of CNS infection with *E. coli* and other gram-negative organisms has remained stable. Some studies report similar outcomes while other studies have found a worse prognosis with gram-negative infection compared with GBS[10,11] Meningitis complicates a proportion of early-onset sepsis cases with significant morbidity and mortality.

Imaging features in neonatal meningitis vary based on the pathogen, stage of infection and age of the patient and can be predicted by the pathophysiology. An inflammatory vasculitis permits access through the blood–brain barrier which typically occurs at the level of the choroid plexus as well as in both small and large arteries. Subsequent ventriculitis results in CSF dissemination with leptomeningitis, arachnoiditis, and eventually, the parenchyma is accessed leading to cerebritis and cerebral edema. Imaging findings reflect these patterns but vary based on the age of the patient and ability to mount an immune response. If meningoencephalitis is suspected, MRI with contrast is the preferred imaging modality including T2 weighted, SWI, DWI, FLAIR, pre and postcontrast T1-weighted sequences.

As the organism circulates in the bloodstream, inflammation of the smaller intracranial arterial vessels can lead to focal lesions such as microhemorrhages and ischemic foci seen on SWI and DWI imaging, whereas the involvement of larger vessels and diffuse alterations of cerebral blood flow seen in sepsis can cause global hypoxic/ischemic injury visible as large regions of reduced diffusivity involving deep gray matter or vascular territories on DWI imaging (**Fig. 11**). While the ventricles may be normal, characteristic features of ventriculitis include enlargement and hyperenhancement of the choroid plexus, enhancement of the ependymal surface, hydrocephalus with transependymal CSF, and/or periventricular edema and debris layering in the dependent portions of the ventricles, such as the occipital horns. The layering debris may demonstrate reduced diffusivity on DWI in the setting of purulence (**Fig. 12**). Though there is much overlap, in one study comparing CNS imaging features of neonates infected with GBS versus *E. coli*, those with GBS were more likely to demonstrate infarcts and those with *E. coli* were more likely to have early-onset hydrocephalus.[12] As the infection spreads to the leptomeninges, one may see the enlargement of the extraaxial spaces with sterile effusions, enhancement, and thickening of the dura and enhancement and increased FLAIR signal along the leptomeningeal surface of the brain extending into the sulci. Further inflammation can progress to loculations within

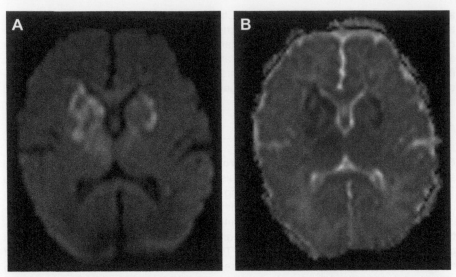

Fig. 11. (*A, B*). 4 days old with GBS meningitis. (*A*). Axial DWI and (*B*) ADC map demonstrating reduced diffusivity in the basal ganglia and thalami bilaterally.

the extra-axial spaces and reduced diffusivity within the collections with frank purulence (**Fig. 13**). These features may be absent in very young neonates who lack the immunologic response leading to the intense leptomeningitis.[13,14] Late in the stage of disease progression, access to the parenchyma leads to cerebritis which can present as either focal or diffuse cerebral edema with hyperintense T2 signal or well-organized abscess with rim enhancement and centrally reduced diffusivity with

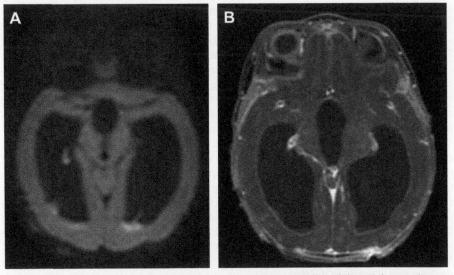

Fig. 12. (*A, B*). 7 days old with GBS meningitis and ventriculitis. (*A*). Axial DWI demonstrating reduced diffusivity within material layering in the occipital horns. (*B*). Axial postcontrast T1-weighted imaging demonstrating the enhancement of the ependymal surfaces of the ventricles and diffuse leptomeningeal enhancement.

surrounding edema. Associated mass effect can present as local sulcal effacement, partial ventricular effacement, midline shift, or frank herniation with a reduction in associated fatality due to the distensibility of the neonatal calvarium.[11] Gram-negative organisms such as Proteus and Citrobacter, while less prevalent overall, are the most common causative organism of cerebral abscesses in the perinatal and early neonatal period, especially in premature neonates, with different organisms responsible after 1 month of age.[13,15] Abscesses may develop rapidly in neonates and are often large at the time of diagnosis and lack a complete capsule.[15] **(Fig. 14)** Despite early antibiotic treatment, survivors of perinatal bacterial meningoencephalitis frequently have neurologic complications at discharge including developmental delay, seizures, and hydrocephalus among others[13]

Listeria. Neonatal CNS listeriosis is rare with most early-onset cases involving infants born prematurely in the third trimester, usually before 29 weeks, to infected mothers.[16] The predilection for rhomboencephalitis in adult Listeria infection is not seen in the fetus and neonate with early-onset perinatal infection presenting as single or multiple macro or micro-abscesses and late-onset infection as meningitis with hydrocephalus, gliosis and encephalomalacia potential complications in both groups.[13,17,18]

Viral

Herpes simplex virus, parechovirus, enterovirus, and rotavirus
Neonatal viral sepsis is less common than bacterial sepsis with HSV including both HSV-1 and HSV-2, being the most common viral agent.[15] Antepartum transplacental transmission is rare but seen occasionally with HSV-2. In utero infections can cause microcephaly, cerebral malformations, ventriculomegaly, chorioretinitis, skin lesions, hepatosplenomegaly, and intrauterine growth retardation. Neonatal infection is diagnosed when the infection manifests more than 48 hours after delivery. Both congenital

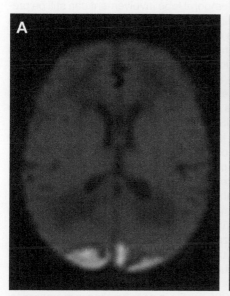
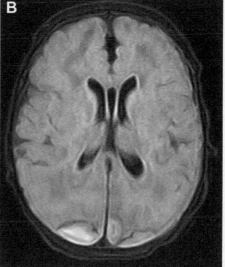

Fig. 13. (*A, B*). 5 days old with *E. coli* empyema. (*A*). Axial DWI demonstrates reduced diffusivity with the extra-axial space in both occipital regions with corresponding hyperintense signal on (*B*) axial FLAIR imaging.

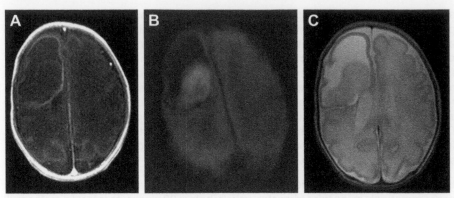

Fig. 14. (A–C). 2 days old with enterobacter abscess. (A). Postcontrast axial T1 demonstrating a rim enhancing cavity in the right frontal lobe with centrally reduced diffusivity contents on (B). Axial DWI and hypointense signal on (C). axial T2.

and neonatal HSV infections are classified into 3 levels of disease; skin, eye, and mouth; encephalitis with or without skin, eye, and mouth infection and disseminated disease with high mortality rates. The pathogenesis of this neurotropic virus also predicts patterns of involvement with direct invasion of parenchymal tissue, spread along meningeal nerves, and diffusion across vasculature all permitting entry. Symptoms are often nonspecific and skin lesions are absent in one-third of neonates with HSV encephalitis;[19] therefore, one should have a low threshold for imaging and treatment of suspected cases. CT and ultrasound are insensitive to detect all potential sites of involvement and therefore MRI with and without contrast should be obtained in these patients. In contrast to childhood and adult presentations of herpes encephalitis, in neonates, the presentation is more variable lacking the same characteristic predilection for the medial temporal lobes[20] though temporal lobe involvement can still be present.[21] The disease may be multifocal involving the cerebral hemispheres, can involve the cerebellum and brainstem as well as the deep gray and periventricular white matter. Involved regions demonstrate hyperintense signal on T2-weighted imaging which can be difficult to appreciate in the background of unmyelinated brain. DWI imaging is, therefore, essential for demonstrating early and more extensive involvement than is visible on the additional anatomic sequences[21] (**Fig. 15**). Ischemic changes may be present in the watershed regions as well as in the cortex[20,21] (**Fig. 16**). Hemorrhage is less frequently a component of neonatal HSV encephalitis compared with older children and adults and postcontrast imaging is typically normal or demonstrates only mild leptomeningeal enhancement[15] As the disease progresses, cystic encephalomalacia and atrophy may ensue with gyriform calcification manifested as T1 shortening on MRI (**Fig. 17**). There is poor long-term neurologic sequela for those infected with HSV-2 in the perinatal period compared with HSV-1.[22]

Additional viral entities which can cause meningitis and meningoencephalitis in the perinatal period include enterovirus, rotavirus, echovirus, and parechovirus. Symptoms are variable but may include fever, seizures, irritability, and diarrhea with a large number of asymptomatic cases.[15] The clinical presentation and imaging features of these entities overlap and thus they are grouped together in this review. If suspected clinically, MRI with and without contrast should be performed and can play an important role in suggesting the diagnosis as the CSF profile is nonrevealing in many cases. The neuroimaging features of these viruses overlap with the characteristic involvement of the periventricular white matter and callosum on DWI with restricted diffusion.

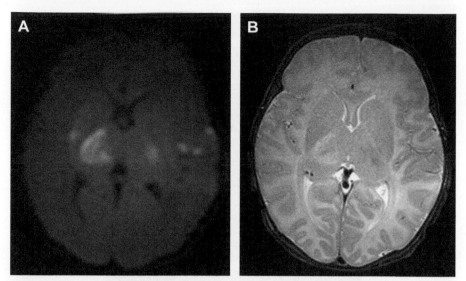

Fig. 15. (*A*, *B*). 7 days old with HSV encephalitis and ischemia. (*A*). Axial DWI demonstrates several foci of reduced diffusivity in both thalami, the right basal ganglia and the left temporal cortex/subcortical white matter that are much less conspicuous on the corresponding (*B*). Axial T2-weighted image.

Enterovirus has been reported to involve the brainstem, cerebellum, and deep gray matter with hyperintense signal seen on T2-weighted imaging and reduced diffusivity on DWI.[23] (**Fig. 18**). In human parechovirus, imaging typically demonstrates reduced diffusivity within the corpus callosum and subcortical white matter with a frontoparietal predominance as well as thalamic involvement and sparing of the basal ganglia and posterior fossa.[24] (**Fig. 19**) One study demonstrated T1 and T2 shortening in the white matter along the deep medullary veins suggesting venous ischemia as potential

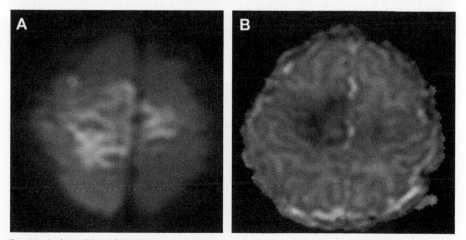

Fig. 16. 5 day old with HSV2 encephalitis and ischemia. (*A*). Axial DWI and (*B*). ADC map demonstrating reduced diffusivity in the right more extensive than left frontal and parietal lobes.

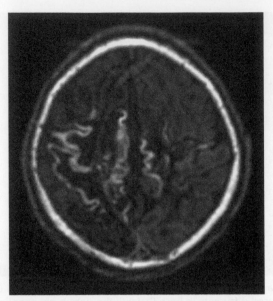

Fig. 17. Follow-up examination in a 25 days old with prior HSV encephalitis demonstrating serpiginous T1 hyperintense signal in the cortex of both frontal and parietal lobes on pre-contrast axial T1-weighted imaging compatible with gyriform calcification.

pathogenetic mechanism to injury.[24] Long-term imaging follow-up in these viral entities demonstrates variable findings ranging from normal without visible sequela on MRI, to gliosis, parenchymal volume loss and cystic encephalomalacia.[15,23,24]

Fungal–candida, aspergillus

Perinatal CNS fungal infections primarily involve those with compromised immune systems including premature and/or low birth weight neonates, typically in the ICU setting, and those with primary immunodeficiency disorders. The primary invasive fungal infections affecting neonates are caused most by Candida species and less frequently by Aspergillus with CNS involvement representing a major complication. Imaging plays an important role in what can often be a challenging diagnosis due to misleading CNS analysis and nonspecific clinical presentation.[25] In the first days of candidemia, imaging may be normal with findings appearing closer to 1 week.

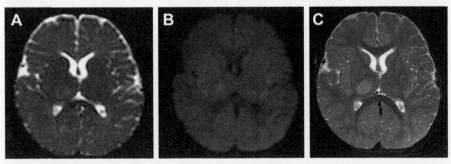

Fig. 18. (*A–C*). 12 months old with enterovirus encephalitis. (*A*). Axial DWI and (*B*). ADC map demonstrating reduced diffusivity in the right thalamus with corresponding edema on the (*C*). Axial T2-weighted sequence.

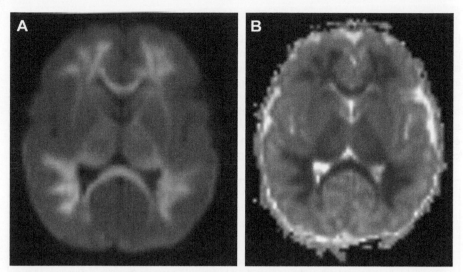

Fig. 19. (*A*, *B*). 6 days old with parechovirus encephalitis. (*A*). Axial DWI and (*B*). ADC map demonstrating symmetric reduced diffusivity in the thalami, callosum, and periventricular white matter.

Ultrasound can be a useful first modality in suspected cases demonstrating numerous small foci of parenchymal increased echogenicity in the case of micro-abscesses.[26] (**Fig. 20**A) Ultrasound also permits easier serial and portable imaging in these frequently fragile patients. MRI with and without contrast is useful to document the full extent of disease depicting multiple foci of signal abnormality throughout the cerebral and cerebellar hemispheres. The micro-abscesses vary in their appearance based on the stage of infection and may demonstrate susceptibility effect on GRE or SWI sequences (**Fig. 20**B), T1 shortening on precontrast T1 sequence, reduced diffusivity on DWI, and enhancement on postcontrast T1-weighted sequences which can range from punctate to ring like in morphology (**Fig. 20**C).[27,28] Survivors of CNS candida infection have generally poor outcome with potential long-term sequela including developmental delay and hydrocephalus though perhaps because of earlier diagnosis and improved treatment, outcomes recently are more favorable.[26]

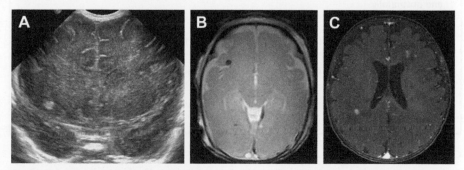

Fig. 20. (*A–C*). 6 days old with disseminated Candidiasis and microabscesses. (*A*) Ultrasound coronal plane image demonstrates a round focus of increased echogenicity in the right frontal lobe. (*B*) Axial SWI image demonstrates the corresponding susceptibility. (*C*) Axial postcontrast T1 demonstrates additional enhancing foci elsewhere in the brain parenchyma.

SUMMARY

Imaging plays an important role in evaluating patients with suspected intrauterine and perinatal infections. Advances in fetal imaging including both ultrasound and MRI allow for increasingly more specific diagnoses if the radiologist is familiar with specific imaging features and patterns. Early imaging of neonates with suspected CNS infection is valuable to permit early treatment and differentiate infection from other conditions which can clinically present similarly. Ultrasound is a useful initial modality to screen for abnormalities; however, MRI with and without contrast remains the optimal examination to characterize the infection, evaluate for potential surgical targets and provide prognostic information for clinicians and families.

Best practices

What is the current practice for imaging congenital and perinatal infections?

Best Practice/Guideline/Care Path Objective(s): For Imaging Fetuses and Neonates Suspected of Having CNS Infection
- Congenital Infection
  Anatomic ultrasound is useful to evaluate for CNS and abdominal calcifications, perform serial follow-up of IUGR and amniotic fluid index, and perform Doppler evaluation of the middle cerebral arteries in certain instances.
  Fetal MRI including targeted imaging of both neuro and body structures provides a more detailed delineation of parenchymal abnormalities including the detection of dysmyelination, migration anomalies, and destructive changes.
- Perinatal Infection
  Screening ultrasound can be a useful initial modality to detect hydrocephalus and to exclude pathologies that may present similarly (ie, hemorrhage)
  MRI with and without contrast including DWI and SWI imaging can be performed in neonates often without the need for sedation using a feed and wrap technique. It is the best modality to detect ischemia, cerebritis, empyema, and ventriculitis. It is also useful for following the course of the infection to detect the need for potential surgical interventions and provide prognostication.

What changes in current practice are likely to improve outcomes?

- Heightened awareness of the variety of appearances of CNS infection in fetuses and neonates to identify those who should be evaluated for the possibility of infection.

- Communication of concern promptly to clinical teams to initiate potential therapies without delay

- Continued advances in neuroimaging allow for earlier and more specific diagnoses in utero and postnatally.

Bibliographic Source(s):

ACR-SPR Practice Parameter for the safe and optimal performance of Fetal Magnetic Resonance Imaging (MRI) Revised 2020 (Resolution 45).

ACR-AIUM-SPR-SRU Practice Parameter for the performance of neurosonography in neonates and infants. Revised 2019 (Resolution 28).

ACR-ASNR-SPR Practice Parameter for the performance and interpretation of Magnetic Resonance Imaging (MRI) of the Brain. Revised 2019 (Resolution 17)

CLINICS CARE POINTS

- Both established and emerging infectious diseases continue to impact fetuses and neonates despite medical advances

- Imaging plays an important role in identification of potential congenital and neonatal infection to aid in clinical decision making regarding the management of the pregnancy, prognosticaion, birth plan and can facilitate early treatment when available.
- In both congenital and perinatal infection, ultrasound continues to play an important role in screening.
- With continued advancement in technology, MRI is used with increasing frequency to image fetuses suspected or at risk of congenital infection.
- Fetal MRI can demonstrate abnormalites that are not apparent or not specific on antenatal ultrasound.
- Expanded capabilities of MRI also extend to use in neonates with faster sequences, pediatric specific hardware such as dedicated head coils, higher field strengths and child life teams at major pediatric centers all aiding in improved image quality and diagnostic yield.

DISCLOSURE

The authors have nothing to disclose.

REFERENCES

1. Jodicke CD, Singh P, Maulik D. Congenital infections. In: Kline-Fath B, Bulas DI, Lee W, editors. Fundamentals and advanced fetal imaging ultrasound and MRI. 2nd edition. Philadelphia: Wolters Kluwer; 2021. p. 948–65.
2. Available at: https://www.cdc.gov/DiseasesConditions/. Accessed on 9 20, 21.
3. Bascietto F, Liberaty M, Murgano D, et al. Outcome of fetuses with congenital parvovirus b19 infection: systematic review and meta-analysis. Ultrasound Obstet Gynecol 2018;52(5):569–76.
4. Von Kaisenberg CS, Jonat W. Fetal parvovirus B19 infection. Ultrasound Obstet Gynecol 2001;18(3):280–8.
5. Yazigi A, De Pecoulas AE, Vauloup-Fellous C, et al. Fetal and neonatal abnormalities due to congenital rubella syndrome: a review of literature. J Matern Fetal Neonatal Med 2017;30(3):274–8.
6. Neuberger I, Garcla J, Meyers ML, et al. Imaging of congenital central nervous system infections. Pediatr Radiol 2018;48:513–23.
7. Gupta Suruchi, Gupta Nikhil. Short-term pregnancy outcomes in patients with Chikungunya infection: an observational study. J Fam Med Prim Care 2019; 8(3):985–7.
8. Afsharpaiman S, Torkaman M, Saburi A, et al. Trends in incidence of neonatal sepsis and antibiotic susceptibility of causative agents in two neonatal intensive care units in tehran, I.R Iran. J Clin Neonatol 2012;1(3):124–30.
9. Cortese F, Scicchitano P, Gesualdo M, et al. Early and late infections in newborns: where do we stand? A review. Pediatr Neonatal 2016;57(4):265–73.
10. Schrag SJ, Farley MM, Petit S, et al. Epidemiology of invasive early-onset neonatal sepsis, 2005 to 2014. Pediatrics 2016;138(6):e20162013.
11. Schneider JF. Neonatal brain infections. Pediatr Radiol 2011;41(Suppl 1).3143–8.
12. Kralik SF, Kukreja MK, Paldino MJ, et al. Comparison of CSF and MRI findings among neonates and infants with E coli or group B streptococcal meningitis. AJNR Am J Neuroradiol 2019;40(8):1413–7.
13. Blaser S, Jay V, Becker LE, et al. Neonatal brain infection. In: Rutherford M, editor. MRI of the neonatal brain. 2021. Available at: http://mrineonatalbrain.com/ch04-10.php. Accessed on June 14, 2021.

14. Maisey HC, Doran KS, Nizet V. Recent advances in understanding the molecular basis of group B Streptococcus virulence. Expert Rev Mol Med 2008;10:e27.
15. Schneider JF, Hanquinet S, Severino M, et al. MR imaging of neonatal brain infections. Magn Reson Imaging Clin N Am 2011;19(4):761–75.
16. Tai YL, Chi H, Chiu NC, et al. Clinical features of neonatal listeriosis in Taiwan: a hospital-based study. J Microbiol Immunol Infect 2020;53(6):866–74.
17. Hsu CC, Singh D, Watkins TW, et al. Serial magnetic resonance imaging findings of intracerebral spread of listeria utilising subcortical U-fibres and the extreme capsule. Neuroradiol J 2016;29(6):425–30.
18. Teixeira AB, Lana AM, Lamounier JA, et al. Neonatal listeriosis: the importance of placenta histological examination-a case report. AJP Rep 2011;1(1):3–6.
19. de Vries LS. Viral infections and the neonatal brain. Semin Pediatr Neurol 2019; 32:100769.
20. Soares BP, Provenzale JM. Imaging of herpesvirus infections of the CNS. AJR Am J Roentgenol 2016;1:39–48.
21. Vossough A, Zimmerman RA, Bilaniuk LT, et al. Imaging findings of neonatal herpes simplex virus type 2 encephalitis. Neuroradiology 2008;50(4):355–66.
22. Baskin HJ, Hedlund G. Neuroimaging of herpesvirus infections in children. Pediatr Radiol 2007;37:949.
23. Shen WC, Chiu HH, Chow KC, et al. MR imaging findings of enteroviral encephalomyelitis: an outbreak in Taiwan. AJNR Am J Neuroradiol 1999;20(10):1889–95.
24. Sarma A, Hanzlik E, Krishnasarma R, et al. Human parechovirus meningoencephalitis: neuroimaging in the era of polymerase chain reaction–based testing. AJNR Am J Neuroradiol 2019;40(8):1418–21.
25. Drummond RA, Lionakis MS. Candidiasis of the central nervous system in neonates and children with primary immunodeficiencies. Curr Fungal Infect Rep 2018;12(2):92–7.
26. Pahud B, Greenhow T, Piecuch B, et al. Preterm neonates with candidal brain microabscesses: a case series. J Perinatol 2009;29:323–6.
27. Mao J, Li J, Chen D, et al. MRI-DWI improves the early diagnosis of brain abscess induced by Candida albicans in preterm infants. Transl Pediatr 2012;1(2):76–84.
28. Lai PH, Lin SM, Pan HB, et al. Disseminated miliary cerebral candidiasis. AJNR Am J Neuroradiol 1997;18(7):1303–6.

Imaging of Congenital Craniofacial Anomalies and Syndromes

Jing Chen, MD, Sangam Kanekar, MD*

KEYWORDS

- Facial clefting • Craniostenosis • Midface anomalies • CHARGE syndrome
- Branchial arch syndromes

KEY POINTS

- Craniofacial malformation is one of the most commonly encountered birth defects in the prenatal and postnatal period.
- Facial clefting, cleft lip (CL) with or without cleft palate (CP), is the most common congenital craniofacial malformation.
- Craniofacial syndromes commonly associated with craniostenosis include Apert syndrome, Crouzon syndrome, and Pfeiffer syndrome, which are secondary to mutations of fibroblast growth factor receptor (FGFR).
- Higher-resolution and 3D antenatal ultrasonography and multidetector CT scan with 3D reformatted images have improved the definition of the soft tissue and bone structures of the craniofacial anatomy and its malformations.

INTRODUCTION

Craniofacial malformation is one of the most commonly encountered birth defects in the prenatal and postnatal periods. Early diagnosis of these malformations has vital clinical significance because some may present as acute emergencies in the postnatal period, whereas others may require long-term treatment. Craniofacial malformations can be either isolated or part of a defined genetic syndrome. Some may also be associated with brain anomalies. For the past 2 decades, our understanding of the genetic basis and embryologic development of the head and face has significantly improved. Higher-resolution and 3D antenatal ultrasonography (US) and multidetector computed tomographic (CT) scan with 3D reformatted images have improved the definition of the soft tissue and bone structures of the craniofacial anatomy and its malformations. These techniques have helped in better characterizing the malformation and have

Radiology Research, Division of Neuroradiology, Penn State Health, Penn State College of Medicine, Mail Code H066 500 University Drive, Hershey, PA 17033, USA
* Corresponding author.
E-mail address: skanekar@pennstatehealth.psu.edu

Clin Perinatol 49 (2022) 771–790
https://doi.org/10.1016/j.clp.2022.04.005

greatly helped surgical planning. This article focuses on the imaging findings of commonly encountered craniofacial malformations. These malformations are discussed under the following headings: facial clefting, cleft lip with or without cleft palate (CLP); craniofacial syndromes with major chromosomal anomalies; craniofacial syndromes with craniosynostosis (upper face pathologies); midface anomalies; lower face pathologies/branchial arch syndromes (BAS); and fetal alcohol syndrome (FAS). When these malformations are diagnosed via imaging, appropriate genetic testing is suggested to confirm the specific gene deletion or underlying syndrome.

Craniofacial Embryology and Genetics

The facial and nasal structures arise from the ectodermal, neural crest, and mesodermal cells, developing during the fourth to eighth week of gestation.[1–4] The first sign of facial development begins as a depression below the developing brain called stomodeum; this is surrounded by the frontonasal prominence, the paired maxillary prominences, and the paired mandibular prominences that give rise to the development of midfacial structures.[1–4]

The nose is derived from the single median frontonasal prominence and the paired maxillary prominences; these arise from the proliferation and migration of neural crest cells early in the fourth week of gestation. By the end of the fourth week of gestation, the frontonasal prominence gives rise to bilateral nasal placodes, which then proliferate and create the nasal pits and the medial and lateral nasal prominences.[1–4]

During the fifth week of gestation, the nasal pits deepen toward the oral cavity to form the primitive nasal cavity, which grows dorsally and is separated from the oral cavity by the bucconasal membrane of Hochstetter.[1–4] The bucconasal membrane is an epithelial plug that normally ruptures by the seventh week of gestation to allow communication between the oral and nasal cavities. This membrane normally resorbs during the third trimester resulting in posterior choanae. It has been hypothesized that choanal atresia may be attributed to the failure of bucconasal membrane rupture.

During the sixth and seventh weeks of gestation, the medial nasal prominences migrate medially as the maxillary prominences extend medially toward each other. As the fusion occurs at the junction of these prominences, the upper lip, nasal tip, philtrum, primary palate, and columella are formed.[1–4] The medial nasal prominences fuse and form the primary palate, whereas the lateral nasal prominences fuse with the maxillary prominences and form the lateral bones of the piriform aperture. It has been hypothesized that deficiency in the primary palate or bony overgrowth of the nasal processes of the maxilla may result in horizontal narrowing of the lateral walls of the piriform aperture, triangular-shaped palate, and single central incisor seen in congenital nasal piriform aperture stenosis.

At the end of the sixth week of gestation, surface ectoderm migrates from the nasooptic fissure within the nasolacrimal grooves to form the epithelial cords, which eventually develop into the nasolacrimal ducts (NLDs) and sacks. At the seventh to eighth week of gestation, the cartilaginous capsule surrounding the nasal cavity extends from the chondrocranium of the skull base and preturbinates begin to form from this capsule. At the 9th to 10th week of gestation, the cartilage penetrates the preturbinates and the precursor of the uncinate process forms.

The nasal and frontal bones are separated by the fonticulus frontalis superiorly. A dural extension extends between the anterior cranial fossa and the foramen cecum where the frontal bone articulates with the ethmoid bone into a prenasal space; this separates the nasal bone from the cartilaginous nasal capsule framework. As the nasal and frontal bones grow, the fonticulus frontalis and the prenasal space are obliterated and the frontonasal suture forms.[1–4]

The embryonic development of the head, neck, and face requires complex coordination of cell growth, migration, differentiation, and apoptosis.[5–8] These embryonic events involve many factors such as fibroblast growth factors, sonic hedgehog proteins, bone morphogenetic proteins, homeobox genes Barx1 and Msx1, distal-less homeobox (Dlx) genes, and local retinoic acid gradients.[5–8] It is now known that multiple genes are involved in the formation of the face. In addition, single genes seem to influence the development of different parts of the face. For example, PRDM16 is linked to the length and the prominence of the nose as well as the width of the alae, SOX9 is thought to be related to the shape of the ala and nose tip, and PAX3 is associated with eye to nasion distance, prominence of the nasion, eye width, side walls of the nose, and prominence of nose tip.[5–8] Any major or minor disturbances in these processes will result in abnormalities involving a wide spectrum of anomalies. The causes of craniofacial syndromes are complex. Many are related to abnormal migration and malformation of facial and skull base structures and are associated with central nervous system (CNS) anomalies. Common genes and locuses associated with facial malformations are illustrated in **Table1**. Detail facial genetics is beyond the scope of this article because this article predominately focuses on the imaging of various malformations and developmental anomalies

Facial Clefting, Cleft Lip with or Without Cleft Palate

Facial clefting, CLP, is the most common congenital craniofa0cial malformation.[9–11] Facial clefting is seen in more than 300 different syndromes and has an estimated incidence of approximately 1 of 2000.[10,11] Higher-resolution and 3D fetal US and fetal MRI can diagnose CLP during the antenatal period. However, identifying a cleft in the secondary palate or an isolated cleft palate on the antenatal US is challenging. Early diagnosis of a facial cleft is critical because it can guide surgical, dental, orthodontic, speech, hearing, and psychological management during childhood.

Cleft lip occurs due to a failure of fusion of the medial frontonasal process with the maxillary process of the first pharyngeal arch. A cleft of the secondary palate is due to lack of fusion of the palatal shelves of the maxillary processes. Pathologically they are classified into CLP and isolated cleft palate.[9–11] This distinction is important because CLP is more common than isolated cleft palate and is less likely to be associated with a congenital syndrome. The most common syndrome associated with isolated cleft palate is Stickler syndrome, which consists of ocular abnormalities, maxillary hypoplasia, and isolated cleft palate.

An isolated cleft palate is more difficult to detect at fetal imaging than CLP because the lip and alar base are not involved in an isolated cleft palate. Clefts of the lip can be classified as unilateral or bilateral and as complete or incomplete. A complete cleft implies clefting of the lip and alveolar process that extends through the nasal sill, whereas an incomplete cleft involves part of the alveolus but does not extend through the nasal floor.[9,10] On the coronal US, cleft lip is typically seen as a hypoechoic region in the upper lip. On 2D planar US images, the uvula can be seen as a linear echogenic structure surrounded by parallel anechoic spaces, giving rise to an "equals sign" appearance.[12] Failure to visualize this normal appearance has been termed the "absent equals sign" and may indicate a cleft palate. When a cleft of either the lip or palate is identified on prenatal US, it is imperative to look for associated anomalies, particularly midline defects. Postnatal imaging plays a vital role in identifying dentofacial deformities secondary to the cleft, including missing or supernumerary teeth, oronasal fistulas, velopharyngeal insufficiency, hearing loss, maxillary growth restriction, and airway abnormalities.[13] Postnatal CT and MRI help in defining the extent of the cleft and other associated facial, dental, and brain anomalies (**Fig. 1**).

Table 1
Common genes and locuses associated with facial malformations

	Chromosome Locus	Genes
Facial clefting, cleft lip with or without cleft palate	9q21, 10q25, 17q22.6 22q11 deletion syndrome	trisomy 13, trisomy 18, and trisomy 21), microdeletion syndromes
Craniofacial syndromes/ malformations due to chromosomal anomalies	Chromosome 21 Chromosome 18 Chromosome 21	
Crouzon syndrome	10q25–10q26	FGFR2
Velocardiofacial syndrome	22q11.2 (del syndr)	TBX1
Apert syndrome	10q26	FGFR2
Pfeiffer syndrome	8p11.22-p12 10q25-q26	FGFR1 FGFR2 genes
CHARGE syndrome	22q11.2	CHD7 gene
Hemifacial microsomia	14q32 3q29 3q29 20q13.33	OTX2 ATP13A3 XXYLT1 MYT1
Treacher Collins syndrome	5q32 13q12.2 6p21.1	TCOF1 POLR1D POLR1C
Pierre Robin sequence	17q24.3	SOX9

Craniofacial Syndromes with Major Chromosomal Anomalies

Craniofacial syndromes/malformations due to chromosomal anomalies are rare. Antenatal diagnosis of symmetric intrauterine growth retardation, hypotonia, multiple major and minor anomalies congenital malformations, and a history of recurrent miscarriage should lead to the suspicion of chromosomal anomalies.[14,15] All dysmorphic neonates should be karyotyped. A skeletal survey should be requested in neonates with evidence of limb shortening or disproportionate short stature on antenatal scans or at birth. Antenatal US or fetal MRI may be helpful in identifying the CNS malformation and facial anomalies. Postnatal imaging will largely depend on the clinical examination.

Trisomy 21: Down syndrome

Down syndrome (DS), or trisomy 21, is the most frequently encountered chromosomal abnormality at birth. The World Health Organization estimates an incidence of about 1 in 1000 to 1 in 1100 live births.[14,15] About 95% of patients have free trisomy 21, about 3% to 4% have an unbalanced Robertsonian translocation between the long arms of chromosome 14 and chromosome 21, and 1% to 2% have mosaic trisomy 21.[14,15]

Antenatal US is sensitive for the diagnosis of fetus with DS. Sonographic markers pointing toward DS include thickened nuchal fold, cystic hygroma, hydrops, ventriculomegaly, echogenic intracardiac focus, congenital heart disease (particularly atrioventricular septal defect), duodenal atresia, mild renal pyelectasia, and talipes.[15–18] The craniofacial dysmorphisms associated with trisomy 21 include microcephaly and brachycephaly (widening of the transverse diameter of the calvarium) without craniosynostosis of the coronal and lambdoid sutures. Other craniofacial morphologies include midface hypoplasia, malocclusion with posterior cross-bite and anterior

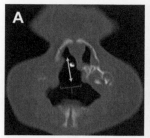
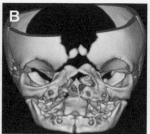
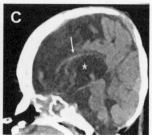

Fig. 1. Cleft Palate with congenital malformation of the brain. Coronal CT scan (A) and 3D reformatted (B) images show large right cleft lip and palate (red brace) with nasal cavity communicating with the oral cavity (orange arrow). Sagittal T1 WI (C) shows microcephaly, dilated ventricles (yellow star) and severely thinning of the corpus callosum (white arrow).

open bite, and macroglossia. DS is associated with flattening of the skull base or platybasia. Almost two-thirds of patients with DS present with hearing loss. Conductive hearing loss is secondary to stenotic external auditory canal, chronic otitis media, or ossicular chain abnormalities.[15–17] Sensorineural hearing loss is due to the spectrum of lateral semi circular canal (LSCC) dysplasia and semicircular canal dehiscence. In addition there may be stenosis of the cochlear nerve canal, stenosis of internal auditory canal, with aplasia or hypoplasia of the cochlear nerve.

MRI of the brain may show microcephaly with reduced brain volume and progressive brain atrophy. In addition, there may be basal ganglia calcifications and corpus callosum malformations.[16,17] Radiograph or CT scan of the cervical spine may show craniocervical instability, flattened surface of the occipital condyles, bifid anterior or posterior C1 arches, atlanto-occipital assimilation, and congenital os odontoideum.

Trisomy 18: Edward syndrome
Most cases of the Edward syndrome show free trisomy 18, and a minority are due to mosaicism. Antenatal findings include growth retardation, increased nuchal thickness with cystic hygroma, microretrognathia, small mouth, sloping forehead, and dysplastic and low-lying ears.[14,19] In addition, there may be prominent occiput with bifrontal narrowing. US or MRI of the brain may show cleft palate, choroid plexus cysts, and posterior fossa abnormalities such as Dandy-Walker malformation, clenched hands with overlapping fingers, and congenital heart disease (**Fig. 2**). The best clues to the diagnosis are overlapping fingers with hypoplastic nails, and the diagnosis can be confirmed by chromosome analysis on a blood sample.

Trisomy 13: Patau syndrome
More than 80% of those with Patau syndrome have free trisomy 13, and about 20% have Robertsonian translocations between chromosomes 13 and 14. Antenatal screening is highly sensitive and can diagnose this condition in almost 90% to 100% of the cases.[19–21] There is a wide range of dysmorphism in trisomy 13 ranging from a simple median incisor to cyclopia.

Commonly associated craniofacial dysmorphism include microcephaly with sloping forehead, microphthalmia with coloboma and retinal dysplasia, dysplastic ears, cleft lip, and cleft palate.[19–21] In addition, fetal sonography or fetal MRI may show other features of trisomy 13 such as alobar, semilobar, or lobar holoprosencephaly. Additional features include Dandy-Walker malformation, hydrocephalus, agenesis of the corpus callosum, neural tube defects, and cardiac anomalies.

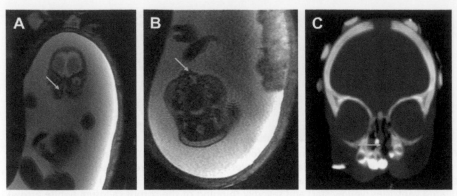

Fig. 2. Trisomy 18 with cleft palate. Fetal MRI, axial (A) and coronal (B) views of the fetus head shows cleft palate (orange arrows) and polyhydramnion. Post-natal CT scan (C) of the paranasal sinus confirms the defect. (*Image courtesy* Dr. Hisham Dahmoush, Stanford University).

Craniofacial Syndromes with Craniosynostosis (Upper Face Pathologies)

Dysmorphisms associated with craniostenosis result from the premature fusing of one or several sutures. This premature closure of the suture results in an abnormal skull shape. Most cases of craniostenosis are sporadic and of uncertain cause. Craniostenosis may be one feature of a larger recognized syndrome of chromosomal or genetic abnormality. Craniofacial syndromes commonly associated with craniostenosis include Apert syndrome, Crouzon syndrome, and Pfeiffer syndrome, which are secondary to mutations of fibroblast growth factor receptor (FGFR).

Apert syndrome

Apert syndrome is one of the most common craniosynostosis syndromes and is associated with multisuture craniosynostosis, midfacial hypoplasia, abnormal skull base development, and syndactyly/symphalangism of all extremities. The incidence of Apert syndrome is estimated to be 1 of 65,000[14]; its inheritance is autosomal dominant with incomplete penetrance and is associated with an FGFR2 gene mutation at 10q26.[22–24] This mutation causes an upregulated response of the androgen end-organ receptors, leading to diffuse early epiphyseal fusion and thereby craniosynostosis, short stature, vertebral fusion, and syndactyly.

CT and 3D reconstructed images of the brain and face show brachycephaly due to coronal synostosis with a wide midline defect and widened metopic and sagittal sutures extending from the glabella to the posterior fontanelle[25] (**Fig. 3**). There may be associated skull base hypoplasia, leading to multiple cranial neuropathies due to foraminal stenosis. Sections through the base of the skull may also reveal nasopharyngeal and oropharyngeal airway compromise and posterior choanae hypoplasia or choanal stenosis.

MRI of the brain is useful in diagnosing primary and secondary CNS malformations of Apert syndrome. The most common primary CNS malformation is ventriculomegaly, which presents in 60% of patients with Apert syndrome.[26] Abnormalities of midline development such as agenesis of the corpus callosum, septo-optic dysplasia spectrum, and isolated absence of the cavum septum pellucidum are also commonly associated. MRI may reveal megalocephaly, gyral abnormalities, generalized reduction in the white matter, and heterotopic gray matter.[26]

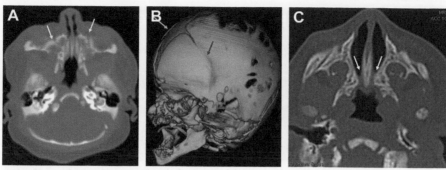

Fig. 3. Apert Syndrome. Axial CT scan of the face (A) and 3D reconstruction (B) images show severe maxilla hypoplasia (yellow arrows), bilateral coronal suture synostosis (red arrow), and widening of the metopic and anterior fontanel (orange arrow). Axial CT scan (C) at the nasal level shows bilateral choanal atresia (white arrows).

Most of the secondary CNS manifestations of Apert syndrome are due to the osseous deformity/malformation. Premature closure of the sutures causes cephalocranial disproportion leading to tonsillar herniation. Other anomalies include frontal encephalocele, kleeblattschädel, and cleft palate.[25,26] There is also a high prevalence of otitis media and eustachian tube dysfunction. Conductive hearing loss is common due to external and middle ear malformations. In addition, the inner ear may show nonspecific but typical inner ear anomalies such as a common cavity malformation of the lateral semicircular canal and vestibule with an absent bone island.

Crouzon syndrome
Crouzon syndrome is a rare genetic disorder characterized by a triad of craniosynostosis, midface hypoplasia, and ocular abnormalities usually manifesting as exophthalmos.[22,27] Morphologically, Crouzon syndrome is akin to Apert syndrome without the extremity anomalies.[28] The inheritance is autosomal dominant with variable penetrance and is related to mutations in the FGFR2 gene on 10q25–10q26[23,28]; its incidence is estimated to be 1 of 25,000 live births.[28]

On imaging, facial dysmorphism is characterized by craniosynostosis, maxillary hypoplasia, shallow orbits with exophthalmos, bifid uvula, and cleft palate (**Fig. 4**). There is premature fusing of the coronal sutures leading to brachycephaly. There may be associated midface hypoplasia, beaked nose, and straight mandible.[19,22,23] Besides the facial dysmorphic features, neuroimaging may show progressive hydrocephalus, anomalous venous drainage, and Chiari I malformations. Noncranial manifestations of the syndrome include calcification of the stylohyoid ligament, craniovertebral junction abnormalities, butterfly vertebrae, and cervical spine fusion anomalies.

Pfeiffer syndrome
Pfeiffer syndrome is also called acrocephalosyndactyly type V and is characterized by acrocephalic skull, regressed midface, syndactyly of hands and feet, and broad thumbs and big toes. With an estimated incidence of around 1 of 100,000 live births, Pfeiffer syndrome is an autosomal dominant syndrome with incomplete penetrance and is linked to FGFR1 and FGFR2 gene mutations.[28–30] Clinically severity is classified into 3 types: type 1, or classic Pfeiffer, where most patients have normal intelligence and lifespan; type 2, which presents with classic cloverleaf skull (kleeblattschädel), occurs sporadically, and has a poor prognosis with severe neurologic compromise; and

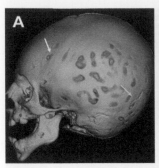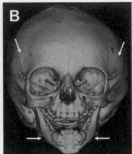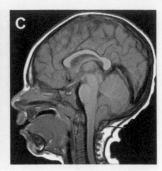

Fig. 4. Crouzon Syndrome. 3D reformatted images of the CT scan (A and B) of the face shows craniosynostosis of the bilateral coronal (yellow arrows) and lambdoid sutures (orange arrow), bilateral maxillary and mandibular hypoplasia (white arrows). Sagittal T1 WI (C) shows mild microcephaly and tonsillar herniation below the basal line, suggestive of Chiari I malformation (red arrow).

type 3, which includes craniosynostosis and severe proptosis, occurs sporadically, and has poor prognosis.[29,30]

CT and 3D reformatted images shows craniosynostosis of the coronal and lambdoid, giving a turribrachycephaly shape to the skull. Severe multisutural synostosis leads to classical kleeblattschädel (cloverleaf skull)[29–31] (**Fig. 5**). This deformity leads to headaches and visual changes caused by increased intracranial pressure. 3D evaluation of the calvarium also shows severe bulging of the calvarium and scalloping of the inner skull table caused by pressure erosion from underlying brain parenchyma.

The most common facial features are a regressed midface and shallow orbits. Maxillary hypoplasia results in shallow orbits and exophthalmos. Patients can also present with a small larynx and pharynx leading to breathing difficulties. Most patients present with moderate to severe conductive hearing loss due to stenosis and/or atresia of the external auditory canal or hypoplasia of the middle ear cavity.

Midface Anomalies

Midface anomalies may be classified depending on the involvement of the anatomic region: nasal cavity (eg, choanal atresia and pyriform aperture stenosis), nasofrontal region (mostly congenital midline nasofrontal masses such as nasal glioma, nasal encephalocele, nasal dermoid cyst, nasal epidermoid cyst, hemangioma, or lymphangioma), nasolacrimal apparatus (eg, NLD stenosis and dacryocystoceles), and craniofacial syndromes (eg, Apert syndrome, Crouzon syndrome, and Treacher Collins syndrome).[22]

Nasal cavity and midface (choanal atresia and stenosis)

Choanal atresia is the most common cause of neonatal nasal obstruction with an incidence of 1 of 8000 to 1 of 5000.[22,32,33] Unilateral choanal atresia is twice as common as bilateral choanal atresia. Bilateral choanal atresia is life threatening and can present with neonatal respiratory distress in infants. Unilateral choanal atresia may go unrecognized until later in life and may present with stuffiness, rhinorrhea, or infection. Clinically, failure to pass a nasogastric tube beyond 32 mm is considered to be diagnostic and requires further evaluation with imaging.

CT remains the imaging modality of choice and is to be performed after vigorous suctioning and administration of topical decongestants. Choanal atresia is classified into osseous (90% of cases), membranous (10%), or osseomembranous

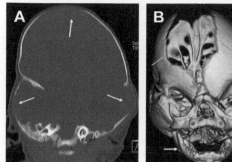
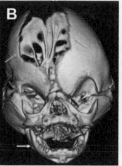
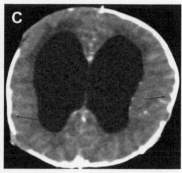

Fig. 5. Pfeiffer Syndrome. Coronal (a) and 3D reconstructed images (b) of the CT scan of the face shows premature fusion of lambdoid and coronal sutures giving appearance of 'cloverleaf skull'(yellow arrows). There is splaying of the sagittal and metopic sutures (green arrows) with protrusion of cerebral parenchyma through the defect. Axial CT scan of the brain (c) shows gross hydrocephalus and scalloping of the inner skull table (red arrows). Also seen is mandibular hypoplasia (white arrow).

(rare).[22,32,33] Osseous obstruction is due to incomplete canalization of the choanae, whereas membranous obstruction is due to incomplete resorption of epithelial plugs. Diagnostic features of high-resolution CT (HRCT) include narrowing of the posterior choanae to a width of less than 3 mm (done at the reference level of the pterygoid plates in the axial plane), inward bowing of the posterior maxilla, fusion or thickening of the vomer, and the presence of a bone or soft tissue septum extending across the posterior choanae.[22,32,33] The nasal cavity is usually filled with air, soft tissue, fluid, or hypertrophied inferior turbinates. Choanal atresia may be seen in multiple syndromes, so a skeletal survey is suggested for confirmed cases.

Congenital nasal pyriform aperture stenosis. Pyriform aperture stenosis is the result of early fusion and hypertrophy of the medial nasal processes. The exact incidence is unknown, but unlike choanal atresia, it is a rare cause of airway obstruction. This condition can occur in an isolated form or may be associated with other craniofacial anomalies such as lobar and semilobar holoprosencephaly, facial hemangioma, and central megaincisor (in 75% of the cases).[34,35]

HRCT remains the imaging modality of choice; it needs to be performed in planes angled along the hard palate with a section thickness of 1 to 1.5 mm and should include the maxillary spines. Imaging features of pyriform aperture stenosis include inward bowing and thickening of the nasal processes of maxilla and narrowing of the pyriform aperture measuring less than 8 mm (normal: >11 mm).[34,35] In confirmed cases using CT of the face, MRI of the brain is suggested to rule out intracranial malformations of the brain such as holoprosencephaly.

Nasofrontal region (congenital midline nasofrontal masses)
Congenital midline nasofrontal masses result from abnormal regression of the embryologic dural diverticulum from the prenasal space. The mass can be intranasal, extranasal, or both, depending on the nature of the faulty regression.[36] Intranasal masses are due to the extension of dura mater through the foramen cecum into the prenasal space and nasal cavity. Glabellar masses are due to the extension of the diverticulum through the foramen cecum and fonticulus frontalis. Imaging plays an important role in characterizing the lesion, defining its extension, and helping surgical

planning. Common lesions in this group include nasal glioma, nasal encephalocele, nasal dermoid cyst, nasal epidermoid cyst, hemangioma, and lymphangioma.[36,37]

Dermal sinus tract results from no involution or partial involution of the dural diverticulum extending through the foramen cecum to the columella.[36,37] Dermoid and epidermoid cysts can form anywhere along the dermal sinus tract. Dermoid and epidermoid cysts occur when skin elements are pulled into the prenasal space along with the regressing dural diverticulum. Dermoid cysts contain ectoderm with skin appendages, are usually paramidline, and tend to occur near the columella. Dermoid cysts are also usually midline with a tendency to occur at the glabella, whereas the epidermoid cysts contain ectodermal elements without skin appendages.

In most cases, a sinus tract opening, dimple, or tuft of hair may be present on the skin surface. Both dermoid and epidermoid cysts are firm, nonpulsatile lesions that do not transilluminate and do not change in size with crying or the Valsalva maneuver. CT and MRI show a sinus tract anywhere from the nasal bridge to crista galli along with large foramen cecum, with bifid or deformed crista galli or cribriform plate.[36,37] The sagittal plane is useful in displaying the course of the sinus tract from the nasal dorsum to skull base. The tract is hypodense to isodense on CT and shows low signal on T1-weighted MRI. On CT, a dermoid cyst shows a fatty density, whereas an epidermoid cyst shows water density; both are commonly found along the dermal tract. On MRI, a dermoid cyst appears as a well-defined hyperintense mass on T2-weighted imaging (T2WI) with variable signal intensity on T1-weighted MRI. An epidermoid cyst is hypointense on T1-weighted imaging (T1WI), hyperintense on T2WI, and shows restricted diffusion on diffusion-weighted imaging-apparent diffusion coefficient.[36,37]

Nasal neuroglial heterotopia. Nasal neuroglial heterotopia (NGH) is a sequestered, dysplastic, nonneoplastic, neurogenic brain tissue that consist of astrocytes and neuroglial fibers with a fibrovascular connective tissue stroma.[38,39] NGH results from the extension of ectodermal tissue through the foramen cecum into openings in the nasofrontal region, without any connection with the subarachnoid space. NGH presents as a soft tissue mass that is most often midline, intranasal or extranasal at the nasal dorsum, or a combination of both. On T1- and T2-weighted MRI of the face and nose, this mass is isointense to the brain parenchyma without evidence of restricted diffusion (**Fig. 6**). The mass does not show any intracranial extension, but a fibrous stalk is sometimes present. Although MRI is sensitive, CT may be complementary in assessing the anterior skull base lesions, with better demonstration of the adjacent osseous structures.

Nasal glioma is a misnomer, because it does not have any neoplastic features. Nasal glioma is also known as nasal cerebral heterotopia, which consists of dysplastic, sequestered, neurogenic tissue that has become isolated from the subarachnoid space due to failed regression of the dural diverticulum. About 30% of nasal gliomas are intranasal, 60% are extranasal, and 10% are a combination of the 2.[36,40,41] Clinically, extranasal gliomas present as firm, red to bluish skin-covered masses that do not exhibit pulsations or increase in size with the Valsalva maneuver. Intranasal gliomas present as large, firm, submucosal masses that extend inferiorly toward or near the nostril; they present with obstruction to the nasal passages, obstruction of the NLD, epistaxis, cerebrospinal rhinorrhea, and, rarely, meningitis.

MRI is the imaging modality of choice for diagnosis, but CT can be used as well. On noncontrast CT scan extranasal glioma is seen as a well-circumscribed, soft tissue mass, isodense to the brain. The mass is commonly located at the glabella, superficial to the point of fusion of the frontal and nasal bones (fonticulus frontalis). Intranasal glioma is seen as a soft tissue density mass within the nasal cavity, typically high in nasal

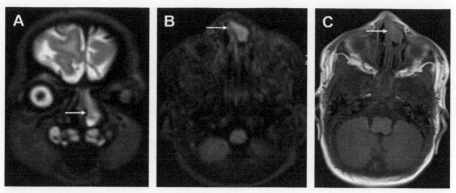

Fig. 6. Nasoglial heterotopia. Coronal T2, (A) axial FLAIR (B) and T1 weighted (C) images show intranasal soft tissue mass on the left side (yellow arrow), with signal intensity almost matching the normal brain parenchyma on all the sequences.

vault[36,40,41] (**Fig. 7**). A third of the patients show defects in the cribriform plate. On MRI, nasal gliomas are isointense to hypointense relative to gray matter on T1WI and are hyperintense on T2WI. Nasal gliomas may also show a faint intracranial stalk. There is no enhancement of the dysplastic tissue seen on the postcontrast scans. The fibrous pedicle may be seen extending toward skull base but without intracranial component.

Cephalocele results from herniation of intracranial contents through a defect in the skull. Depending on the herniated contents, the cephalocele is termed as mengingocele (meninges and cerebrospinal fluid [CSF]) or meningoencephalocele (meninges, CSF, and brain herniates).[36,37,40,41] Cephaloceles are classified based on location as occipital, sincipital (frontoethmoidal), or basal. The frontoethmoidal encephalocele involves the midface, and is due to failed detachment of the cutaneous ectoderm and neuroectoderm of the anterior neuropore in the third week of fetal life. Depending on the location there are 3 types of sincipital encephalocele: frontonasal cephaloceles, which protrude through the fonticulus nasofrontalis into the glabella; nasoethmoidal cephaloceles, which protrude through the foramen cecum into the nasal cavity; and naso-orbital cephaloceles, which protrude into the orbit through the lacrimal bone.[36,37,40,41] The frontonasal cephalocele is the most common among the 3.

Basal cephaloceles are due to failed ossification of the base of the skull, with extension of neural crest cells through the osseous defect. Basal cephalocele may contain pituitary tissue, optic nerves, or vascular structures along with brain and meninges. Examples of midline basal cephaloceles include the transethmoidal, sphenoethmoidal, and sphenopharyngeal types.[37,40,41] Nasopharyngeal cephaloceles are uncommon, occult, and can extend through the ethmoid bone, sphenoid bone, or basiocciput into the nasal cavity or nasopharynx.

Clinical manifestation largely depends on site and size of the cephalocele. Most cephaloceles are diagnosed either antenatally or at birth, exception being basal cephaloceles (nasopharyngeal cephaloceles), which are mostly occult and are diagnoosed in the postnatal period. Nasopharyngeal cephaloceles may manifest as airway obstruction or CSF leak; they can be pulsatile, increasing in size during crying, the Valsalva maneuver, or jugular compression. Biopsy of such masses is contraindicated due to the potential risk of CSF leaks, seizures, or meningitis.

CT and MRI complement each other in showing the bony and soft tissue details, respectively. nonenhanced CT (NECT) shows a heterogeneous, mixed density mass

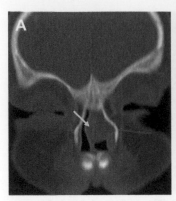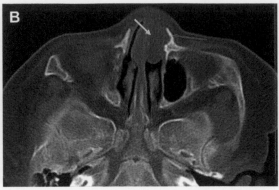

Fig. 7. Nasal glioma. Coronal (A) and axial (B) CT scan of the paranasal sinus in bone window shows well defined mass lesion in the left side of the nasal cavity (orange arrow) causing smooth scalloping of the nasal bone (red arrow), biopsy proven case of nasal glioma. There was no intracranial communication of this mass.

extending intracranially through bony defect (**Fig. 8**). In the frontonasal cephalocele bone, window images show superior displacement of the frontal bones and inferior displacement of the nasal bones and frontal processes of maxillae. There is anterior bowing of the nasal bone, bifid or absent crista galli, and deficient or absent cribriform plate in nasoenthmoidal cephalocele.[37,40–42] MRI is superior in revealing the size, extent, and contents of the encephalocele as well as uncovering the presence of associated intracranial anomalies. Signal intensity in T1- and T2-weighted images usually match the developing brain or may be slightly hyperintense due to congestion.[37,40–42] A herniated brain is usually hyperintense on T2WI due to gliosis. There is surrounding T2-hyperintense CSF rim surrounding the herniated soft tissue parenchyma, which is contiguous with intracranial parenchyma extending through bony defect.

MRI of the brain is always indicated in a suspected case of nasal or basal enecphalocele to look for associated intracranial anomalies such as callosal agenesis, interhemispheric lipoma, facial clefts, optic nerve hypoplasia, midline facial anomalies, hypothalamic-pituitary axis dysfunction, and schizencephaly[42] (**Fig. 9**). Encephaloceles are treated with immediate complete surgical resection to prevent CSF leakage, meningitis, or increase in mass size.

Nasolacrimal apparatus

Congenital nasolacrimal duct mucocele is the cystic dilatation of the NLD that is caused by obstruction of the duct's distal opening. When the obstruction is in the distal end of the NLD, the classic triad presents with a dacrocystocele, which appears as a medial canthal mass; a dilated NLD with expansion of its osseous canal; and an intranasal mass (mucocele) below the inferior turbinate, which is the inferior extension of the dilated duct.[38] When the obstruction is proximal, it results in a dilated nasolacrimal sac (classic dacrocystocele). Dacryocystoceles are the second most common cause of neonatal nasal obstruction after choanal atresia and require prompt attention. Dacryocystoceles commonly present as a tense, blue-gray mass at the medial canthus or in the nasal cavity. It is not uncommon for dacryocystoceles to get infected or present as an abscess with surrounding cellulitis.

Imaging of dacrocystocele shows NLD dilatation with well-circumscribed round cystic lesions with a thin rim in the medial canthus.[38,43] On CT, noninfected dacrocystocele is a low-attenuating cyst, with sharp, well-defined surrounding walls. MRI

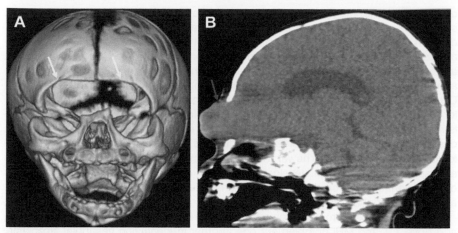

Fig. 8. Frontal cephalocele. Sagittal (A) and coronal (B) 3D reformatted images show large bony defect (arrows) in the frontal and nasal bone with herniation of the brain parenchyma, encephalocele (arrow).

shows a well-defined tubular fluid structure extending from the medial canthus into the inferior nasal cavity, which is hyperintense on T2WI (**Fig. 10**). On contrast-enhanced study, dacryocystitis shows enhancement and swelling of the adjacent soft tissue. Further assessment should be made for complications such as periorbital cellulitis and abscess formation.[44]

Midface anomalies associated with other anomalies
Various other syndromes or skeletal malformations may cause midface or combined facial malformations, including CHARGE syndrome, achondroplasia, maxillofacial dysplasia (Binder syndrome), thanatophoric dysplasia, Prader-Willi syndrome, otopalatodigital syndrome, and DiGeorge syndrome (now called 22q11 deletion syndrome)

CHARGE syndrome
CHARGE is an acronym for clinical features of coloboma of the iris, congenital heart defects, choanal atresia, mental retardation, genital hypoplasia, and ear abnormalities. The incidence of CHARGE is estimated between 1 of 8500 and 1 of 12,000.[45,46] Nearly two-thirds of these patients have been found to have mutations

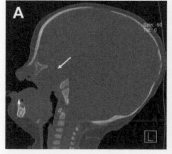
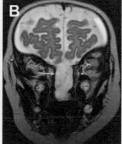
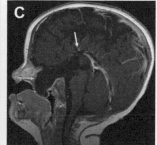

Fig. 9. Nasopharyngeal cephalocele. Sagittal reconstructed CT image (A) through the base of the skull shows large bony defect in the anterior base of the skull (yellow arrow). Coronal T2 (B) and Sagittal T1 (C) weighted images show herniated sac (meningocele-orange arrow) with absent corpus callosum (white arrow).

of the CHD7 gene, which is mostly sporadic. Mutations of the CHD7 gene in CHARGE syndrome seem to affect a broader range of craniofacial development than 22q11.2 deletion syndrome.[46] The craniofacial features in the neonatal period include asymmetrical facies, unilateral facial palsy, iris colobomas, malformed ears, small mouth, and cleft palate. The disease is associated with middle ear dysplasia, suggesting abnormal development of the first and second pharyngeal arches. The diagnosis of CHARGE syndrome should be considered in any neonate with 4 major criteria or 3 major and 3 minor criteria. Major criteria include coloboma; choanal atresia; characteristic abnormalities of the external, middle, or inner ear; and cranial nerve dysfunction (anosmia, facial nerve palsy, deafness and vestibular problems, or swallowing problems).[45–47] Two newer major criteria include olfactory complex anomalies and abnormal basiocciput development. Minor criteria include genital hypoplasia, developmental delay, cardiovascular abnormalities, short stature, cleft lip or palate, and tracheoesophageal defects.

On imaging, most common anomalies are seen involving the ear, orbit, nasal cavity, and brain. CT and MRI complement one another in identifying vestibular dysplasia, semicircular canal (SCC) dysplasia, cochlear dysplasia, absence of the cochlear aperture, cochlear nerve deficiency, internal auditory canal dysplasia, and enlarged vestibular aqueduct (**Fig. 11**). HRCT of the temporal bone is sensitive in diagnosing dysplastic ossicles with ankyloses, absent stapedius, pyramidal eminence, sinus tympan, and aberrant course of the facial nerve.[45,46] Other possible findings include choanal atresia, coloboma, and cleft lip/palate. Besides temporal bone anomalies, MRI is sensitive in demonstrating the olfactory bulb and sulcal hypoplasia/aplasia, basiocciput hypoplasia resulting in shortening of the clivus, and basilar invagination. MRI of the brain may reveal hypoplasia of pons with cerebellar malformation, ventriculomegaly with hypoplasia, or aplasia of cranial nerves I, VII, and VIII.

Lower Face Pathologies/Branchial Arch Syndromes

BAS involving the first and second branchial arches represent the second most common craniofacial malformation after cleft lip and palate. BAS manifest as combined tissue deficiencies or hypoplasias of the face, external ear, middle ear, and maxillary and

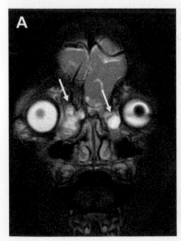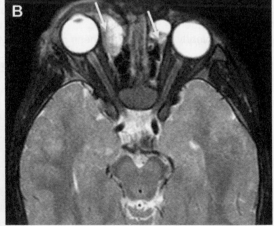

Fig. 10. Dacryocystocele. Coronal (A) and axial (B) T2 weighted images show bilateral well defined, cystic lesions extending from medial canthus to the inferior nasal cavity. dilation of the.

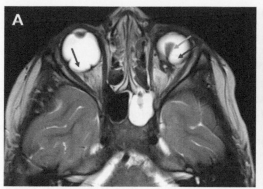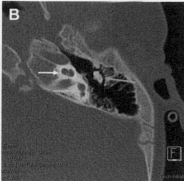

Fig. 11. CHARGE syndrome. Axial T2 WI (A) shows bilateral colobomas (red arrows) and left retinal detachment (blue arrow). HRCT of the temporal bone (B) shows ossicular (green arrow), cochlear (white arrow) and vestibular and semicircular canal dysplasia (orange arrow).

mandibular arches. Depending on the dominance of the dysplastic development, BAS is classified as hemifacial microsomia, mandibulofacial dysostosis, branchio-oto-renal syndrome, Pierre Robin sequence, or Nager acrofacial dysostosis. The most important sectors involved in otomandibular dysplasias are the sphenotemporozygomandibular, linguomandibulohyovertebral, and alveolodental areas.[48]

The wide spectrum of otomandibular dysplasias is classified by the OMENS classification representing 5 dysmorphic manifestations: O, orbital asymmetry; M, mandibular hypoplasia; E, ear (auricular) deformity; N, nerve involvement; and S, soft tissue deficiency.[49] Otomandibular dysplasias can be divided into symmetric, or bilateral, forms and asymmetric, or unilateral, forms.[48,50] Isolated symmetric forms include mandibulofacial dysostosis, Franceschetti syndrome, or Treacher-Collins syndrome. Nonisolated symmetric forms include acrofacial dysostosis and Nager or Miller syndromes with limb anomalies.[50] Isolated asymmetric forms include hemifacial microsomy, first arch syndrome, or first and second arches syndrome, whereas nonisolated asymmetric forms include Goldenhar syndrome.[50] Facial dysmorphisms of these syndromes share the characteristic external ear anomalies, lower face anomalies at the mandibular level, and midface anomalies at the malar level.

Craniofacial microsomia

Hemifacial microsomia, now referred to as craniofacial microsomia, is an entity of the oculoauricular-vertebral spectrum, affecting the first and second brachial arches and resulting in poor growth of the cranium, facial skeleton, and facial soft tissues.[51,52] The incidence of the oculoauricular-vertebral spectrum is estimated to be about 1 of 20,000 births[51] with the mode of inheritance being thought to be autosomal or X-linked dominant in most cases.

The craniofacial anomaly is characterized by notable growth and asymmetry in the mandible, mandibular hypoplasia, restricted growth of the maxilla, zygomatic arch hypoplasia, and hypoplasia of the muscles of mastication and parotid gland. There may be associated microtia, external auditory canal (EAC) atresia/stenosis, middle ear hypoplasia, and ossicular anomalies. In addition, the inner ear may show oval window atresia, CN7 anomaly/hypoplasia, or anomalies of the vestibule, cochlea, and semicircular canals.

Goldenhar syndrome is an oculoauricular-vertebral spectrum disorder derived from developmental malformation of the first and second branchial arches. When epibulbar

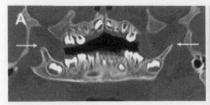
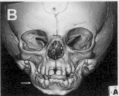
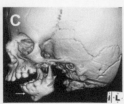

Fig. 12. Goldenhar syndrome. Sagittal (A) and coronal 3D reformatted images (B,C)show marked hypoplasia of the mandible, especially the mandibular condyles and condylar head as well as the temporomandibular joints. Patient also had severe hypoplasia of the internal auditory canals (not shown).

dermoids and vertebral anomalies are seen along with hemifacial microsomia (HFM), the syndrome is called Goldenhar syndrome.[53] Goldenhar syndrome occurs sporadically in most cases. In rare cases, its inheritance is autosomal or X-linked dominant linked to an EYA1 gene mutation on chromosome 8.

Otolaryngologic manifestations are similar to craniofacial microsomia, which include hypoplastic mandibular ramus and condyles; unilateral hypoplasia of the maxilla, malar, and temporal bones; and underdeveloped mastoid air cells[53,54] (**Fig. 12**). Approximately a third of cases demonstrate bilateral involvement with right side dominance. Macrostomia, parotid gland agenesis, and cleft palate/lip are other associated features. Microtia, ossicular anomalies, abnormal course of the facial nerve, and conductive hearing loss are frequently associated findings. Cervical spine CT may show hemivertebrae and fused vertebrae.

Mandibulofacial dysostosis or Treacher-Collins syndrome
Mandibulofacial dysostosis is also referred to as Treacher Collins syndrome; its incidence is estimated to be 1 of 50,000, and it is autosomal dominant in 40% of cases and sporadic in the remaining 60%. About 60% of cases are related to a de novo mutation at 5q32, and expression can vary within a family.[55]

Prominent manifestations of mandibulofacial dysostosis include hypoplasia of the malar bone, mandibular ramus, condyle, and zygomatic complex.[55] An antimongoloid slant of the palpebral fissures is common in these patients. 3D CT reconstructed images are helpful in documentation of mandibular hypoplasia. HRCT images through the temporal bone are recommended to evaluate for associated ear anomalies such as absent external auditory canal, pinna deformity, middle ear malformation, and internal ear anomalies such as deficient cochlea and vestibular apparatus. CT scan of the face can reveal coloboma and ankylosis of the temporomandibular joint.

Pierre Robin sequence
Pierre Robin syndrome is a triad comprising hypoplasia of the mandible (micrognathia), glossoptosis, and posterior U-shaped cleft palate or high-arched palate.[56,57] The Pierre Robin sequence may be associated with other malformations and syndromes such as velocardiofacial syndrome, Stickler syndrome, and Treacher Collins syndrome. The Pierre Robin sequence occurs as an isolated finding in about 40% to 65% of the cases. The exact cause of the Pierre Robin sequence remains unknown. Various theories include pressure on the mandible secondary to fetal positioning, teratology effects of medications, and genetic causes. Chromosomal aberrations in patients with Pierre Robin syndrome include 2q duplication, 2q deletion, 4q deletion, 11q deletion, 17q deletion, and 18q deletion.[56,57] The primary cause is thought to be the growth defect of the embryonic mandible due to a mutation in the SOX9 gene.

Imaging shows variable mandibular morphology, the most common being symmetric hypoplasia of the mandible. There may be associated condylar and coronoid hypoplasia. Lateral radiography of the face may show abnormal dorsal position of the tongue (glossoptosis) resulting in glossopharyngeal-laryngeal respiratory obstruction. In addition, various severities of cleft palate are seen, possibly involving both the primary and secondary palates, leading to open communication between the nasal and oral cavities. There may also be associated teeth agenesis.

Fetal Alcohol Syndrome

Prenatal alcohol exposure has a toxic effect on the developing brain, face, and soft tissues of the fetus. Toxic metabolites from alcohol may lead to congenital malformation of the brain leading to CNS dysfunction, prenatal and postnatal growth deficits, and specific craniofacial features. Neurodevelopmental abnormalities related to prenatal alcohol exposure can span over several categories, including FAS, partial FAS, alcohol-related neurodevelopmental disorders, and alcohol-related birth defects.[58,59] Clinically, a child may present with lowered intelligence quotient, hyperactivity, behavioral and adaptive difficulties, and deficits in motor function, attention, verbal learning, expressive and receptive language, executive function, and visuospatial skills.

On imaging, a common finding seen with FAS is microcephaly or reductions in the volume of frontal, temporal, parietal, and to a lesser degree, occipital lobes.[58,59] There is a disproportionate decrease in white and gray matter volumes in the occipital-temporal region along with corpus callosum agenesis/dysgenesis. Characteristic facial dysmorphology associated with FAS includes short palpebral fissures, a thin vermilion border of the upper lip, short lower face, retrognathia, a long-domed philtrum, and midfacial hypoplasia.[59,60]

CLINICS CARE POINTS

- Higher-resolution and 3D antenatal ultrasonography and multidetector CT scan with 3D reformatted images have improved the early diagnosis of the craniofacial anatomy and its malformations.

- These imaging techniques have helped in better characterizing the malformation and have greatly helped surgical planning.

DISCLOSURE

The authors have nothing to disclose.

REFERENCES

1. Johnson JM, Moonis G, Green GE, et al. Syndromes of the first and second branchial arches, part 1: embryology and characteristic defects. AJNR Am J Neuroradiol 2011;32(1):14–9.

2. Stone JA, Figueroa RE. Embryology and anatomy of the neck. Neuroimaging Clin N Am 2000;10:55–73, viii.

3. Som PM, Naidich TP. Illustrated review of the embryology and development of the facial region, part 1: early face and lateral nasal cavities. AJNR Am J Neuroradiol 2013;34(12):2233–40.

4. Som PM, Naidich TP. Illustrated review of the embryology and development of the facial region, part 2: late development of the fetal face and changes in the face from the newborn to adulthood. AJNR Am J Neuroradiol 2014;35(1):10–8.

5. Yoon AJ, Pham BN, Dipple KM. Genetic screening in patients with craniofacial malformations. J Pediatr Genet 2016;5(4):220–4.

6. Marazita ML. The evolution of human genetic studies of cleft lip and cleft palate. Annu Rev Genomics Hum Genet 2012;13(1):263–83.

7. Twigg SR, Wilkie AO. New insights into craniofacial malformations. Hum Mol Genet 2015;24(R1):R50–9.

8. Richmond S, Howe LJ, Lewis S, et al. Facial genetics: a brief overview. Front Genet 2018;9:462.

9. Abramson ZR, Peacock ZS, Cohen HL, et al. Radiology of cleft lip and palate: imaging for the prenatal period and throughout life. Radiographics 2015;35(7): 2053–63.

10. Mulliken JB, Benacerraf BR. Prenatal diagnosis of cleft lip: what the sonologist needs to tell the surgeon. J Ultrasound Med 2001;20(11):1159–64.

11. Johnson DD, Pretorius DH, Budorick NE, et al. Fetal lip and primary palate: three-dimensional versus two-dimensional US. Radiology 2000;217(1):236–9.

12. Wilhelm L, Borgers H. The "equals sign": a novel marker in the diagnosis of fetal isolated cleft palate. Ultrasound Obstet Gynecol 2010;36(4):439–44.

13. Rosen H, Chiou GJ, Stoler JM, et al. Magnetic resonance imaging for detection of brain abnormalities in fetuses with cleft lip and/or cleft palate. Cleft Palate Craniofac J 2011;48(5):619–22.

14. Suri M. Craniofac syndromes. Semin Fetal Neonatal Med 2005;10:243–57.

15. Inglis A, Hippman C, Austin JC. Prenatal testing for Down syndrome: the perspectives of parents of individuals with Down syndrome. Am J Med Genet A 2012;158A(4):743–50.

16. Rodrigues M, Nunes J, Figueiredo S, et al. Neuroimaging assessment in Down syndrome: a pictorial review. Insights Imaging 2019;10(1):52.

17. Radhakrishnan R, Towbin AJ. Imaging findings in Down syndrome. Pediatr Radiol 2014;44(5):506–21.

18. Stoll C, Dott B, Alembik Y, et al. Associated congenital anomalies among cases with Down syndrome. Eur J Med Genet 2015;58(12):674–80.

19. Jean-Marc L, Jean-Philippe B, Benoit B, et al. Normal and abnormal fetal face atlas. ultrasonographic features. Springer; 2017.

20. Schinzel A. Catalogue of unbalanced chromosome aberrations in man. Berlin: Walter de Gruyter; 2001.

21. Shipp TD, Benacerraf BR. Second trimester ultrasound screening for chromosomal abnormalities. Prenat Diagn 2002;22:296–307.

22. Lisa LH, Booth TN, Joglar JN, et al. Midface anomalies in children. RadioGraphics 2000;20(4):907–22.

23. Ketwaroo PD, Robson C, Estroff J, et al. Prenatal imaging of craniosynostosis syndromes. Semin Ultrasound CT MR 2015. PMID: 26614129.

24. Yu K, Herr AB, Waksman G, et al. Loss of fibroblast growth factor receptor 2 ligand-binding specificity in Apert syndrome. Proc Natl Acad Sci U S A 2000; 97:14536–41.

25. Computed tomography assessment of apert syndrome. marco antônio portela albuquerque 1, marcelo gusmão paraíso cavalcanti. Braz Oral Res 2004; 18(1):35–9.

26. Tan AP, Mankad K. Apert syndrome: magnetic resonance imaging (MRI) of associated intracranial anomalies. Child's Nervous Syst 2018;34:205–16.

27. Grover SB, Bhayana A, Grover H, et al. Imaging diagnosis of Crouzon syndrome in two cases confirmed on genetic studies - with a brief review. Indian J Radiol Imaging 2019;29(4):442–7.

28. Buchanan EP, Xue AS, Hollier LH Jr. Craniofacial syndromes. Plast Reconstr Surg 2014;134(1):128e–53e.

29. Nieuwenhuyzen-De Boer GM, Hoogeboom AJ, Smit LS, et al. Pfeiffer syndrome: the importance of prenatal diagnosis. Eur J Obstet Gynecol Reprod Biol 2014; 181:339–40.

30. Cohen JrMM. Pfeiffer syndrome update, clinical subtypes, and guidelines for differential diagnosis. Am J Med Genet 1993;45(3):300–7.

31. Duggal N, Omer A, Jupalli S, et al. Pfeiffer syndrome in an adult with previous surgical correction: a case report of CT findings. Radiol Case Rep 2021;16(9): 2463–8.

32. Burrow TA, Saal HM, de Alarcon A, et al. Characterization of congenital anomalies in individuals with choanal atresia. Arch Otolaryngol Head Neck Surg 2009; 135(6):543–7.

33. Hsu CY, et al. Congenital choanal atresia: computed tomographic and clinical findings. Acta Paediatr Taiwan 1999;40(1):13–7.

34. Osovsky M, Aizer-Danon A, Horev Gadi, et al. Congenital pyriform aperture stenosis. Pediatr Radiol 2007;37(1):97–9.

35. Belden CJ, Mancuso AA, Schmalfuss IM, et al. CT features of congenital nasal piriform aperture stenosis: initial experience. Radiology 1999;213(2):495–501.

36. Hedlund G. Congenital frontonasal masses: developmental anatomy, malformations, and MR imaging. Pediatr Radiol 2006;36(7):647–62, quiz 726-7.

37. Paller AS, et al. Nasal midline masses in infants and children. dermoids, encephaloceles, and gliomas. Arch Dermatol 1991;127(3):362–6.

38. Rodriguez DP, Orscheln ES, Koch BL. Masses of the nose, nasal cavity, and nasopharynx in children. Radiographics 2017;37(6):1704–30.

39. Adil E, Robson C, Perez-Atayde A, et al. Congenital nasal neuroglial heterotopia and encephaloceles: an update on current evaluation and management. Laryngoscope 2016;126(9):2161–7.

40. Barkovich AJ, Vandermarck P, Edwards MS, et al. Congenital nasal masses: CT and MR imaging features in 16 cases. AJNR Am J Neuroradiol 1991;12(1): 105–16.

41. Huisman TA, Schneider JFL, Kellenberger CJ, et al. Developmental nasal midline masses in children: neuroradiological evaluation. Eur Radiol 2004;14(2):243–9.

42. Connor SE. Imaging of skull-base cephalocoeles and cerebrospinal fluid leaks. Clin Radiol 2010;65(10):832–41.

43. Yazici Z, Kline-Fath BM, Yazici B, et al. Congenital dacryocystocele: prenatal MRI findings. Pediatr Radiol 2010;40(12):1868–73.

44. Wong RK, VanderVeen DK. Presentation and management of congenital dacryocystocele. Pediatrics 2008;122(5):e1108–12.

45. Hoch MJ, Patel SH, Jethanamest D, et al. Head and neck MRI findings in CHARGE syndrome. AJNR Am J Neuroradiol 2017;38(12):2357–63.

46. Jongmans M, Admiraal R, van der Donk KP, et al. CHARGE syndrome: the phenotypic spectrum of mutations in the CHD7 gene. J Med Genet 2006;43: 306–314 Medline.

47. Verloes A. Updated diagnostic criteria for CHARGE syndrome: a proposal. Am J Med Genet A 2005;133A:306–8.

48. Senggen E, Laswed T, Meuwly JY, et al. First and second branchial arch syndromes: multimodality approach. Pediatr Radiol 2011;41(5):549–61.

49. Vento AR, LaBrie RA, Mulliken JB. The O.M.E.N.S. classification of hemifacial microsomia. Cleft Palate Craniofac J 1991;28:68–76.
50. Levaillant Jean-Marc BJ-P, Bernard B, Gérard C. Normal and abnormal fetal face atlas - ultrasonographic features. Switzerland: Springer International Publishing; 2017.
51. Swibel Rosenthal LH, Caballero N, Drake AF. Otolaryngologic manifestations of craniofacial syndromes. Otolaryngol Clin North Am 2012;45(3):557–77.
52. Charrier JB, Bennaceur S, Couly G. Hemifacial microsomia. embryological and clinical approach. Ann Chir Plast Esthet 2001;46:385–99.
53. Maryanchik I, Nair MK. Goldenhar syndrome (oculo-auriculo-vertebral spectrum): findings on cone beam computed tomography-3 case reports. Oral Surg Oral Med Oral Pathol Oral Radiol 2018;126(4):e233–9.
54. Saccomanno S, Greco F, D'alatri L, et al. Role of 3D-CT for orthodontic and ENT evaluation in goldenhar syndrome. Acta Otorhinolaryngol Ital 2014;34:283–7.
55. Magalhães MHCG, Barbosa da Silveira C, Moreira CR, et al. Clinical and imaging correlations of Treacher Collins syndrome: report of two cases. Oral Surg Oral Med Oral Pathol Oral Radiol Endod 2007;103(6):836–42.
56. Holder-Espinasse M, Abadie V, Cormier-Daire V, et al. Pierre robin sequence: a series of 117 consecutive cases. J Pediatr 2001;139:588–90.
57. Printzlau A, Andersen M. Pierre robin sequence in Denmark: a retrospective population-based epidemiological study. Cleft Palate Craniofac J 2004;41:47–52.
58. Norman AL, Crocker N, Mattson SN, et al. Neuroimaging and fetal alcohol spectrum disorders. Dev Disabil Res Rev 2009;15(3):209–17.
59. Guerri C. Mechanisms involved in central nervous system dysfunctions induced by pre-natal ethanol exposure. Neurotoxicit Res 2002;4:327–35.
60. Johnson VP, Swayze VW II, Sato Y, et al. Fetal alcohol syndrome: craniofacial and central nervous system manifestations. Am J Med Genet 1996;61:329–39.

Special Article

Congenital Anomalies of the Kidneys and Urinary Tract

Deborah Stein, MD, Erin McNamara, MD, MPH

KEYWORDS

• CAKUT • Postnatal assessment • Nephrology • Urology

KEY POINTS

• Congenital anomalies of the kidneys and urinary tract are common.
• Postnatal assessment is critical to ensure that severe anomalies are detected and addressed early.
• Neonates may require additional monitoring in the neonatal period depending on the degree of anomalies present and the perinatal course.
• Children with CAKUT require long-term specialty care to assess both urologic and renal function.
• Many children will require support from both nephrology and urology specialists.

INTRODUCTION

Congenital anomalies of the kidneys and urinary tract (CAKUT) are some of the most common abnormalities detected on prenatal imaging assessment. It is estimated that CAKUT comprises 20% to 30% of all major birth defects.[1–3] More than 200 clinical syndromes currently include CAKUT as a component of the phenotype.[1]

Typical renal development results in each individual born with 2 kidneys, each of which should have upwards of 1 million nephrons, although there is a significant variation among populations.[2] Early insults, especially those involving the lower urinary tract, result in the maldevelopment of nephrons and subsequent renal insufficiency.

Prenatally, the fetal bladder may be first visible at 10 to 12 weeks gestation and by mid-gestation, fills and empties every 30 to 60 minutes. Corticomedullary differentiation should be apparent by 20 weeks of gestation. Fetal urine production begins by 9 to 10 weeks of gestation and increases by 14 to 16 weeks, such that after this point the bulk of amniotic fluid is made of fetal urine.[1,4] Hence, oligohydramnios may be a marker for severe fetal renal anomalies including CAKUT. To date, there are no studies demonstrating accurate prediction of postnatal renal function or postnatal lung function despite improvement in prenatal imaging techniques.

The author has nothing to disclose.
Department of Pediatrics, Harvard Medical School, Boston, MA, USA
E-mail address: deborah.stein@childrens.harvard.edu

Clin Perinatol 49 (2022) 791–798
https://doi.org/10.1016/j.clp.2022.06.002   **perinatology.theclinics.com**

Antenatal urinary tract dilation is diagnosed in 1% to 5% of all pregnancies. Between 36% and 80% of these will resolve postnatally. The risk of postnatal pathology increases with the increasing severity of urinary tract dilation. *HNF1B* is the gene encoding hepatocyte nuclear factor 1B, and dominant mutations in this gene are the most frequently identified monogenic cause for renal anomalies, although 50% of detected mutations are de novo.[2,5] Mutations result in a wide spectrum of disease, not restricted to renal anomalies, and including both mild and severe kidney disease, which varies even within affected families. Other frequently detected genetic mutations include those in PAX2, EYA1, and others.

PATHOPHYSIOLOGY AND CLINICAL FEATURES

Unilateral renal agenesis is common and may be multifactorial. Most cases of a solitary functioning kidney result from the involution of a multicystic dysplastic kidney (MCDK) or unilateral renal agenesis. Additional causes include inadequate vascular supply or an involuted unilateral dysplastic kidney that is not detected with typical imaging techniques. Outcomes for neonates with a solitary functioning kidney are generally favorable if other forms of CAKUT are absent. Individuals with solitary kidneys are at risk for hyperfiltration injury[6] and require long-term follow-up. In most individuals with a solitary functioning kidney, the kidney will undergo compensatory hypertrophy, thought to be related to nephron hypertrophy and not an increase in nephron number, as nephrogenesis is typically complete by 36 weeks gestation.

Bilateral renal agenesis is considered a form of CAKUT. Historically this was considered to be a fatal condition, incompatible with extrauterine life. There are reports of amnioinfusion to support lung development, and studies are currently underway to assess this intervention and its outcomes. It is critical to note that even if lung development is adequate, the neonate will have end-stage renal disease, and amnioinfusion increase the risk for preterm delivery, both of which will contribute to morbidity and mortality.[7,8]

Renal ectopia is a condition for which the kidney is located anywhere besides the typical renal fossa, and may be diagnosed prenatally, postnatally, or later in childhood or life if imaging is obtained for another purpose. Ectopic kidneys are most commonly located in the pelvis, but very rarely are found in the thorax.[1] Horseshoe kidney results from the fusion of the 2 kidneys connected by an isthmus usually associated with the lower poles. Crossed-fused renal ectopia is also a fusion anomaly and results in both kidneys being located on one side. The ureter of the ectopically located kidney inserts orthotopically into the bladder, on the original side.[1]

Multicystic dysplastic kidney is composed of noncommunicating cysts without intervening normal renal tissue. These do not have function and typically involute over time, although some persist. They are not believed to pose an increased risk of malignancy.[9] In some cases, it is unclear whether a dilated kidney represents severe obstruction that could be addressed or an MCDK. In these cases, functional imaging such as dimercaptosuccinic acid (DMSA) scan or mercaptoacetyltriglycine (MAG3) scan can be used to determine whether intervention is appropriate.

Renal dysplasia may result from other causes of CAKUT, or occur independently. Dysplastic kidneys have abnormal development and may contain cysts as well. They can be large or small and may be unilateral or bilateral.

Ureteropelvic junction obstruction (UPJO) results from intrinsic stenosis, fibrosis, or a crossing vessel leading to ureteral compression. Severe cases may result in a urinoma, caused by rupture of the fornix. Less severe cases are often asymptomatic and may be found later in childhood or even adulthood. It is very unusual to require surgery in the neonatal period, except in severe cases without a normal contralateral kidney, or in cases of bilateral UPJO. Criteria for surgery include poor or decreasing renal function, symptoms which may result from pain or the size of the kidney, and drainage parameters worsening over time. The best practice for unilateral cases with a normal contralateral kidney is still not defined. Some cases may be due to genetic abnormalities and in cases with familial CAKUT, the patient may be evaluated for such.[5]

Primary megaureter refers to an enlarged ureter secondary to an intrinsic cause. They may be an obstructed primary megaureter, a refluxing primary megaureter, or a nonrefluxing unobstructed primary megaureter. While many resolve by 1 to 3 years of age, infants with megaureter are still at risk for pyelonephritis and renal scarring. Thus, in the case of vesicoureteral reflux accompanying megaureter, prophylactic antibiotics are commonly prescribed. Secondary megaureter may result from a more distal abnormality including neurogenic bladder or urethral issues such as posterior urethral valves.

Ureterovesical junction obstruction may result from a primary obstructive process, or secondarily in cases of bladder hypertrophy, often associated with bladder outlet obstruction.

Vesicoureteral reflux (VUR) is the retrograde flow of urine from the bladder upwards into the ureters and kidneys, resulting from the failure of the antirefluxing anatomy of the ureterovesical junction. VUR is graded by voiding cystourethrogram (VCUG) on a scale of 1 to 5, with 1 being the most mild and 5 the most severe. The degree of vesicoureteral reflux is poorly correlated with the degree of urinary tract dilation seen on ultrasound, thus voiding studies are required to assess this.[10] VUR leads to an increased risk for pyelonephritis if bacteria enter the bladder, and pyelonephritis may result in renal scarring. High-grade VUR can also lead to bladder dysfunction over time even if the bladder was normal early in infancy. VUR is a significant risk factor for chronic kidney disease in children.

Duplex kidneys have an increased risk for abnormal urinary drainage. The Weigert-Meyer rule explains the anatomic development and insertion of the upper pole and lower pole ureters and the most likely associated findings. In the case of a duplex kidney with a dilated upper pole, the Weigert-Meyer rule describes an upper pole ureter ending in ureterocele, which is often obstructing, and a refluxing lower-pole ureter.[11] A ureterocele is a thin-walled cystic dilation of the ureter as it enters the bladder.[12]

Prune-belly syndrome is also known as Eagle–Barrett syndrome and includes the absence of the rectus abdominis leading to outpouching of the abdominal wall, undescended testes as well as anomalies including CAKUT and sometimes gastrointestinal, cardiac, pulmonary, and musculoskeletal anomalies. VUR is common.[12] Associated findings include megaureter, a dilated bladder and urethra (megalocystis and megalourethra), and abnormal bladder function which sometimes requires catheterization or other drainage modalities.

Posterior urethral valves (PUV) are the most common cause of lower urinary tract obstruction and have a higher mortality rate than most other forms of CAKUT due to the potential for pulmonary hypoplasia in the setting of oligohydramnios in utero, as well as the higher risk for end-stage renal disease in the neonatal period.[13,14] Classically, the bladder will develop a keyhole appearance, with the dilation of the posterior urethra visible prenatally in many cases. Theoretically, these result from a mucosal membrane that has failed to involute or an overgrowth of tissue in the posterior urethra. PUV are frequently associated with VUR and dysplasia. Assessment of outcomes for infants with PUV reveals that a nadir serum creatinine $\geq$ 1 mg/dL is associated with progression to end-stage renal disease in childhood.[15]

Cloacal anomalies refer to those for which the urinary, genital, and gastrointestinal systems open into a common channel to the perineum, rather than distinct orifices. Many of the aforementioned forms of CAKUT may be present.

Included in the category of CAKUT are bladder anomalies. The bladder may not be visualized prenatally in the case of a bilateral severe renal anomaly resulting in absent renal function. In such cases, a bladder is often present but empty. A large bladder typically results from either bladder outlet obstruction or is the result of being neurogenic with poor emptying capacity.[9]

Cystic diseases, as well as syndromes resulting in abnormal appearing kidneys, will be reviewed in another article.

EVALUATION WITH IMAGING

Anomalies associated with CAKUT include cardiac, genital, skeletal, colorectal and others (**Box 1**). Thus, all infants with CAKUT warrant close examination, including a complete physical examination and attention to any anomalies detected on imaging, such as spinal dysraphism, or vertebral anomalies. Associated birthmarks, branchial cleft cysts, or skeletal anomalies may offer insight into a potential underlying genetic condition.

In most cases, postnatal imaging should be delayed for 48 hours to avoid underestimating the severity of findings due to typical newborn physiologic dehydration. In cases with severe prenatal findings, or in any case suspicious for lower urinary tract obstruction or anuria, imaging and possibly intervention will occur soon after birth. In 2014, a consensus statement was released including recommendations for the classification of prenatal and postnatal urinary tract dilation and includes general guidelines for postnatal assessment based on the findings.[16] Infants with suspicion of high-grade vesicoureteral reflux or obstruction should receive prophylactic antibiotics to prevent urinary tract infections.

Postnatal imaging modalities include ultrasound, voiding cystourethrogram, radionuclide cystogram, magnetic resonance urography (MRU), MAG3 scan, and DMSA scan.

Ultrasound is commonly used to follow abnormalities longitudinally. Ultrasound poses no risk, with no radiation, and no need for sedation. It is typically the first test

---

Box 1
Evaluation

Imaging
- Ultrasound (with or without contrast)
- Voiding cystourethrogram
- Radionuclide cystogram
- MAG3
- DMSA
- MRU

Laboratories
- Complete blood count
- Electrolytes
- BUN
- Creatinine
- Parathyroid hormone
- 25-hydroxyvitamin D
- Urinalysis

performed in infants with confirmed or suspected CAKUT, as it can be conducted even in an unstable patient, often bedside, and can offer substantial information to guide potential interventions (**Box 2**). Voiding contrast-enhanced ultrasound can often give similar detail to VCUG but is only offered in institutions with this expertise.

VCUG is conducted to assess for VUR, PUV, and possibly ureteroceles and bladder diverticula. Radionuclide cystogram is used to follow vesicoureteral reflux but will not give anatomic detail of the urethra, ureterovesical junction, or bladder. Thus, when suspecting posterior urethral valves, ureterocele, or other anatomic anomalies, VCUG is preferred as the initial study. MRI/MRU can be used to evaluate for obstructive lesions, anomalies external to the urinary tract, and detail regarding cysts and other anomalies. MRI/MRU can be useful in duplex kidneys to evaluate the insertion of upper pole ureters and have also been used to determine the renal differential function and drainage/obstructive parameters. Sedation is often not required if conducted in the first 3 months of life as a "feed and wrap" study.[17]

A MAG3 scan is a nuclear medicine test used to evaluate for obstruction. This test also provides split differential renal function. It may also be used in cases of potential renal trauma to detect a urinary leak. A DMSA scan consists of administering a short-lived radioisotope that is taken up by kidneys. This test provides information regarding the size, function, shape, and position of the kidneys. It is typically used to detect renal scarring but can also be used to evaluate for pyelonephritis and infarction and to determine whether a kidney is nonfunctioning. Because both MAG3 and DMSA depend on the uptake of the kidneys, which requires a degree of maturity, these tests are both typically not undertaken until after 3 months of age.

Cystoscopy and retrograde studies are conducted to treat posterior urethral valves and further evaluate vesicoureteral reflux, bladder anomalies, intravesical masses and ureteroceles, and sometimes obstruction.

CLINICAL EVALUATION AND MANAGEMENT

Infants with one normal kidney and one abnormal kidney rarely require urgent evaluation or intervention. Those with bilateral anomalies have increased risk of renal insufficiency and complications, therefore, requiring a higher level of monitoring and assessment.

Box 2
Potential interventions for patients with CAKUT

Surgeries
• Pyeloplasty
• Ureteral reimplantation
• Valve ablation

Lower urinary tract drainage techniques
• Urethral catheter
• Suprapubic tube
• Vesicostomy

Upper urinary tract drainage techniques
• Percutaneous nephrostomy tube
• Ureterostomy

Long-term bladder management
• Medications
• Continence/continent catheterizable stoma
• Augmentation

Infants with unilateral renal agenesis or a unilateral MCDK with normal contralateral kidney rarely require urgent evaluation. Most may undergo postnatal ultrasound at some point after 48 hours. Infants with any degree of urinary dilation should be evaluated based on the algorithms described in the multidisciplinary consensus.[16] Those with renal ectopia also rarely need urgent evaluation. All of these patients should undergo a postnatal ultrasound, the timing of which depends on the severity of the prenatal findings. Decision regarding additional studies, including VCUG, depends on the concern for reflux or obstruction.

Ureteropelvic junction obstruction frequently improves over time in those detected prenatally. Infants with unilateral UPJO do not commonly require intervention, unless there is obstruction of other organs, or resultant urinoma causing compression of the ureter. In such cases, a nephrostomy tube or other intervention to drain the renal pelvis may be required. Those with bilateral UPJO require monitoring for oliguria, renal insufficiency, and electrolyte derangements. If such complications develop, drainage or diversion may be required.

As discussed above, ureterovesical junction obstruction is more often seen secondary to bladder thickening in the setting of bladder outlet obstruction. Less commonly, this may be due to primary megaureter or other mechanisms. Similar to those with bilateral UPJO, if there is oliguria or renal insufficiency, intervention may be warranted, and may include ureterostomy or nephrostomy tube placement.

Management of VUR includes antibiotic prophylaxis in many cases, to prevent urinary tract infections. Many cases of VUR will improve over time, and not all children require surgical repair. Indications for repair typically include infections despite receiving antibiotic prophylaxis, family refusal of prophylaxis, and no improvement, or worsening of VUR, by age 4 to 6 years.

Duplex kidneys often require no intervention and may be monitored by renal ultrasound. In cases that involve a ureterocele, and in infants with a ureterocele without a duplex kidney, incision of ureterocele is often required to avoid obstruction within the bladder.

Infants with prune belly syndrome should not be catheterized unless absolutely necessary. They may have issues with bladder emptying given the lack of musculature; however, infection and degree of hydronephrosis will determine the need for intervention. These patients may also require additional procedures to correct reflux and/or megaureters, as well as orchidopexy for undescended testes.

Infants with suspected PUV should have a urinary catheter placed soon after birth. If a urinary catheter cannot be placed, access to the bladder should be obtained either by suprapubic tube or vesicostomy. If the bladder cannot be drained, in some cases upper urinary tract drainage may be required.

MEDICAL MANAGEMENT

Infants with CAKUT are at risk for renal insufficiency, significant metabolic derangements, and progression of chronic kidney disease. Manifestations of chronic kidney disease include metabolic acidosis, anemia, mineral and bone disorder leading to secondary hyperparathyroidism, hypertension, growth impairment, and others. Laboratory assessment will include a combination of electrolytes, blood urea nitrogen, creatinine, complete blood count, parathyroid hormone, 25-hydroxy vitamin D level, and iron stores. Serum creatinine is often used to estimate renal function, although equations developed for this are not validated in the neonate. Additional testing such as cystatin C may be used. Cystatin C is a low molecular weight protein produced by all nucleated cells. It is freely filtered and less affected by muscle mass, age, and gender than serum creatinine.[9] The frequency of laboratory assessment will depend on the severity of the findings and any metabolic derangements that require attention. The frequency of outpatient assessment is guided by the degree of chronic kidney disease and complications from this. Children with CAKUT require long-term assessment of voiding function, which may change over time.

Newborns with CAKUT must be monitored closely as urine output may be inappropriately high or low. Overall volume status should be assessed frequently and if the anatomic findings are more than mild, laboratory assessment may be required as well.

Infants with low urine output may require fluid restriction and electrolyte management. Such infants may require feeds to high higher caloric density as well as medications to manage electrolyte disturbances. In some cases, the urine output may increase within several days after birth and frequent adjustments may be required.

Infants with high urine output may require fluid resuscitation and supplemental fluids or feeds to avoid prerenal physiology and subsequent dehydration. These infants may also require manipulation of feeding regimens to ensure good metabolic balance.

Anuric infants who have undergone appropriate decompression of any potential urinary tract obstruction should be challenged with diuretics. If there is no response, the infant requires assessment for renal replacement therapy.

Long-Term Outcomes

The long-term outcome for individuals with CAKUT varies widely. As noted, CAKUT is the most common cause of ESRD in children, but also contributes substantially to chronic kidney disease. These children should be monitored regularly with ultrasounds and additional studies when appropriate. All children with CAKUT should be evaluated by pediatric specialists to determine the need for laboratory tests as well as the assessment of voiding and bladder function. Many forms of CAKUT can worsen over time (UPJO, VUR, dysplasia) and lead to worsening renal function. Families must be counseled regarding these risks, and appropriate follow-up established.

CLINICS CARE POINTS

- Infants and children with CAKUT may require multi-specialty care.
- Children require longiitudinal assessment of kidney function and bladder function.
- All children with CAKUT should undergo regular blood pressure screening as they may be at risk for hypertension.

REFERENCES

1. Mileto A, Itani M, Katz DS, et al. Fetal urinary tract anomalies: review of pathophysiology, imaging, and management. AJR Am J Roentgenol 2018;210(5): 1010–21.
2. Rosenblum S, Pal A, Reidy K. Renal development in the fetus and premature infant. Semin Fetal Neonatal Med 2017;22(2):58–66.
3. van der Ven AT, Vivante A, Hildebrandt F. Novel Insights into the Pathogenesis of monogenic congenital anomalies of the kidney and urinary tract. J Am Soc Nephrol 2018;29(1):36–50.
4. Aulbert W, Kemper MJ. Severe antenatally diagnosed renal disorders: background, prognosis and practical approach. Pediatr Nephrol 2016;31(4):563–74.
5. Bockenhauer D, Jaureguiberry G. HNF1B-associated clinical phenotypes: the kidney and beyond. Pediatr Nephrol 2016;31(5):707–14.

6. Schreuder MF. Life with one kidney. Pediatr Nephrol 2018;33(4):595–604.

7. Sugarman J, Anderson J, Baschat AA, et al. Ethical considerations concerning amnioinfusions for treating fetal bilateral renal agenesis. Obstet Gynecol 2018; 131(1):130–4.

8. Huber C, Shazly SA, Blumenfeld YJ, et al. Update on the prenatal diagnosis and outcomes of fetal bilateral renal agenesis. Obstet Gynecol Surv 2019;74(5): 298–302.

9. Geary DF, Schaefer F. Comprehensive pediatric nephrology. Philadelphia (PA): Mosby/Elsevier; 2008.

10. Nelson CP, Johnson EK, Logvinenko T, et al. Ultrasound as a screening test for genitourinary anomalies in children with UTI. Pediatrics 2014;133(3):e394–403.

11. Meyer R. Normal and abnormal development of the ureter in the human embryo; a mechanistic consideration. Anat Rec 1946;96(4):355–71.

12. Chow JS, Littooij AS. Urogenital pathologies in children revisited. In: Hodler J, Kubik-Huch RA, von Schulthess GK, editors. Diseases of the abdomen and pelvis 2018-2021: diagnostic imaging - IDKD book. Cham (CH): Springer; 2018. p. 67–73. Copyright 2018 The Author(s).

13. Malin G, Tonks AM, Morris RK, et al. Congenital lower urinary tract obstruction: a population-based epidemiological study. BJOG 2012;119(12):1455–64.

14. Yulia A, Winyard P. Management of antenatally detected kidney malformations. Early Hum Dev 2018;126:38–46.

15. Coquillette M, Lee RS, Pagni SE, et al. Renal outcomes of neonates with early presentation of posterior urethral valves: a 10-year single center experience. J Perinatol 2020;40:112–7.

16. Nguyen HT, Benson CB, Bromley B, et al. Multidisciplinary consensus on the classification of prenatal and postnatal urinary tract dilation (UTD classification system). J Pediatr Urol 2014;10(6):982–98.

17. Antonov NK, Ruzal-Shapiro CB, Morel KD, et al. Feed and wrap MRI technique in infants. Clin Pediatr (Phila) 2017;56(12):1095–103.

Printed and bound by CPI Group (UK) Ltd, Croydon, CR0 4YY

03/10/2024

01040406-0010